Healthy Boundaries

Rochester Studies in Medical History

Senior Editor: Theodore M. Brown
Professor of History and Preventive Medicine
University of Rochester

Additional Titles of Interest

The Lobotomy Letters
Mical Raz

Plague and Public Health in Early Modern Seville
Kristy Wilson Bowers

Medicine and the Workhouse
Edited by Jonathan Reinarz and Leonard Schwarz

Stress, Shock, and Adaptation in the Twentieth Century
Edited by David Cantor and Edmund Ramsden

Female Circumcision and Clitoridectomy in the United States:
A History of a Medical Treatment
Sarah B. Rodriguez

The Spanish Influenza Pandemic of 1918–1919:
Perspectives from the Iberian Peninsula and the Americas
Edited by María-Isabel Porras-Gallo and Ryan A. Davis

Infections, Chronic Disease, and the Epidemiological Transition: A New Perspective
Alexander Mercer

Save the Babies: American Public Health Reform
and the Prevention of Infant Mortality, 1850–1929
Richard A. Meckel

Intrusive Interventions: Public Health, Domestic Space,
and Infectious Disease Surveillance in England, 1840–1914
Graham Mooney

The Antivaccine Heresy: "Jacobson v. Massachusetts" and
the Troubled History of Compulsory Vaccination in the United States
Karen L. Walloch

A complete list of titles in the Rochester Studies in Medical History series
may be found on our website, www.urpress.com.

Healthy Boundaries

Property, Law, and Public Health in England and Wales, 1815–1872

James G. Hanley

UNIVERSITY OF ROCHESTER PRESS

First published 2016

University of Rochester Press
668 Mt. Hope Avenue, Rochester, NY 14620, USA
www.urpress.com
and Boydell & Brewer Limited
PO Box 9, Woodbridge, Suffolk IP12 3DF, UK
www.boydellandbrewer.com

ISBN-13: 978-1-58046-556-4
ISSN: 1526-2715

Library of Congress Cataloging-in-Publication Data

Names: Hanley, James G. (James Gerald)
Title: Healthy boundaries : property, law, and public health in England and Wales, 1815–1872 / James G. Hanley.
Description: Rochester, NY : University of Rochester Press, 2016. | Series: Rochester studies in medical history, ISSN 1526-2715 ; v. 35 | Includes bibliographical references and index.
Identifiers: LCCN 2016000569 | ISBN 9781580465564 (hardcover : alk. paper)
Subjects: LCSH: Public health—England—History—19th century. | Public health—Wales—History—19th century. | Public health—Social aspects—England—History—19th century. | Public health—Social aspects—Wales—History—19th century. | Public health—Political aspects—England—History—19th century. | Public health—Political aspects—Wales—History—19th century.
Classification: LCC RA418.3.G7 H35 2016 | DDC 362.10942—dc23 LC record available at http://lccn.loc.gov/2016000569

A catalogue record for this title is available from the British Library.

This publication is printed on acid-free paper.
Printed in the United States of America.

For Amy

Contents

Acknowledgments   ix

Abbreviations   xi

Introduction   1

1   The Laws of Nuisance before 1846: Property, Health, and Democracy in the Age of Reform   17

2   Private Benefit and Public Service: Paying for Sewers before 1848   39

3   The Boundaries of Health, 1848–70   65

4   The Benefits of Health: London, 1848–65   89

5   Healthy Domesticity, 1848–72   111

Conclusion   132

Notes   137

Bibliography   229

Index   253

Acknowledgments

Two conference papers provided an important early impetus for the research presented in this book. The first was a closing lecture delivered to the Annual Meeting of the Canadian Association for the History of Nursing (2001) and the second was a paper delivered at a London School of Hygiene and Tropical Medicine conference on "Healthy Towns, Healthy Cities: Public Health in British Cities, 1844–2004" (2004). I am grateful to the organizers of both conferences for the invitation and stimulus they provided. Audiences at the annual meetings of the Canadian Society for the History of Medicine, the American Association for the History of Medicine, the Western Conference on British Studies, and the Victorian Studies Association of Western Canada in Winnipeg, Montreal, Toronto, Saskatoon, Ottawa, Fredericton, Halifax, Kansas City, Austin, and New Haven have helpfully responded to different iterations of this work over the years, as have wonderful colleagues in Winnipeg's medical history community, including Esyllt Jones, Chris Dooley, and Marion McKay.

This project could not have been completed without the financial support of several private and public sources. A major part of the research was conducted during a sabbatical leave funded by Associated Medical Services (Hannah Institute for the History of Medicine) in 2005–6, and a major part of the manuscript was written during another leave in 2010, funded by a Social Sciences and Humanities Research Council of Canada Standard Research Grant. I am deeply grateful to both organizations. I am also grateful that the University of Winnipeg Faculty Association's Collective Agreement provides Members with the opportunity to pursue regular sabbatical leaves and to the university's Research and Study Leave Committee, Dean of Arts, Vice-President (Academic), President, and Board of Governors for supporting them. The university's Research Office provided essential support through its Discretionary Grant and Major Research Grant programs.

The archival research for this book could not have been completed without the efficient and expert assistance of archivists across England and Wales. In London, I would like to thank the archivists at the National Archives, the Parliamentary Archives, the London Metropolitan Archives, and the Tower Hamlets, Camden, Greenwich, Southwark, and Wandsworth local history libraries and archives. Outside London, I have depended on archivists at the Surrey, Worcestershire, Buckinghamshire, Hertfordshire, Shropshire, Gloucestershire, and Caernarfon county record offices and the Hull and Liverpool city archives.

Staff at the British Library, especially the Newspaper Library at Colindale, were particularly helpful.

Earlier versions of parts of chapter 1 were included in "Bye Laws, the Environment, and Health before Chadwick, 1835–1840," in *Lawyers' Medicine: The Legislature, The Courts and Medical Practice, 1760–2000*, edited by Imogen Goold and Catherine Kelly (Portland, OR: Hart Publishing, 2009), 39–59; and in "Parliament, Physicians, and Nuisances: The Demedicalization of Nuisance Law, 1831–1855," *Bulletin of the History of Medicine* 80, no. 4 (2006): 702–32; and are reprinted with permission from Bloomsbury Publishing PLC and the Johns Hopkins University Press, respectively. An earlier version of part of chapter 2 was included in "The Metropolitan Commissioners of Sewers and the Law, 1812–1847," *Urban History* 33, no. 3 (December 2006): 350–68, and is reprinted with permission from Cambridge University Press. And an earlier version of part of chapter 4 was included in "Public Health, London's Levels and the Politics of Taxation, 1840–1860," *Social History of Medicine* 20, no. 1 (April 2007): 21–38, and is reprinted with permission from Oxford University Press and the Society for the Social History of Medicine. I wish to thank the proprietors of these works for their kind permission to reuse this material.

Simon Szreter and Martin Daunton kindly read chapters, and I am very grateful to them for their comments, even if I failed to respond adequately to their careful suggestions. Two referees for the University of Rochester Press provided the kind of feedback for which authors can only hope. I would like to thank Graham Mooney for providing a proof of his *Intrusive Interventions: Public Health, Domestic Space, and Infectious Disease Surveillance in England, 1840–1914*. I would like to record my appreciation of long-standing friends and colleagues in New Haven and Winnipeg, including Greg Anderson, Alexander Freund, and Nolan Reilly. Working with the University of Rochester Press has been a pleasure, and I especially thank Barbara Curialle for her patience and careful work in editing the book. Finally, this project would never have been completed without the loving support provided by Amy Richmond, to whom I am grateful for so very many things.

Abbreviations

BL	British Library
DBW	District Board of Works
HALS	Hertfordshire Archives and Local Studies
HO	Home Office
HOTC	Health of Towns Commission
LBH	Local Board of Health
LJ (MC)	Law Journal (Magistrates Cases)
LMA	London Metropolitan Archives
LRO	Liverpool Record Office
MBW	Metropolitan Board of Works
MCS	Metropolitan Commission of Sewers
MMA	Metropolis Local Management Act
MOH	Medical Officer of Health
NA	The National Archives
PA	Parliamentary Archives
PHA	Public Health Act
PP	Parliamentary Papers
QB	Queen's Bench
SKCS	Surrey and Kent Commissioners of Sewers
SRO	Surrey Record Office
THLHLA	Tower Hamlets Local History Library and Archives
UCL	University College London
V	Vestry
WCRO	Worcestershire County Record Office
WCS	Westminster Commissioners of Sewers

Introduction

In 1815, the boundaries of health were very narrowly drawn, and property owners had little to fear from concerns about health. Individuals could not easily be forced to clean up their property, to pay for healthy infrastructure *intended* to benefit others, or to open their homes to sanitary inspection. By 1872, they could be forced to do all of these things, and many more. This book describes the evolution of the laws that permitted these developments in nineteenth-century England and Wales, and its argument may be simply stated. Between 1815 and 1872, local public servants and commissioners of one kind or another, using public health as their rationale, stimulated a threefold transformation in the nature of property, redefining its salubrity, liability, and sanctity. These changes displayed themselves in the creation of a statutory health hazard (chapter 1), in the minute control of private domestic arrangements (chapter 5), and most important, in a revolution in the financial responsibility for the health of others (chapters 2–4). Redefining the liability of property itself stimulated new and highly controversial ideas of community. Public health thus became an important, if contradictory, site in the creation of communities, enhancing the right to health for some while simultaneously restricting the privacy rights of others in the name of health. These transformations have been studied before, but not, I believe, in such a way as to highlight their common institutional and ideological roots, nor to highlight the way in which they build on recent changes in our understanding of the nature, locus, chronology, and legacy of early English and Welsh public health.

In the earliest and most conventional telling, the English public health movement dated from 1838 and was a story of bureaucratic and parliamentary initiatives, often under utilitarian inspiration. In that year, Edwin Chadwick, secretary to the Poor Law Commission and former secretary to Jeremy Bentham, ordered several pilot inquiries into the health of London's poor. These inquiries triggered a national study, the results of which Chadwick published in 1842 in his *Report on the Sanitary Condition of the Labouring Population of Great Britain*. Following two royal commissions and various false starts, and spurred on by the vigorous propaganda of metropolitan sanitary activists, Parliament took action in 1847 with the creation of a new local authority for London (a process it repeated in 1855) and in 1848 with the creation of new local authorities for the rest of England and Wales. The 1848 Public Health Act (PHA) was the first national, if permissive, comprehensive public health statute. The act was usually seen as a failure, thwarted by some combination of ratepayer parsimony and anticentralizing sentiment. But the progressive narrative resumed with the appointment of Sir John Simon as medical officer to the Privy Council. Thereafter, central state bureaucrats and national political developments and actors figure prominently in accounts of the subsequent evolution of early English and Welsh public health, culminating in the 1875 Public Health Act, not superseded until 1936.[1]

This interpretation, regardless of its faults, was at least an advance on studies that saw the early development of public health as an unplanned, uncoordinated reaction to bad conditions.[2] The model had wide appeal, in part as a result of its congruence with the post–World War II welfare state.[3] Historians of medicine and public health by and large embraced this framework, and studies of the poor law medical service, the Metropolitan Asylum Board's hospitals, and the medical profession all connected health, broadly construed, to the growth of state provision.[4] Historians of government in turn saw public health as one of the prime examples of the Victorian revolution in government.[5] Debate surrounded the motor for this revolution in government, but all parties accepted the fact of the expansion of state capacity; the phenomenon was a natural complement to the anticentralization dynamic that inspired so many early public health historians.[6] Royston Lambert's biography of Sir John Simon merged the history of medicine and of the growth of government, using the career of this distinguished medical bureaucrat to illuminate the dynamics of central government growth.[7]

One context for the growth of public health in most of these studies was demography, aided and abetted by disease. England and Wales experienced a significant demographic transformation over the course of the nineteenth century, with population increasing significantly and shifting from countryside to city.[8] The urban population, estimated at 22 percent in 1801, rose to 77 percent by 1901.[9] Individual cities grew dramatically. London is an example, though it is hardly typical. Its estimated population of 1.4 million in 1815 rose to 6.5 million by the end of the century.[10] But the numbers alone do not tell the whole story, and the way in which population was distributed even within urban areas altered. Though the roots of this process are certainly visible even in eighteenth-century London, suburbanization escalated significantly in the early nineteenth century.[11] And suburbanization was linked to the deterioration of inner-city areas, another development that exacerbated the effects of population expansion in an underserviced environment.[12] The effects of these interlinked changes were deadly, even without the added burden caused by epidemics.

Notwithstanding the widespread acknowledgment of the importance of cities, urban history itself was poorly integrated into the traditional interpretation. When they appeared at all, local authorities were usually condemned, for not only were conditions bad but localities supposedly resisted improving them.[13] The history of the Victorian city as told by urban historians, however, presented a different picture. Urban historians naturally shifted the focus from public health to urban reform more generally, and from the center to the locality, highlighting different dynamics for change and resistance to it.[14] Peter Hennock's influential study of Birmingham connected sanitary reform to changes in the religious and political life of the city, not in the central government. Derek Fraser's analyses of cities as middle-class political and social battlegrounds also directed attention away from the center and simultaneously reformulated local support for and opposition to public health reform; there was no simple dichotomy between clean and dirty parties.[15] Various historians drew attention to the difficulties of sanitary reform and highlighted the sometimes bewilderingly complex financial, technical, and legal choices local governments faced.[16] Without justifying the slow pace of change, historians of nineteenth-century cities increasingly drew attention to what local authorities did instead of what they did not do, challenging the traditional dismissal.[17]

An increasing volume of work on public health history simultaneously fleshed out and reinforced the limitations of the traditional model.[18] A comprehensive review of this literature is beyond the scope of this introduction, but this work highlighted the diversity of health activity undertaken by the state.[19] In the Victorian period alone, the state was in part responsible for conventional sanitary work;[20] epidemiology and medical statistics;[21] the monitoring and institutional, prophylactic, and therapeutic management of infectious diseases;[22] the quality of food;[23] the health of workers, workplaces, and work practices;[24] health visiting and the well-being of mothers and infants;[25] the control of immigrant populations;[26] and the regulation of housing.[27] These studies revealed that different domains had distinctive chronologies, logics, and dynamics, thus complicating any simple narrative about increasing central involvement. They also illuminated neglected dimensions of "public health" as it was constructed in the early Victorian period and reproduced in early postwar historical studies. And constructed it was. Christopher Hamlin analyzed Chadwickian sanitarianism, at one time seen as an all but inevitable and wholly desirable solution to the health problems created by urbanization, as an ideologically loaded disciplinary tactic.[28] There were other models of "public health," he argued, and environmental reductionism was not determined by the data.

Scholars interested in the history of government also revisited the genesis and disciplinary legacy of the Victorian interest in health.[29] Peter Baldwin's magisterial comparative study convincingly argued that European preventive policies in the century after cholera were an important element in the formation of liberal regimes.[30] Inspired by Foucault's later turn to liberal subjectivities and governmentality, others examined public health as one of the constitutive elements of liberal self-governance.[31] Classical liberalism, with its preference for limited state involvement, low taxes, and market mechanisms, was traditionally seen as an obstacle to tax-funded, state-based activity in the interest of health, and the growth of public health was conversely presented as a paradigmatic instance of collectivist provision. Turning this idea on its head, Patrick Joyce reinterpreted statistics, sewers, and slaughterhouses—all public health perennials—within the governmentality paradigm.[32] In Joyce's analysis, each represented strategies or technologies of governance designed to produce liberal, self-governing subjects.

For Joyce, public health was not locked in conflict with liberalism; indeed, it was one of liberalism's crucial supports.

                                  ❧ ❧ ❧

Revisionist scholarship has thus comprehensively challenged the premises of traditional understandings of the history of public health.[33] The presumed beneficence of the state and its agents has come in for particular scrutiny, echoing in many ways, as Martin Wiener noted, the disillusionment with the state manifested by both the political left and right.[34] There is, of course, no consensus on the significance of these new interpretations, particularly "governmental" approaches. Peter Mandler noted that the behavioral norms and patterns essential to liberal subjectivity may be seen as a legacy of the varied and unrelated responses to some of the manifest challenges of urban society identified by social historians. Simon Gunn likewise highlighted potential analytical limitations of governmentality, suggesting that it may leave some questions around agency and the motor for change unanswered.[35] It can also be somewhat silent on conflict, and Joyce's claim that agreement on the need for intervention in the construction of freedom was "widespread and increasingly consensual" as the nineteenth century progressed does not do justice to the extent of internecine conflict around these issues.[36] Public health projects, for example, deeply divided the property-owning class.

This book highlights these divisions through an analysis of legal conflict. The legal system was the accepted framework within which all public health was carried out: establishing permissible activities, defining the conditions under which they might be carried out, and, most crucial, stipulating who should pay for them. Legal history in medicine is an increasingly important study,[37] yet with the exception of a limited number of instances, public health historians have shied away from interdisciplinary legal history.[38] Taggart's analysis of a celebrated late-nineteenth-century Bradford water-supply case is a fine example of the way in which Parliament responded to case law with statutory modification, and historians have pursued this line of inquiry productively in the analysis of industrial nuisances.[39] The legal scholar Jamie Benidickson's important three-nation study illustrates that the courts in Britain had a significant impact on the implementation of public health legislation, and the geographer Peter Atkins has analyzed the importance of the common law in the making of milk.[40] These studies show the promise of interdisciplinary legal history.[41]

My own interest in the legal history of public health emerged over time. My dissertation work on public health activity in five smaller towns convinced me of the importance of domestic regulation in shaping nineteenth-century attitudes to property and public health. A postdoctoral project led to an encounter with Chambers' *Digest of the Law Relating to Public Health*, a massive late-century compendium of more than twelve hundred cases, the vast majority of which of course fell after mid-century.[42] The analytical taxonomy of the cases illustrated the extent to which the law forged new spheres of state action and social concern, some of which appear to me to be crucial for the development of modern liberal urban society. The regulation of property and financial responsibility for public health were two such areas, and this book emerged as I followed the threads of these concerns and their cases before and after the mid-century legislative watershed marked by the 1848 Public Health Act (PHA) and the 1855 Metropolis Local Management Act (MMA).

In this book I focus on the making of the laws of public health, broadly considered. Law making in this study includes several related but distinct processes: the forging of public acts, local acts, and local bylaws; and the creation of a body of case law around them. Three types of legal source material are particularly important in this study and merit brief descriptions. The first is case law. Victorian property owners jealously guarded their rights and frequently pursued their cases all the way to the superior courts; the published reports of these cases are an essential source. I do not restrict myself to the authoritative published reports, produced as they were for a particular purpose and audience.[43] Case reports came in a variety of forms, ranging from newspaper accounts to semipopular legal journals (such as the *Justice of the Peace*) to the authoritative reports. The content and thus the utility of these reports varies, and reports of the trial may be more detailed in newspapers than published reports, where the emphasis was on the facts, the holding, and the judicial reasoning. I use all forms of case reports and where possible and appropriate supplement them with relevant archival records such as legal opinions on controversial decisions, briefs, affidavits, and occasionally trial transcripts from private shorthand reporters, which can be far more detailed and which can provide essential context for the case.

The existence of a body of case law surrounding public health is of interest because statutes could not anticipate every contingency. As local authorities tested the limits of their powers, judges created, in their rulings, guidelines that structured the behavior of parties not involved in the original action. As Albert Venn Dicey said, "Many statutory enactments . . . have been the subject of so much judicial interpretation as to derive nearly all their real significance from the sense put on them by the Courts."[44] Thus, the limits of public health legislation often were established when parties contested at the local level and judges ruled on their action.[45] Of course, the judges were not the only important parties in this process. Equally important was the role that local authorities played in driving this judicial lawmaking. The judges could rule only on cases brought before them, but the importance of local authorities extended beyond providing the occasion for a ruling, for they significantly influenced, I argue, the specific direction in which the law moved and the specific character of the decisions reached; their arguments mattered. To be sure, what parties argued in court was often determined by the legal strategy associated with the law and the facts, but the documentary record of these cases reveals the political and ideological dimension of their positions as well.

Case law also has the advantage of allowing us to recover the agency and significance of local institutional bodies that often escape historical attention. The cases obviously were fought in particular places, but the outcomes were generally applicable. The Epsom Local Board of Health's victory at Queen's Bench in 1855, for example, had ripple effects around the country. I must stress that these cases did not necessarily tell local authorities what to do (though sometimes they did), and they are not evidence of what happened in other places, any more than the existence of a statute is evidence of its implementation. Yet if a case was deemed to be significant, it was reported widely and the holding quickly found its way into handbooks or manuals produced for clerks of local authorities.[46] In order to determine how these cases influenced local practice, it is necessary to study the records of local authorities in detail. I have not undertaken that task, and my interest lies rather in the fashioning of judge-made law than in its implementation, although I have explored the impact of select cases in a few instances in order to illustrate how case law could influence local practice.

Statutes, especially but not exclusively local acts, are a second important legal source, and I focus on them as works in progress. Local acts, or private bills as they were called while they were before Parliament, were, depending on when they passed, subject to multiple levels of scrutiny. In the late 1840s, at a pivotal moment in the history of English public health, Parliament briefly required on-site public hearings on private bills. The transcripts, newspaper accounts, and official reports of these hearings, infrequently studied by historians of public health, are a valuable register of changing conceptions of health, property, and duty.[47] Parliamentary select committees on private bills, the hearings and reports of which were usually unpublished, provided similar occasions though with far less democratic participation.[48] Both sets of proceedings were conducted like trials, with the bills' promoters and opponents or their counsel calling witnesses who were examined and cross-examined at some length. Neither local nor parliamentary reports on private bills were binding on Parliament, but select committee reports had powerful persuasive power, not least because of parliamentary confidence in the thoroughness of their proceedings. In 1860, for example, a House of Commons select committee examined the rating clauses of the Metropolis Local Management Amendment Bill over ten days, far longer than the full House did, and this process is a window on contesting conceptions of benefit and burden.

Local bylaws are the third major legal source. English municipal authorities received bylaw-making authority through the 1835 Municipal Reform Act (MRA). In the first five years after the act, more than one hundred town councils passed fresh bylaws, some several times. Historians have not paid sufficient attention to these early bylaws even though they reveal much about the depth and breadth of sanitary sentiment across the country after the 1831–32 cholera epidemic; one of the most common features of these bylaws was a concern with sanitary nuisances.[49] Local authorities consulted widely with one another about desirable practices and policies, and I also approach these local laws not just as finished documents but rather as works in progress, tracking successive draft bylaws as councillors formulated their own definition of a health hazard. Councils were not at complete liberty to develop bylaws, and parliamentary control over legislation was mirrored in bylaws by official oversight, often through the Home Office or the General Board of Health. This oversight was unevenly exercised but was, at times, astonishingly detailed and illuminates the contested and negotiated character of early public health law.[50]

◦ ◦ ◦

My analysis of the legal history of public health leads me to three principal reconsiderations of the history of early nineteenth-century public health. First, it amplifies an ongoing shift in the chronology and locus of early English and Welsh sanitary reform, moving it back in time and shifting it to both provincial and metropolitan local authorities.[51] Among historians interested in early Victorian public health, the local state does not have a reputation for energetic activity, though there is no consensus on the extent of or explanation for its lethargy. Simon Szreter's is the most widely noticed structural account of the evolution of local public health over the century. Szreter argues that the unreformed municipal corporations had a variable but not utterly lamentable record. The reformed municipal corporations elected in the aftermath of the 1835 MRA were dominated by a petty capitalist class, long seen as an obstacle to sanitary reform.[52] This led, Szreter argues, to a significant deterioration of urban conditions in the second quarter of the century. Changes in the franchise during the late 1860s opened up space for a cross-class alliance such as that seen in Birmingham, where newly enfranchised voters supported a newly interventionist neoliberal patrician class led by Joseph Chamberlain.[53] Other general developments, such as changes in the availability of funds for capital projects, also were critical, allowing localities to access capital at favorable rates.[54] By the end of the century, local debt had risen to alarming levels, but mortality had fallen significantly for some groups.[55]

Szreter's political sociology is a persuasive synthesis and has been taken up in several recent treatments, yet I am also impressed with local authority activity both before and after the 1835 reform act. Much of the driving force for national public health legislation and thus national sanitary reform came, I argue, from the periphery, not the center. Historians of public health have noted that local initiatives often preceded national legislation.[56] Yet the local stimulus extended, as I hope to show, well beyond mere legislative example: local acts, bylaws, and legal challenges—in short, local lawmaking—shaped the character of central understanding and the meaning of parliamentary legislation more, I think, than we have reckoned. The main players in this story were local town councils (chapter 1), improvement and sewer commissions (chapter 2), local boards of health (chapter 3), and metropolitan local authorities (chapter 4). These were not dominated by the "statesmen in disguise" who allegedly carried the Victorian "revolution in government" to fruition. The key actors were in fact statesmen, albeit local statesmen, making law in various ways, some of which decisively influenced parliamentarians and judges.

Any claim about the importance of local authority initiative in Britain obviously needs to be qualified. Local authorities could only do what statutes permitted them to do, and Parliament thus completely controlled their action; anything they did, they did because Parliament told them or permitted them to do it.[57] Local authority autonomy was also compromised by the central government, particularly the oversight functions given to the Home Office and, to a lesser extent, the General Board of Health (GBH).[58] In the 1835 Municipal Reform Act, the 1848 Public Health Act, and the 1851 Common Lodging Houses Act, Parliament gave these central departments authority to reject bylaws produced at the local level. Exercised somewhat erratically before 1840, by mid-century this process had tightened up considerably, and in important ways the oft-described era of local autonomy was circumscribed.[59] These qualifications are obviously true, but the fact remains that local authorities had significant influence over the final form their local acts took. The liability for rates that the Metropolitan Board of Works (MBW) collected after 1858 was significantly different from the liability given in the statute that Parliament had passed in 1855, and the difference was the result of the MBW's determination to change the law.[60]

Second, my analysis highlights the differential significance of medicine and disease in the early development of English public health.[61] A generation of scholarship has established the critical role that some medical men played in the formative period of English public health. By the middle of the nineteenth century, medical participation in state-based public health projects was increasingly common.[62] Dr. Thomas Southwood Smith, one of Chadwick's early collaborators, was appointed to the General Board of Health in 1848 and was succeeded by Sir John Simon. They were the first two in a long line of medics holding continuous central government public health posts.[63] William Farr likewise towers over the history of population and vital statistics from his perch at the General Register Office.[64] Provincial medical officers of health could be appointed under the 1848 PHA, and as W. H. Duncan's example in Liverpool shows were locally influential even before the 1848 PHA passed.[65] Medical officers of health (MOH) were also compulsory in London under the 1855 MMA. Anne Hardy's work powerfully illustrates their significance in the decline of mortality rates in the metropolis over the second half of the century.[66] Nuisance procedures in 1832 and after 1846 relied on medical participation, and after mid-century Parliament increasingly solicited medical opinion at select committees dealing with public health legislation.[67]

But this was, of course, a process, not an event, and the unevenness of medical participation in public health matters around mid-century is equally striking.[68] When town after town developed its own definition of what constituted a health hazard after 1835, the work was done by town councilors acting primarily in conjunction with their legal advisers. When the central government developed procedures for conducting hearings on private bills in 1847, there is no evidence that physicians were consulted or were expected to be involved. Even their participation at the local level, though common, did not reflect an unambiguous acceptance of medical authority.[69] Although parliamentarians heard evidence from some physicians in hearings on public health bills, no physicians

testified at the parliamentary hearings in 1860 dealing with the health benefits and costs of metropolitan drainage, several years after metropolitan medical officers of health were first appointed.[70] Most of the legal cases that I will
describe did not include medical witnesses, even after mid-century.[71] This is a
story about healthy property and the legal costs and benefits of it, and physicians play a supporting, though by no means dominant, role in the crucial early
phase. As Dorothy Porter notes, medical knowledge was only one component of
public health expertise.[72]

Disease, in contrast, was fundamental. The nineteenth century is often identified as an age of epidemics, but the significance of these epidemics is more elu-
sive. Epidemics such as cholera were not so demographically significant as, say,
tuberculosis.[73] And they did not have the kind of revolutionary political impact
that historians at one time looked for.[74] Part of the problem with assessing epidemic impacts was, as Gilbert has noted, that the bar had been set too high;
when historians shifted their gaze, other effects came into focus.[75] I share the
view that epidemic disease was a critical influence, although I examine its initial effects less in the realm of action than that of ideas, especially legal ideas.[76]
Disease, I argue, forced local authorities to think about how they could act. Even
if they had some vaguely defined idea that undrained streets or heaps of fester-
ing refuse were unhealthy, local authorities needed to work out what had to be
done. They had to establish which piles of refuse were dangerous and why, and
under what circumstances; they had to decide who would decide that; they had
to figure out ways of paying for any enhanced drainage that they might provide;
in short, they had to rethink the boundaries of healthy property. In the pre-1848
period, they could not have easily remedied the situation.[77] This was work, and
typhus and cholera made the work happen.

The medical theory that local authorities relied on was miasmatism, the
notion that effluvia from decaying animal and vegetable matter were implicated
in disease. Miasmatism, as Hamlin argues, was flexibly interpreted by medics,
and its meaning for lay people involved in aspects of local governance was, I
suggest, similarly underdetermined.[78] For some of them, miasmatism was a theory less of disease than of property and its qualifications, and the way in which
they deployed it varied over time and with the context of application.[79] Starting
during the postwar typhus epidemic, the Westminster Commissioners of Sewers
used miasmatism to legitimate a new taxation regime for sewers.[80] According
to statute and case law, no property could be taxed for drainage that did not
directly benefit from it. By relying on miasmatic explanations and identifying
health as an indirect benefit of drainage, the commissioners extended that benefit at the very least beyond individuals whose property was connected to sewers. But they did not extend it very far, and the commissioners did not initially
believe that miasma theory obliged them to build new works. Cholera was critical
in this regard. In response to it in 1831–32, they wrestled with the implications
of building sewers in streets and neighborhoods hitherto unprovided with them.
Provincial municipal corporations formed in 1835, in contrast, were not usually responsible for sewers, but they were responsible for creating local nuisance

bylaws. In the aftermath of the 1831–32 cholera outbreak they too deployed miasmatism in their construction of the sanitary health hazard in local bylaws, redefining property's salubrity.

Local bodies responsible for the urban environment thus made miasmatism do political and legal work.[81] This work evolved over time, but it had its limits. In Westminster in 1831–32, miasmatism legitimated building sewers but provided no help in paying for them. Even if we assumed that miasma in poor neighborhoods could transmit disease to middle-class ratepayers and that expenditure on sanitary reform was thus in the middle class's self-interest, that was not an argument for forcing ratepayers to pay to improve property occupied by people too poor to do so; it was merely an argument for the reasonableness of voluntarily doing so. Donations to voluntary hospitals, to take an analogous case, might benefit middle-class subscribers psychologically and financially, but that did not mean that the middle classes were compelled to support them.[82] Fear of disease did not easily translate into love of taxation or even the power to tax.

My third reconsideration concerns the intersection of health and property in the making of "public health." This is, again, hardly new. I share Kearns's belief that "Private property was the crucial political and ideological bloc to public health reform."[83] We can see property at work in multiple ways. In the most obvious sense, a propertied electorate and its even more propertied parliamentary representatives determined the character of healthy laws, and at the local level the property-weighted Local Board of Health (LBH) franchise structured their implementation.[84] Christopher Hamlin also illustrated the way in which sewers and water public health was designed explicitly to protect capitalist wage relations. The inability of central and local governments to deal with housing for most of the century further reflects the ideological and political power of private property.[85]

In what follows I build on these analyses, emphasizing the legal transformation of property. I frame the analysis in terms of boundary shifts between different kinds of private property and rights. In particular, I demonstrate the intersection of health and property in the shifting boundaries between public and private nuisances, between public and private services, between rateable and unrateable property, between city and suburb, between the state and the individual, and among different kinds of individuals. These boundary-making processes were themselves inflected by different material, political, and ideological developments; demography, disease, democracy, and domesticity, in particular, shaped the legal limits of public health.[86]

Though I examine several different kinds of shifts in public and private boundaries, a major focus of this book is on changes in property's liability, particularly to taxation. My thinking on this matter has been strongly influenced by Martin Daunton's work on the history of taxation. Daunton argues that over the nineteenth century, Britain, in contrast to many of its Continental rivals, created a system of revenue generation and expenditure that built up trust among taxpayers. That trust allowed the British government to raise revenue at the end of the century to levels that its rivals struggled to match.[87] The situation at the local level was both similar and different. Local governments needed to establish mechanisms of trustworthy accountability so as to ensure that local taxation could be made responsible and adequate.[88] Yet Daunton also notes that ratepayers, too, had to be redefined, because the prevailing philosophy of local taxation did not define them as investors in collective goods but rather as consumers of local services.

I have demonstrated what I believe is one of the important ways in which ratepayers became investors in collective goods, via a locally developed and judicially sanctioned interpretation of the doctrine of benefit.[89] After 1815, local actors of various kinds promoted the idea that drainage provided not only direct benefits—property got drained—but indirect benefits as well, and the principal indirect benefit was the health of the people who lived in the vicinity of sewers even if their homes were not connected to them. As local actors contemplated drainage schemes, however, they were deterred by cost. In order to finance appropriate works, they developed a novel extension of the idea of benefit, shifting from notions of indirect benefit *as* health to notions of indirect benefit *of* health, from health as a benefit to health as a provider of benefit. Shifting attention to the benefits of healthy places and persons sanctioned a much wider extension of taxation than did the miasmatically determined notion of health as an indirect benefit of drainage. Under this inspiration, local actors in particular places proposed significant intra- and interparochial transfers, redistributing the costs and benefits of public health in significant ways. By the early 1860s, this tandem of public health and indirect benefit secured for provincial and metropolitan authorities a series of victories in Parliament and the courts. Those victories permitted the financing of health infrastructure on a broader scale than would have been possible without them.

It is clear that in this process, public health promoters created not just a new ratepayer but a new kind of community with a distinctive bundle of quasi rights and duties.[90] Only in the most nominal sense were these communities of ratepayers. More important, they were communities of health, united by a shared financial liability.[91] The redistribution of rates from wealthier areas to poorer ones in the name of public health, a feature in several of the cases considered in this book, was a novel and important part of this community making. Rates could not legally be redistributed from the rich to provide for the poor except through the Poor Law, an ancient responsibility.[92] In forcing some ratepayers to improve other people's property and indirectly their health, public health promoters implicitly argued that freedom from preventable epidemic disease was a (qualified) right[93] of those unable to pay for it, just as poor relief was a right for those unable to maintain themselves, and thus redistributive taxation was appropriate.[94] I do not want to overstate this development. We know that inclusion within a boundary does not imply membership in a community.[95] Public health was not always an inclusive force; people with cholera or who were susceptible to smallpox, women with syphilis, and even common lodgers were in one way or another stigmatized and restricted in the enjoyment of their bodily and civil liberties.[96] Yet healthy boundary making was not only about exclusion; health was one of the key, if contradictory, sites in constructions of community and citizenship.[97]

❧   ❧   ❧

I begin with a fresh narrative of a key feature of the movement: its environmental theory of disease. In the first chapter I explore the prehistory of the statutory health hazard, first created by Parliament in 1846. Relying on local acts of Parliament before 1831, I show that local elites often sought nuisance control authority in their acts, but the kind of nuisances on private land which would shortly be identified as health hazards did not feature prominently. The cholera epidemic of 1831–32 transformed this situation, and local elites pushed the boundaries of health onto private land. The inclusion of bylaw making power in the 1835 Municipal Reform Act accelerated the change and multiple corporations introduced the control of nuisances on private land into their bylaws. There was, however, no unanimity about this; local authorities disagreed about the things that were hazardous, about the conditions that made them so, and, most importantly, about the inevitably political processes for identifying them.[98] Different local authorities thus reconciled danger, democracy, and property in quite different ways. All of this diverse activity was challenged by the central government, which effectively preempted further local experimentation with its own statutory health hazard in 1846.

In chapter 2, I analyze the delivery, scope, and financing of urban drainage in terms of its status as a municipalized service. Urban drainage rarely features in narratives of municipalization, and to some extent that makes sense. Urban drainage was often (but not always) provided by public bodies, so in that sense sewers already were municipalized, even at the start of the nineteenth century. But public delivery of this service was only one aspect, and not the most interesting one, of municipalization. Municipalized drainage services, I argue, required particular strategies of financing, principally the taxation of all property within a district, that were not possible in the first half of the century. According to both statute and case law, property could not be taxed for sewers unless it derived a benefit (or avoided damage) from them. Notwithstanding its public delivery, drainage was essentially a private good, and this fact seriously interfered with the provision of drainage in London. Using the example of the Westminster Commission of Sewers, I illustrate the way in which commissioners used typhus and cholera outbreaks to reformulate the benefits of drainage, shifting them from property onto people and redistributing the costs among people so presumed to benefit. This agenda was incompletely realized when the commission was abolished in 1847, largely as a result of parliamentary and judicial resistance.

For other metropolitan and provincial authorities, the attempt to reframe liability for drainage arose in the context of struggles over its geographic scope. In the late 1840s, the battle over equitable taxation shifted to the suburbs. The central government again thwarted local desire to spread the costs of drainage widely, but in chapter 3 I show that the passage of the 1848 Public Health Act created new possibilities for redistribution. Some local boards of health formed under the act, such as that in Epsom, aggressively pushed their boundaries of drainage, capturing property hitherto exempt from contribution. As was the case in London, local ratepayers challenged these decisions in the courts, but the Epsom LBH succeeded in convincing the court that properties not directly benefiting from drainage works were nonetheless liable to pay for them. This victory permitted the Epsom LBH to finance its operations by taxing property owners even though they had escaped to the suburbs. The ruling in Epsom's case—the most important change to the law of sewers in two hundred fifty years—could be applied in jurisdictions all over the country, permitting the costs of drainage to be spread much more widely than in the past. The Epsom ruling, for example, emboldened local authorities in Swansea to tax profitable industrial property outside the town, and those in Cheltenham to tax wealthy enclaves within it. The PHA thus permitted a significant redistribution of the burdens of healthy infrastructure, but this potential was realized only as a result of local authority initiative.

The Epsom LBH's case echoed arguments that metropolitan commissioners had been making for years, but the ruling in Epsom's case did not apply to London. In London, the subject of chapter 4, the Metropolitan Board of Works and its second-tier partners also fought numerous legal battles over taxation, and in the early years the courts ruled repeatedly against them. These early losses convinced the MBW that the legislation under which it operated had to be amended. The MBW sought to change its operating act six times between 1858 and 1862, scoring two major successes in 1858 and 1862. Rating was a central feature, if not the central feature, of the whole series of attempted amendments. Concurrent with this parliamentary struggle, metropolitan authorities fought further court battles, securing a series of victories from 1860 to 1865 that cemented their ability to raise revenue for sewerage as they saw fit and to redistribute its costs locally as seemed to them just. In a sense, the story in London replicated that in the provinces, yet the circumstances in London gave the story a particular political valence. As a result of the excessively parochial character of nineteenth-century metropolitan governance, the boundaries that the MBW forged were those within which rates were effectively equalized. All parties recognized that the stakes in this battle were high. The MBW's success linked the story of drainage to the longer and broader movement toward equalized local rates in London and the nation.

In the final chapter, I examine two new kinds of private/public boundaries that central and local authorities helped redraw as they focused on healthy domesticity. The first derived from the state's entry onto private property. The key pieces of public health legislation passed at mid-century gave local authorities the compulsory power to drain private property and to ensure sufficient sanitary accommodation on it, thereby establishing a new threshold of privacy.[99] Some local authorities aggressively interpreted this brief, but Victorian property owners jealously guarded their rights and appealed to the central government and the courts, both of which took their objections very seriously.[100] The boundaries of these local health powers, like all statutory powers, were thus established by parties on the ground. The second boundary was drawn as control was exercised over "common lodging houses." All kinds of people lodged in all kinds of situations in Victorian Britain, but only certain kinds of lodger and lodging house were controlled before 1866. The places and people controlled, furthermore, were subject to an extremely intrusive inspectorial regime. The boundary drawn in this case was between people, demarcating those entitled to certain privacy rights from those who were not. Although most of the people denied these privacy rights were the very poor, the control over lodging was about more than class, and the regulations demonstrated a complex intersection of sex, health, class, and property.

In one sense, the control of common lodging houses brings this book full circle. The first chapter is a story of local bylaws around sanitary nuisances, the last around common lodging houses. But there the similarity ends. Chapter 1 is a story of local initiative and of the way in which the central government reacted to it, with the passage of the Nuisances Removal Act effectively preempting local experimentation. The last chapter shows the next phase in the evolution of central local relations, with the central government holding all the cards. The control of lodging houses was promoted by the central government, which also essentially compelled local authorities to accept its vision of regulation. Health was an arena for the negotiation of central-local boundaries, and lodging house regulation confirmed and amplified the shift in power that nuisances had triggered.

✒ ✒ ✒

Finally, let me add a few words about my self-imposed boundaries. Geographically, the project is rooted in England and Wales.[101] It moves between London (for which Parliament always made separate legislative provision and which thus had a distinct body of common-law jurisprudence) and selected provincial locales. In this study, London functions as both center and periphery: the center of the national government and its bureaucracy, London's government was locally controlled and bitterly resisted any central intervention.[102] Because this book is largely case driven, I will not attempt to select provincial locations on the basis of their functional character (resort, market town, and so on). In any event, such an attempt would not necessarily be productive, because quantitative analyses of sanitary reform yield no clear-cut evidence that activity varied according to size or functional character. Indeed, Bill Luckin's recent survey highlights the different and asymmetrical paths that different towns and places took to sanitary salubrity.[103]

The time frame of this book extends from 1815 to 1872. Early post–World War II histories of public health took the 1830s as their starting point, reflecting the central bias in such studies.[104] The publication of two such studies in 1952 triggered a brief response from Bryan Keith-Lucas in which he attempted to draw attention to developments in the late eighteenth century, although this initiative was not well received.[105] Part of the problem was one of periodization. If we define public health merely as a collective concern, or even as a state-based concern, with the health of a population, we can trace such efforts back quite some time.[106] Yet most historians see something distinctive about the kind of public health that developed in the 1830s.[107] All observers connect Victorian public health in one way or another with industrialization, urbanization, and epidemic disease.

I pick up the story in 1815, just as political dissatisfaction was reenergized and as urban development and disease gave a new prominence to health matters. Modern scholarship has made clear that the early decades of the nineteenth century were a nadir in the economic condition of the working classes and the physical well-being of the population.[108] Certainly the 1817–18 typhus outbreaks in London were part of a wider economic and political crisis in the postwar period. The 1831 cholera outbreak, too, coincided with intense conflict around political reform, agricultural and factory labor, poor relief, and the antislavery movement.[109] Populations thrown together in housing utterly unfit for accommodating them were, in the context of intense economic dislocation and political dissatisfaction, an increasing focus of concern for provincial, metropolitan, and national elites during the postwar period.[110] If the growth of urban infrastructure was one of the ways that English and Welsh elites came to grips with the massive medical challenges associated with urbanization and industrialization, it was also one of the ways that they came to grips with their social and political challenges.[111] Edwin Chadwick's role in formulating and implementing the controversial 1834 New Poor Law prior to his movement into public health in 1838 and his appointment to the General Board of Health in 1848 illustrates particularly clearly the way in which public health represented more than simply a response to terrible urban conditions.[112]

There were, however, additional pathways to a public health, such as those forged by various local bodies with responsibility for one or another aspect of the local environment. That is not to say that these bodies were insulated from the wider context of social conflict; they were not.[113] The work of municipal corporations in formulating a health hazard was powerfully structured by contemporaneous democratic politics. Improvement commissions, metropolitan sewers commissions, local boards of health, and the Metropolitan Board of Works were likewise concerned with and engaged in prolonged conflict over the implications of residential segregation and suburbanization for the provision of healthy infrastructure.[114] It is this consistent effort to forge the legal instruments with which to make public health that gives the period its coherence. All these developments took place in a context of concern over poverty and social conflict, even if the New Poor Law was not always the primary focus.

My terminal date does not rest on any particular statutory enactment, though any one of a number of developments suggests that it is a convenient demarcation. The final report of the Royal Sanitary Commission (RSC) and the 1871 Local Government Board Act reintegrated the Poor Law and public health in a new and, from John Simon's perspective, unacceptably subordinate position.

The 1872 Public Health Act transformed the architecture of local public health. At the same time, developments within medical science brought to light new possibilities for interpreting the incidence of disease and the condition of the environment, though bacteriology by no means immediately transformed public health (or medicine).[115] Finally, political and ideological developments—most notably franchise reform in 1867 and 1869 and the rise of new programs of urban renewal as manifested most famously in Birmingham—gave the succeeding period a new impetus. New emphases, such as housing and the control of individuals, were added to the traditional priorities of sanitary work.[116] The period that this book covers was, I believe, a distinct phase in the history of governance, local governance, and public health.

Chapter One

The Laws of Nuisance before 1846

Property, Health, and Democracy in the Age of Reform

The following chapters make three principal claims. First, critical aspects of public health in nineteenth-century Britain, from the initial development of the health hazard to the liability of property for drainage, were driven as much by lay as professional people. Disease, especially epidemic disease, played a fundamental role, but the attempt to avoid disease was directed largely by local elites, only some of whom had medical training or relied on medical knowledge. Second, more important to these early developments than medicine was property. Public health and property were mutually constitutive, and the evolution of laws around public health cannot be understood apart from the concepts of property they were intended to inflect. A third claim is that we hear this health-property dialogue most clearly if we listen to local rather than central government actors, because local actors, including metropolitan actors, made many of the important decisions and forged many of the crucial concepts. Indeed, the central government was ambivalent about local experimentation.

The early development of the statutory health hazard is an example of this picture of public health. In 1846, Parliament created the first national statutory health hazard. The statutory health hazard remains one of the two limbs of British statutory nuisance law today.[1] This law was passed in anticipation of a cholera epidemic and marked the third time Parliament or the central government responded to cholera by identifying a health hazard.[2] Cholera was not the act's sole central inspiration, and passage of the law was also likely linked to a series of developments relating to the establishment of the early English public health movement. Foremost among these developments in the central government was Edwin Chadwick's inquiry (1839–42) into the sanitary condition of the laboring classes.[3] In his *Report on the Sanitary Condition of the Labouring Population of Great Britain*, Chadwick argued that decaying animal and vegetable material was a primary cause of much surplus death, and these materials ended up being identified as health hazards.[4]

In recent years, historians less inclined to take Chadwick's version of public health for granted have challenged this experiential and empirical account of the creation of the sanitary nuisance.[5] Although Chadwick's theory reflected

long-standing medical and popular beliefs about filth as a potential cause of disease, historians have argued that the emphasis that he and some other public
health reformers of the 1840s placed on filth went well beyond medical belief at
the time, and they see strong ideological content in his sanitary program.[6]

I share these authors' belief that the health hazard was not "discovered" in
any straightforwardly empirical sense, though I approach the problem of its construction from a local rather than a central direction.[7] Through an analysis of
local acts and bylaws, I show that the history of the health hazard must also be
sought away from Parliament and Whitehall. In the first forty years of the nineteenth century, local authorities of one sort or another engaged in considerable
experimentation around nuisance definition. First in local acts of Parliament,
but then more fully in bylaws created after 1835, local elites constructed, decon-
structed and reconstructed different kinds of "health hazard." I argue, further,
that all this local experimentation was not merely a prelude to a central ratifica-
tion and generalization. The concept of a health hazard was in fact highly contested between and within local and central governments in the second quarter
of the century. The 1846 statutory health hazard was less Parliament's attempt
to codify provincial practice than to impose a measure of uniformity onto an
increasingly diverse situation.

I also agree with these authors that the health hazard or sanitary nuisance
was ideologically loaded, though again I see it from a local and legal perspective.
Local laws of nuisance, drawing on long-held lay and medical beliefs, invariably
privileged environmental sources of disease, as did Chadwick, yet in the local
case the environmental health hazard emerged out of a distinctive set of structures and concerns. The common law of nuisance, a nonstatutory collection of
precedents (or leading cases) and their underlying principles, was particularly
important here.[8] During the first third of the nineteenth century, the only legal
remedies against nuisances that effectively applied to the entire country were
provided through the common law, and in theory a wide range of nuisances
could be prosecuted under it.[9] In the early part of the nineteenth century, nuisances legally encompassed a broad range of irritants ranging from pig keeping
and chemical manufacture to projecting street signs and dilapidated buildings.[10]
What they had in common was the possibility of causing "hurt, inconvenience,
or damage," in Blackstone's phrase.[11]

Though "noisome smells," which fell under Blackstone's rubric of a nuisance,
could be prosecuted and most closely anticipated the health hazard, nuisances
were by no means limited to dangers to health, nor were health hazards conceptualized separately from nuisances.[12] Nuisance law was intended to protect the
enjoyment of property and not the enjoyment of health; thus, nuisances did not
have to be unhealthy to be nuisances.[13] Nonetheless, nuisance law provided the
most accessible resource available to local elites as they contemplated change
and control in their local environments.

Although common opinion and common law thus led local elites to construct
an environmental health hazard, they determined neither the precise form this
new object would take, nor, more crucial, the way in which it would be identified

and managed. This indeterminacy generated an interesting diversity of local nuisance laws. One thing all these laws shared, however, was a concern with private property as much as health. Indeed, as Daunton argues, tensions over the control of private property in the Age of Reform shaped the construction of nuisance law to a considerable extent.[14] The environment-based health hazard thus had its own locally constructed ideological roots.

In this chapter, I argue that local nuisance law passed through three partially overlapping phases of development from 1815 to 1846. Before 1831, control of what would be called sanitary nuisances on private land was, with a few exceptions, not a priority for local elites. The cholera epidemic, however, gave these nuisances a new relevance in the provinces and in Whitehall, but there was no consensus over the objects or the measures necessary to control them, and central and local ideas were in flux. This early evolution of local nuisance law was transformed by the 1835 Municipal Reform Act. Provincial theoretical interest in the control of sanitary nuisances escalated dramatically as a result of the act's bylaw-making provisions, providing us with an unparalleled opportunity to study provincial elite opinion on protection of health and/from property. I show that nuisance bylaws circulated widely among towns, and the form of nuisance law that town councils developed often reflected the deliberate rejection, modification, or adoption of other towns' models. An important principle structuring their deliberation was a concern over property rights. I do not mean here merely that the rights of property were taken into account when nuisance laws were applied in the courts.[15] I mean rather that the identity of potential nuisances, the features that made them dangerous, and the procedures by which they were so identified were inextricably bound up with the protection of property; the local laws of nuisance that town councils created reflected different local balances among disease, democracy, and property.[16]

In the final section, I examine the central response. Local bylaws, according to the 1835 Municipal Reform Act, had to be reviewed by the Home Office and could be disallowed by the Privy Council. The record of these reviews and rejections reveals considerable provincial and central government conflict over the understanding of hazards to health. The central government often censored local ideas and restricted local actions, imposing its own view of the rights of property. All of this central government review, I suggest, influenced developing central notions of the statutory health hazard. As early as 1839, the central government signaled its own view in a metropolitan police statute of that year. The 1846 Nuisances Removal Act, continuing this central government reaction, thus was not an affirmation of provincial practice but its negation.

Sanitary Nuisances before 1831: Common Law, Local Acts

The institutional landscape of pre-1834 British local government does not lend itself to easy description.[17] The largest divisions of England and Wales were the historic English and Welsh counties. These counties themselves encompassed a further array of often overlapping jurisdictions, including parishes, unions of parishes, manors, hundreds, townships, boroughs, and a variety of what the Webbs called statutory authorities for special purposes, most of which operated over some particular geographic space.[18] These last included but were not limited to improvement commissions, one focus of this chapter, and commissions of sewers, to be discussed at length in the next chapter. In short, only the most well-informed resident could enumerate the variety of jurisdictions under which she or he fell. He or she could easily be simultaneously a resident of a parish, a union, a borough, an improvement area, a sewer commission, and a county.

For the purposes of this chapter, the principal institutions of local governance were municipal corporations and improvement commissions. There were about 180 municipal corporations at the beginning of the nineteenth century.[19] Most of them owed their foundation to a charter, though not all did, and most of their charters were not given to them so that they could provide a range of municipal services.[20] Some did perform such functions, but for many of them, the main functions were to elect the local MP, to manage corporate property, and to participate in the local administration of justice.[21] For places not served by a corporation, and even for some that were, typical governmental functions such as road maintenance and the administration of justice could be performed by parish or county authorities. Poor relief was, of course, the most important local function for which parishes were everywhere responsible; parishes also maintained highways.[22]

Notwithstanding this profusion of authorities, contemporaries often believed that the existing institutions were not always adequate to the task. Beginning in the seventeenth century but accelerating in the second half of the eighteenth century, a significant number of localities acquired local acts of Parliament that authorized a variety of different initiatives.[23] They were often promoted for specific purposes, such as the improvement of a harbor or creation of a turnpike, but sometimes were intended to provide for more quotidian practices of local government.[24] Historians typically call these last cases improvement acts; they often created a novel local body, which historians usually call an improvement commission. These commissions themselves often returned to Parliament to augment their power with fresh acts.[25]

These acts were necessary not just because changing circumstances of the time seemed to demand new management but because of the developing sense in the eighteenth century that local bodies needed specific sanction for actions they proposed to carry out, particularly, as Joanna Innes has shown, if they raised rates, interfered with private property, or breached another statute.[26] Although the specific legal doctrine at issue evolved over time, in the nineteenth century it was associated with the doctrine of *ultra vires*. In general terms, this doctrine stipulated that "the recipient of a statutory power can only do those things which are authorised by the statute to be done."[27] This provided a constitutional brake on local overreach, whether it was exercised by improvement commissions or municipal corporations.[28]

Municipal corporations and improvement commissioners thus were the institutional basis for much, though by no means all, local government of the time, and I use them as a window into the prehistory of the sanitary health hazard. I do not mean to imply that the local management of nuisances in the early nineteenth century was exclusively in the hands of these authorities. An important jurisdiction at the time, as Christopher Hamlin has reminded us, were courts leet, long-standing judicial bodies that policed public spaces. The Manchester Manor Court Leet, for example, was an active local body with records dating back to 1552; this continuous record of local practice would have powerfully shaped local notions of what to do.[29] My focus in this chapter is on the legal construction of what would come to be called sanitary nuisances. Because corporations and commissions specifically needed to seek parliamentary or ministerial approval for their powers, they were important actors in the theoretical construction of local nuisance laws.[30] It is virtually a certainty that any given act or bylaw was an amalgam, reflecting the influence of common-law nuisance, the experiences and examples of other places, and last but not least local experience. I do not explore this record of local experience in order to trace its presence in local acts; I take these acts as starting points for further discussion.

From the perspective of historians of medicine, these local acts are of interest because they contained a wide range of provisions governing what would soon be called sanitary nuisances. According to Frederick Spencer, prior to the 1740s provisions dealing with nuisances in these acts were, except in the case of London, rare. Thereafter, nuisance provisions began to appear with increasing frequency and by the start of the nineteenth century were common.[31] These acts show us that semistandard sanitary nuisance provisions already were in place by the beginning of the nineteenth century. There were, for example, usually regulations about the time at which privies and slaughterhouses could be emptied of their contents and about penalties for spilling those contents as they were moved in the streets.[32] In addition, there were almost always regulations, usually found within the general street code, governing nuisances from slaughterhouses and swine sties running into the streets and from other offensive matter left in the streets.[33] As many historians have noted, local authorities' desire to control what we would call sanitary nuisances was already of long standing before 1831.[34]

In addition to these standard nuisance provisions, many local acts of the pre-cholera period also contained provisions against what were variously called "other nuisances" or "particular nuisances," including, to take one example, a prohibition on any "Slaughter House, Hog Stye, or other noisome Building" that was a nuisance.[35] Given that the general street codes usually permitted local improvement commissioners to control nuisances from slaughterhouses and other comparable premises, one might wonder why these supplementary statutory provisions were necessary. They were necessary in part because the supplementary provisions did not deal with street nuisances but rather with the premises themselves; they concerned not blood running into the street from a slaughterhouse but the slaughterhouse itself. Additional statutory provisions were thus required because the provisions dealt with a different set of facts.

Yet the supplementary statutory provisions also categorized and policed these particular nuisances (as I will for convenience call them) differently. The street code, an often unwieldy list of offensive situations or things sometimes several pages long, usually did not have special procedures attached to it, nor did it always claim that the offense in question had to be legally a "nuisance." The acts usually permitted any constable or commissioner to apprehend any violator of the street code "without any Warrant whatsoever" and bring him or her to the magistrates.[36] The local notables who sponsored the acts and the parliamentarians who approved them appear to have believed that little judgment was required beyond the register of a conviction by the magistrates. The mere fact of the occurrence, such as blood from the slaughterhouse running in the street, was all that was required for conviction.

For the "particular" nuisances, in contrast, the local acts frequently developed additional procedural safeguards. Hastings's 1820 local act required that to be removed, "any Hogpound or Stye, or other public and common or private Nuisance" had to be investigated by the commissioners for the act and identified as such. At least seven commissioners were required to order a direct abatement. No comparable procedure existed for street nuisances. Stockton's 1820 act empowered its improvement commissioners to remove any hog sty or other noisome building provided that it was a nuisance "in the legal Acceptation of that Term," again not a requirement of the street code. Taunton's 1833 act allowed its improvement commissioners to remove any "Slaughter House, Hogsty, Necessary House, Manure Heap, or other noisome or offensive Building, Place, Matter or Thing whatsoever" if, after due investigation which the commissioners were required to conduct, they found it to be a "Nuisance." Taunton and York had in their 1833 acts specific appeal procedures for these "particular" nuisances, again in contrast to their general street codes.[37]

The fact that local acts usually stipulated different and more rigorous procedures for the particular nuisances indicates that the framers saw them differently. It was not just that the slaughterhouse itself was a circumstantially different nuisance from its blood running in the street; it was categorically different and required different standards of proof before it could be abated. The acts did not make explicit the nature of the difference between these two kinds of nuisance. The most obvious distinction between the two kinds of nuisance would have been the common-law distinction between private (affecting an individual) and common or public (affecting the community) nuisances, each of which was defined and dealt with differently.[38] Yet the distinction between general street nuisances and particular nuisances did not correspond to the common-law distinction between common and private nuisances.

The feature that most particular nuisances had in common was that they were nuisances on private land. Under the common law, a nuisance on private land could be a common or a private nuisance, depending on the circumstances. It is difficult to determine from the acts if the particular nuisances were seen as common or private nuisances. The language of the acts generally, but not exclusively, permitted action against particular nuisances if they affected any inhabitant.

However, it was highly unlikely that local acts would have been drafted to permit public monies to be spent on a purely private nuisance, that is, a nuisance affecting one individual only. Rather, the acts appeared to contemplate nuisances on private land that were potentially common, although complaints against them could be initiated by a single individual. The procedural distinction these acts drew was effectively between common nuisances on public land (the street code) and common nuisances on private land (the particular nuisances).

Enter Cholera

By the early 1830s, then, many urban authorities had already begun to regulate nuisances that would one day be considered public health hazards, and in so doing they had begun to develop procedures not commonly presented in expositions of the common law of nuisances.[39] Common nuisances, according to the necessarily simplified presentations of the common law, were all dealt with in one way, by indictment before a quarter sessions grand jury. With parliamentary sanction, local authorities had long since introduced summary procedures for dealing with common nuisances in public streets into the general street codes of local acts. Local authorities also clearly recognized that the common law did not adequately protect the public against common nuisances on private land, and they developed new procedures to deal with them. Yet common nuisances on private land, according to local authorities and Parliament, required a higher degree of procedural scrutiny than common nuisances on public land.

The development of the laws of nuisances was given a major impetus by the cholera epidemic that passed through Britain in 1831–32.[40] During this epidemic, acting in response to frequent local importuning and in recognition of the inadequacy of the common law, the central government issued two different temporary regulations against sanitary nuisances. Both regulations required medical certification of the nuisances as dangerous to health or likely to be so, yet in each case the nuisance itself was somewhat different. In 1831, the object had to be a public nuisance, though the nature of the nuisance was defined no further.[41] In 1832, the objects to be regulated were elaborately described and included swine, slaughterhouses, and corrupt or offensive impurities such as decayed fruits, vegetables and garden stuff, and putrid fish within houses or within twenty yards of any house.[42]

In the wake of the epidemic, some urban areas began to develop new nuisance powers related to the control of what would one day be called statutory health hazards. Cheltenham took an early step in this direction with its 1833 local act, obtained the year after the first cholera epidemic ended in Britain. Cheltenham was already a fashionable location, and local act promoters must have recognized that its salubrity was an important part of its appeal.[43] The act was almost exclusively intended to allow a newly created private company to build sewers in Cheltenham, yet the promoters took advantage of the act's passage to insert a provision covering nuisances in the town. This section of the act applied not to the company at all but rather to the already existing street commissioners (among others) who were explicitly given power to appeal to the justices for removal (s. 46) of any "Muck, Filth, Soil, or other offensive Matter or Thing" deemed (by the commissioners and ratified by the justices) to be a nuisance or dangerous to the health of the inhabitants.[44]

Cheltenham's local act had a certain similarity to the central government's 1831–32 cholera regulations, even though Cheltenham's elite abandoned medical certification and modified the list of nuisances against which commissioners and justices were meant to act. Not all towns, however, chose to model themselves on the central government's temporary cholera regulations even as they confronted similar sorts of nuisances. Liverpool's 1835 local act, for example, permitted summary regulation of any "offensive Matter or Thing" in any public street, which was absolutely standard at the time, but it also regulated the same matter (on private land) whether it was surrounded by a fence or not.[45] If the act had left it at that, all the private land in the borough would have fallen under this provision. That was of course intolerable, and the corporation introduced significant restrictions on the process. Although the Privy Council had adopted a twenty-yard standard for danger in 1832, the Liverpool Corporation decided that only offensive matter within ten feet of any public street was liable to removal.

The Liverpool Corporation's decision to use distance as its standard reflected the difficult balances local authorities struck in regulating this material. The corporation wanted this matter controlled, but there seemed to be only two main options, both of which it evidently rejected. The corporation could have followed the examples of the Privy Council or Cheltenham, identifying health as the rationale for control. In removing the exemption based on fencing, the Liverpool Corporation implicitly acknowledged that the problem was one of effluvia, a health issue. But Liverpool was unwilling to make health the explicit criterion, notwithstanding the recognition in Liverpool of the health effects of bad drainage.[46] The corporation also could have controlled the matter if it was identified as a common nuisance, yet it rejected this approach, too. The rejection of the common-law standard was surprising, particularly because the reformed council returned to it the next year. We can only conclude that the Corporation decided that distance, even if somewhat mechanical, gave it the best chance of securing its objectives. At all events, if the common law was insufficient, and health was not an option, the council had little choice other than distance and its sensory marker, smell.

These four acts and proclamations, passed between 1831 and 1835, hinted at the diversity of local, parliamentary, and official ideas around nuisances on private property. There was, evidently, a measure of consensus that some (decaying) biological material on private land was a problem requiring attention, but consensus ended quickly: the Privy Council had one list of potential objects, Cheltenham another, and Liverpool a third. The Privy Council required nuisances to be dangerous to health, a standard that Cheltenham accepted but did not require, though Liverpool did not mention health at all. The nuisances were explicitly based on proximity in the case of Liverpool (ten feet) and the Privy Council (twenty yards), although Cheltenham made no mention of distance. Neither Liverpool nor Cheltenham employed medical men in the certification of these nuisances, though the Privy Council did, and we must regard that as a deliberate choice. It is inconceivable that Liverpool's drafters, to take that city as an example, were unaware of the regulations that the Privy Council promulgated during the cholera epidemic. There was thus no consensus on the objects, on the circumstances that made them objectionable, or on the process required to determine if they were so.

It is tempting to regard the objects potentially regulated by these four documents as tentative approaches to or preliminary approximations of the statutory health hazard. Yet to see them in this way is to assume that the object was ontologically prior to the laws that described it, that it was "out there" waiting to be found by appropriately insightful and careful drafting. Rather, these documents reveal the way in which the objects were constituted by the very regulations that purported to control them.[47] I do not want to claim that these documents constructed the sanitary nuisance *de novo*. Physicians and lay people had worried about the connection between dirt and disease for centuries, and these documents clearly reflected that anxiety, renewed during and after the cholera epidemic. But the boundaries of that kind of nuisance were not established. By creating laws around it, these legal drafters codified particular, and different, interpretations of the nuisance.[48]

Furthermore, the diversity of ideas around these new objects was not solely or perhaps even primarily a result of diverse medical theories or different ideas about health.[49] The health hazard was not only about what made people sick but also about the conditions under which property could be controlled. The limits of these new nuisances coincided with the limits to the control of property. In 1835, for example, Liverpool's elites (and Parliament) had to define the conditions under which property summarily could be tampered with, and the resulting statute legally created a new object of regulation, the ten-foot nuisance, different from the twenty-yard health hazard that the Privy Council had created in 1832. There is no evidence that the difference between the two was related to any discussion or theory about the diffusion of miasma across space.

The development of nuisance law in local acts initiated by cholera continued long after the epidemic. The central government's refusal—and that is the only way to regard it—to pass a statutory nuisance law suggests that it did not believe that demand for this kind of nuisance-control power existed or that a national standard was required if it did. If new powers were required, Parliament trusted to local initiative to seek them out. In the short term, that is exactly what happened. But to the central government's (and one assumes Parliament's) surprise, that power was sought through the Municipal Reform Act, which transformed local nuisance lawmaking. The powerful mix of disease and democracy would test the central government's faith in local initiative.

Bylaws

The enthusiasm for local acts, discussed in the previous section, continued throughout the nineteenth century. Yet the local act procedure was not without its problems. It consumed an enormous amount of parliamentary time, was potentially expensive, and involved a lot of duplication of effort, with each place potentially reinventing some solutions and strategies already in use in another place.[50] Parliament's longer-term solutions to this problem are described in the next chapter, but a solution for nuisances came in part with the 1835 Municipal Reform Act. The MRA allowed municipal corporations to make bylaws for the suppression of nuisances not summarily provided for by any existing local act.[51] This low-cost mechanism triggered a flurry of bylaw creation in corporate towns and provides us with an excellent opportunity to study in detail provincial thought on sanitary nuisances at a pivotal moment in the conventional history of public health. Although nuisance control was hardly the primary purpose of the act, the creation of bylaws allows us to see how the democracy and nuisance control intersected in interesting ways.

The primary purpose of the MRA was, of course, political. As many historians have taught us, the end of the Napoleonic Wars in 1815 brought a renewed focus on what were perceived to be defects in the British political system, particularly parliamentary representation.[52] The initial response of the state to political and economic protest was coercive: suspension of habeas corpus, incarceration, show trials, transportation, execution, censorship, and the violent suppression of dissent.[53] Parliamentary consideration of the Poor Laws provided the occasion for the only constitutional change during the early postwar period in the case of local government, and it was hardly a concession to radicalism. William Sturges Bourne's Acts of 1818–19 weakened democracy, permitting property owners to take control of parish vestries through what became a widely imitated plural voting scale. Inhabitants were granted votes calibrated to the rateable value of the property they occupied, up to a maximum of six votes.[54]

In the late 1820s, however, even the Tory party, committed to the maintenance of existing institutions, recognized the need for some accommodation. The reform era began in 1828 with the repeal of the Test and Corporation Acts, removing the civil disabilities under which Dissenters labored.[55] In 1829, Catholic emancipation, although structured to disenfranchise many franchised voters, opened the doors to Catholic membership in the House of Commons.[56] The Tories would not, however, compromise on a larger measure of parliamentary reform, but the accession to office of the Whigs in 1830 opened up a space for reform legislation at the national and local levels.[57] The next five years witnessed a small avalanche of reforming legislation. The best-known of the various reform acts—the 1832 Reform Act—amended the parliamentary franchise. But the Whigs did not neglect local government and passed legislation that permitted the amendment of parochial constitutions and required the renovation of parochial Poor Law authorities.[58] The 1835 Municipal Reform Act usually is presented as the last great piece of Whig reforming legislation. It was based on a royal commission that investigated 285 places, 246 of which were considered to be in possession of a valid charter. Of these, 178 were scheduled for survival.[59] They received a new constitution with a uniform ratepayer franchise.

The significance of this Whig reforming legislation for the evolution of democracy is ambiguous at both the national and local levels. The impact of the 1832 Reform Act on numbers of voters is unclear, but it was by no means uniformly positive.[60] On the local level, the promising beginning that came with Sir John Hobhouse's 1831 Vestries Act, which gave single votes to all ratepayers resident for one year and permitted a secret ballot, was weakened by the fact that it was permissive and by the high property qualification for election to the post of vestryman.[61] The 1835 MRA had a seemingly more liberal ratepayer voting clause. However, its effect too was blunted because it required three years' residence and because many properties were of such low value that the landlords negotiated with the town council for payment of some fraction of the rates, thereby disenfranchising tenants.[62] In some cases, the rate-paying municipal electorate was smaller than the parliamentary electorate, which had a much higher voting requirement.[63] The 1834 New Poor Law, perhaps the most significant piece of nineteenth-century social legislation, notoriously relied on the plural scale of voting.[64] The antidemocratic character of these remade institutions is not the only thing that gives historians pause; the powers they were provided with were also limited. The 1835 MRA gave newly constituted town councils only one mandatory power, the striking of a watch committee and the establishment of a police force.[65] The town councils were permitted to assume the functions carried out by local improvement commissions, but only if the latter voluntarily surrendered their powers.[66]

The Whig bills show us that property and the franchise were closely linked, largely because of the conviction that property had to be protected against the depredations of democracy.[67] That same tension between property and democracy structured the next stage of nuisance law evolution. The 1835 MRA permitted newly elected town councils to make bylaws for the good governance of the town and for the prevention and suppression of such nuisances as were not already punishable in a summary manner by virtue of any act then in force in the borough.[68] Newly reformed municipal corporations seized the Municipal Reform Act's bylaw-making power with alacrity. The new councils first met in January 1836, and by December 1837 more than seventy-five corporations submitted bylaws to the home secretary. Most councils revisited these bylaws several times in the future, and quite a number did so in the short term.[69]

In this section, I explore sanitary nuisance bylaws in a small number of locations, some of which became both regional and national models. Furthermore, I focus in detail on the process of bylaw-making. Bylaws did not spring *de novo* and in finished form from any given bylaw committee's collective brain at the first go. Committees often compared and contrasted their needs and desires with other councils' bylaws, explicitly rejecting, adopting, or amending what they found. By adopting their comparative method, and by looking at bylaws as the outcome of a process rather than as finished documents, we see local councils actively constructing different models of sanitary nuisance. This focus on process highlights in particular the inseparable mixing and mingling of health and property in the making of these regulations (let alone their implementation).

The sheer number of bylaws produced in the immediate aftermath of the 1835 Municipal Reform Act suggests that the usual means of regulating the urban environment were not wholly satisfactory, although one of the features of the bylaws passed from 1835 to 1840 was their continuity with what came before, particularly in terms of what might be called health or sanitary nuisances. The regulation of night soil, the control of sanitary nuisances in the streets, and the regulation of "particular nuisances" were found in the earliest bylaws, and their presence only increased over time.[70] Yet in addition to these elements of continuity, the bylaws displayed important discontinuities, especially an increased emphasis on nuisances on private property. The attention paid to nuisances on private land was, furthermore, focused on sanitary nuisances. The nature and timing of this interest was too closely linked to the 1831–32 cholera epidemic to be a coincidence and highlighted a second, related feature of this discontinuity: an increased emphasis on health.[71]

Some of the earliest bylaws revealed the significance of the cholera epidemic quite clearly. We can take Pwllheli, a port and market town in north Wales, as our first example.[72] For present purposes, Pwllheli's 1836 street article is of most interest. As was often the case in bylaws, the street article was by far the longest individual bylaw. It controlled and policed a huge range of actions, things, and circumstances in the streets from fighting, brawling, singing, and swearing to projecting street signs. Included on this list were some of the usual sanitary matters, such as the prohibition against anyone emptying privies outside of the prescribed times. This last was an absolutely standard nuisance provision, found in tens of local acts over the preceding decades.

Yet this standard provision was framed in an unusual way. According to the bylaws, the movement of night soil was controlled because moving it emitted unhealthy effluvia. To the best of my knowledge, this is one of the first times that this practice was legally identified as unhealthy. It was routinely controlled, but not explicitly in the name of health.[73] The Pwllheli council pushed its health concerns, surely stimulated by cholera, even further in a bylaw dealing with nuisances on private land. Pwllheli's council appeared to realize that this was a dangerous power, because they hedged it in with qualifications, restricting the kinds of nuisances to which it applied and the sorts of situations in which it might be used. In 1836, the council ordered that only stagnant water, manure, or decomposing animal or vegetable matter on private land could be removed summarily by justices of the peace, and even then only "for the purpose of preventing or averting any dangerous or malignant disease."[74]

The Worcester Corporation's bylaws were also stimulated by public health concerns likely triggered by cholera. The city of Worcester was governed under a local act passed in 1823.[75] Like so many local acts, Worcester's contained a number of statutory provisions that had the character of bylaws, but the Worcester bylaw committee thought the local act was deficient in two ways. First, the new

1835 corporate boundary was more extensive, the local act being confined to the smaller limits of the old city of Worcester. For that reason alone, the bylaw committee recommended adopting as bylaws eleven provisions from the local act that extended what were effectively the old city bylaws to the new, larger corporate boundaries.[76]

Although the bylaw committee claimed that all they did was extend the relevant sections of the local act to the corporate borough, they actually slightly modified some of the clauses. In one small wording change, the committee prohibited privies or necessary houses if they annoyed the neighborhood by reason of the effluvia they generated, whereas the local act had prohibited them if they annoyed passersby.[77] These apparently trivial modifications were, I would argue, highly significant. The new bylaw conceptualized the problem differently, redefining the spatial dimension and specifying the source of the problem. Decomposing matter did not only annoy passersby because it smelled but also polluted the neighborhood because it produced effluvia. And effluvia did not just annoy people; they made them sick. Though the wording change was small, the change in thought behind it was not. This bylaw was not about comfort but about health.

The deficiency of Worcester's old city local act extended beyond the inherent geographic limitations. The bylaw committee drafted an additional set of bylaws not drawn from or based on the local act. Although Worcester's local act already contained provisions around night soil and general street nuisances, the committee recommended and the council enacted a further bylaw regulating nuisances such as a "pig sty, or any other matter."[78] Some insight into the committee's rationale for the procedure emerged the following year, after the Home Office challenged the bylaw. The phrase "any other matter" was deemed too general, and in response the council stipulated a more defined list of nuisances and required that they be prejudicial to the public health as a nuisance before they could be acted on.[79] That the Worcester council decided to extend its local law after only fourteen years is significant; it was not as though nuisances on private land first appeared after 1823. Since the council intended the new bylaw to permit the control of nuisances to health on private land, we must assume that some event after 1823 convinced the council that they needed to worry about them and that they needed to worry about effluvia. The cholera epidemic is the most obvious candidate; the inability to control nuisances on private land was one of the most common complaints during the epidemic.[80]

Stipulating nuisances and the circumstances that rendered them remediable did not exhaust the Worcester committee's labors. Perhaps the most remarkable feature of Worcester's new nuisance bylaw was the mechanism of enforcement. If any of the items on the list of potential nuisances was presented to two or more justices of the peace, the justices were empowered to empanel a five-member inspection inquest. The inquest members had to be drawn from different municipal wards and had to view and report on the alleged nuisance within three days, failure to serve being met with a fine. The majority verdict of the inquest determined the case. The complainant had to pay to initiate the process but recovered from the respondent if the nuisance was proved. The resemblance to coroners' inquests was striking even without the name, and Worcester's bylaw committee was clearly committed to the institution, itself highly politicized in the 1830s.[81]

The bylaw committee's creation of this mechanism was unusual; the deliberative process by which the committee reached its decision has not survived.[82] That the committee worked through the details of this inspection inquest was, however, an indication of the seriousness with which they viewed these particular nuisances and, just as important, their control.[83] Nothing would have been easier for the Worcester council than to have vested authority for deciding on health nuisances in justices of the peace, as did Pwllheli. Worcester's other twenty-one bylaws all relied on justices of the peace to make decisions, and that is what summary justice was. Yet Worcester's committee and council were clearly unhappy with that prospect. Instead, in what must have been lengthy and contentious committee meetings, they created a complex procedure that vested authority over nuisances on private property in five voters who had only to be ratepayers and not necessarily property owners.[84]

The rationale for the new procedure is unclear, but the selection of the five burgesses provides some insight into the political commitments of the committee and council. It seems unlikely that the committee believed that mere numbers mattered: five members were probably not thought more likely to ensure justice more effectively than two borough justices. If numbers had mattered, the committee might have had twelve jurors, as did the quarter sessions, or twelve to twenty-four, as did the coroner's inquest. But potential inspection inquest members had significantly lower property qualifications than justices of the peace, thereby broadening membership. In addition, unlike regular jurors, inspection inquest members were chosen on a ward basis, again ensuring that different interests in the town (and potentially different classes of people) were reasonably equally represented.[85] The inspection inquest was not solely about justice any more than it was solely about disease prevention. This was an expression of value, an affirmation of democratic participation even if it meant abandoning some of the rigor of the common law. Thus, the construction of the health hazard by the Worcester council was a very careful reconciliation of danger, democracy, and property.

Pwllheli's 1836 and Worcester's 1838 sanitary nuisance bylaws were explicitly based on threats to health even though they differed in other highly significant ways. The relative novelty of Pwllheli's and Worcester's explicit reliance on health is apparent if the two sets of bylaws are compared with other councils' contemporary bylaws. The Liverpool corporation, for example, made no reference to health in its 1836 bylaws, though it clearly considered health important. We have already noted that the relevant section of Liverpool's 1835 local act, restricted to the old city boundaries, prohibited throwing or leaving any offensive matter in any public street. This was a commonly seen provision of local acts of the time, but the Liverpool act also prohibited throwing or leaving the same matter on any open or uncovered place, whether surrounded by a wall or not, if it was within ten feet of any public street.[86] The Liverpool council chose to make bylaws in part because the passage of the Municipal Reform Act gave it the chance to harmonize to some extent the variety of regulations then in force within the various boundaries of the town.[87] Yet the council's bylaws were more than just an exercise in standardization. The opportunity to make corporate bylaws forced councillors systematically to scrutinize their laws' existing provisions. The council's bylaw committee spent weeks preparing bylaws for the full council's consideration, and the full council debated the committee's recommendations over five consecutive meetings.[88] The council's 1836 bylaw code was probably the single most extensive code in the country for the time.

The surprising feature of Liverpool's 1836 bylaw code, at least in terms of sanitary nuisances, was its rejection of the model provided by Liverpool's 1835 local act. The provision governing nuisances on private land discussed above had passed parliamentary scrutiny. It is not surprising that the bylaw committee brought it forward unaltered for inclusion in the 1836 bylaws, but it is remarkable that the council did not adopt the proposed bylaw. The councillors were particularly concerned with the ten-foot rule. "Ultimately," the *Liverpool Mercury* reported, suggesting a rather protracted conversation, council referred the matter back to the committee.[89] In the end, the council turned the local act provision into two bylaws. The prohibition on offensive matter in the public streets remained. A new bylaw governed offensive matter on open private land, which could be acted on only if it was a common nuisance.[90]

The transition from one provision in the local act to two bylaws may seem trivial, but drafting fresh language that was not found in their local act was not something the council undertook lightly. The bylaw committee obviously believed the statutory provision should be incorporated into the bylaw code, the mayor and the clerk drew the council's attention to the fact that it was a statutory provision, and at least one member urged the councillors not to vary the language used in the local act.[91] Furthermore, the bylaw expressed an understanding of the issue that was different from the local act in an important way. We can see from the first bylaw that the councillors believed that nuisances on public streets could be dealt with in a summary fashion without having to be identified as such. They also clearly believed that offensive matter on private property was a problem that required urgent procedural attention, but the 1836 councillors believed that the prohibition that Parliament had sanctioned in 1835 was inappropriate. As they struggled to reconcile their belief that something had to be done about nuisances on private property with their anxiety over the rights of private property, the councillors reached back to one of the elements of the common law. Nuisances on private property had to be common nuisances, even if they were within ten feet of a public passage. Even as the councillors streamlined common-law process, they still wanted common-law protections.

Liverpool's example reveals the ongoing negotiation between the nature of nuisances on private property and the essential role that the protection of property played in the minds of those defining and thereby limiting these nuisances. It is not clear from the council's recorded discussion of the bylaws if the councillors believed that the problem was that the 1835 local act left too much property vulnerable or if they decided that the ten-foot distance was too arbitrary, or if they thought the mechanism for identifying problem nuisances was too vague, or if they thought that the provision did not capture what was really at stake. It is not clear that they could have chosen one of these possible options, so intimately connected were the anxieties over property and health. Given the new bylaw that the council drafted, it appears that all four concerns were at work. According to the bylaw, the proscribed object could be farther away than ten feet and still be bad, or it could be closer than ten feet and acceptable, but it now required the judgment of propertied men. Mere proximity no longer determined the case; distance was irrelevant.[92]

I have dwelt at some length on Liverpool and Worcester because of their different approaches and their importance for future bylaw development. In a process to which historians of medicine pay insufficient attention, town council clerks often wrote to each other, asking for information and advice on a variety of topics.[93] Many other councils consulted with Liverpool concerning bylaws. It is not surprising that they relied on the work Liverpool had done in regulating sanitary nuisances. The basic two Liverpool bylaws covered every sanitary possibility on public and private land, and they were as necessary for a two-thousand-person village as for a two-hundred-thousand-person city such as Liverpool. Many places adopted Liverpool's language, and thus Liverpool's notions, *in toto*. A bylaw governing nuisances on private land, including virtually the same list of nuisances in the same order as Liverpool's, appeared in the bylaws of Newcastle (1837), Sunderland (1837), Stockton (1838) and Carnarvon (1838).[94] Worcester too became something of a regional model, with Tewkesbury and Droitwich modeling their sanitary nuisance bylaws on Worcester's. It is interesting that in both cases the councils adopted the inspection inquest.[95] Thus, towns did create, or not, sanitary bylaws according to the degree of local sanitary enthusiasm.

Yet though possessed of copies of Liverpool's and Worcester's bylaws, other towns did not completely adopt their notions. They actively rejected or modified what Liverpool and Worcester had adopted. These varied responses again illustrate the contested nature of the sanitary nuisance or health hazard. Of the five places in which I found copies of Worcester's 1837 bylaws, for example, only two adopted Worcester's model for nuisances on private land (and even they tinkered with it). The three towns that did not adopt Worcester's model surely had instances of nuisances on private land as did Worcester, yet they did not believe that Worcester's solution was the answer. Because they did not propose other solutions, we are left with the conclusion that either they did not see these nuisances as a problem—and they saw them as a problem on public land—or they were reluctant to step outside of the existing common-law procedures for protecting property, even though those procedures were widely seen as too cumbersome.

Shrewsbury provides direct evidence of the impact of anxiety surrounding private property in the case of sanitary nuisance bylaws. The process of constructing its first draft code occupied Shrewsbury's bylaw committee for a considerable time, and its mode of proceeding is not entirely clear from the record.[96] It appears, though, that Shrewsbury's sanitary nuisance provisions underwent considerable evolution during successive edits. Shrewsbury's drafters initially elected not to have any control of sanitary nuisances on private property; only late in the process did the committee insert a bylaw governing sanitary nuisances.[97] It was not, however, taken from Liverpool's 1836 bylaws code, notwithstanding the committee's overt reliance on the Liverpool code.[98] Rather, Shrewsbury's drafters created a clause akin to but significantly different from Liverpool's 1835 local act, including nuisances on public and private land in the same bylaw and making the mere presence of any of a list of enumerated articles grounds for conviction. Shrewsbury did not even initially make an exception for material farther away than ten feet from any public street.[99]

As it turned out, the Shrewsbury council did not send a bylaw code to the Home Office until 1842, and this clause did not survive the process. The councillors evidently balked at the thought of placing so much private property under control. They modified this provision, stripping away only the subclause dealing with private property. They replaced it with a new bylaw that applied explicitly to private property, changed the list of nuisances to refer only to decaying biological material, and gave the offending party twenty-four hours' notice before fines accumulated. Yet once again Shrewsbury's drafters did not display the kind of concern with private property that those in Liverpool had displayed. They made no requirement that the material be formally identified as a common nuisance. In Shrewsbury, the mere presence of the proscribed material sufficed for a conviction (at least in theory). It is clear that though the Shrewsbury council of course intended this to be a bylaw about health, they did not mention it.[100]

Bewdley's drafters also rejected Liverpool's model of sanitary nuisance management.[101] Whereas Liverpool's 1836 bylaws had separate sections (and procedures) for nuisances on public and private property, Bewdley's drafters combined the two and created a bylaw apparently modeled on Liverpool's 1835 local act, protecting property farther than ten feet away from any public street. Although Bewdley's drafters thus adhered more closely to Liverpool's 1835 local act than Shrewsbury's did, Bewdley's draft, too, was further edited before it passed. The portion of the bylaw dealing with nuisances on private property was struck out; no bylaw for nuisances on private property appeared.[102] Liverpool, Shrewsbury, and Bewdley each experimented with policing these nuisances in a unified manner, whether on public or private property, but each retreated from that formulation. Liverpool and Shrewsbury ended up with separate (and different) provisions for nuisances on private property; Bewdley abandoned the task of controlling nuisances on private property altogether.

In general, the record of bylaws produced in the immediate postreform period illustrates an emerging consensus about sanitary nuisances as causes of disease. Worcester and Pwllheli developed bylaws intended to catch nuisances to health of the sort Chadwick would soon promote. Liverpool, perhaps more cautious about its laws, framed its bylaws more conservatively, explicitly relying on the common law. Yet these councils and others that they influenced each pushed the common law in the direction of summary control, private property, decaying material, and, implicitly and explicitly, health. I do not want to claim that these local initiatives were an inspiration for Chadwick. He may not have known of them at all, at least not in the late 1830s, when he began his own sanitary work. By the same token, they, too, probably were independent of him. They show us that the sanitary movement developed from a variety of inspirations, a fact that may help explain the success the movement enjoyed.

But for all they shared, the towns were not all consistent with one another. The pattern of acceptances and rejections of particular models by the different councils probably does not tell us much about the sanitary condition of these towns; all these places were similarly situated. It does tell us that there was implicit and explicit conflict around the very notion of the sanitary nuisance. Although these various bylaws had obvious similarities, principally in the overlap in some of the things that could be regulated—and it is tempting to see them engaged in the same quest—these different places did not deal with the "same" thing in the same way. The difference extended beyond the typical pattern of differential enforcement we expect to see when different jurisdictions apply the same law. These town councils were talking about different "things." Because they jointly conceptualized process with material, who decided and under what circumstances were as important as what it was.

The inability to reach consensus was only partly, if at all, caused by different local notions of disease. More important, I argue, were local notions around the control of or protection of private property. Pwllheli and Worcester protected property by requiring threats to health, and in Pwllheli's case a dangerous or malignant disease; Liverpool, by requiring the same standards as the common law. The final decision-making authority differed too, and again in important ways. Pwllheli and Liverpool relied on justices of the peace, local propertied men. Indeed, in its 1836 bylaws, Liverpool deliberately modified the language of its 1835 local act to give justices of the peace discretion. Perhaps the most intriguing of the control mechanisms arose in Worcester with its relatively democratic inspection inquest. In sum, Worcester, Liverpool, and Pwllheli and all the places that relied on them did not agree on a sanitary nuisance bylaw. The differences were not just details or mechanics of enforcement but substantive differences of opinion relating to the control of property. Just about the only thing that united these councils was their disregard of medical expertise; they did not seem to care, or know, what the doctors thought.[103]

The Central Government

The diversity of bylaws that councils produced after 1835 did not occur in a local vacuum. As we have seen, the 1835 Municipal Reform Act required councils to submit their bylaws to the Home Secretary for review, and the Privy Council could disallow them within forty days of receipt. Although the Privy Council, at the Home Office's request, often disallowed bylaws in whole or in part, the more usual course of events was for the Home Office to suggest amendments to them. Bylaws around sanitary nuisances were among the laws often, though not always, challenged.[104] The character of these changes suggests, furthermore, that the Home Office was deeply concerned with protecting not just local health but also local property. Indeed, taken together, the Home Office changes provide some context for the specific form that the 1846 Nuisances Removal Act assumed.

As was the case with bylaws in general, those on sanitary nuisances received belated and inconsistent treatment. The earlier a corporation got its bylaw in, the better off it was. For example, there is no record of Liverpool's (1836), Newcastle's (1837), or Sunderland's (1837) bylaws being challenged. The Home Office began to pay careful attention to sanitary bylaws in late 1837.[105] The experiences of Worcester and Droitwich illustrate this increasing vigilance. Worcester did not submit a significant bylaw code until April 1837.[106] The Home Office did not challenge these bylaws, and the Privy Council certainly did not disallow them. In May 1838, relying on Worcester's model, Droitwich sent in its own bylaws. The Home Office suggested substantial revisions to them. Droitwich sent a revised set along with what must have been an expression of surprise that its bylaws had been rejected, given that they were based on the approved Worcester set.[107] This triggered the Home Office's own review of Worcester's set, which quickly resulted in suggested revisions to Worcester's bylaws.[108]

The nature of the Home Office's objections to the sanitary nuisance bylaws varied but seemingly encompassed the things that were hazardous, the circumstances that made them so, and the procedures for identifying them. Loose drafting was a particular concern. Worcester's 1837 bylaw regulated a pigsty or any other matter, and the Home Office was clearly concerned at the scope of "any other matter." Suitably limited, the bylaw passed.[109] It is possible that the Home Office was principally concerned about the threat to local trades implied in such a broad nuisance formulation. Devonport's 1838 bylaws prohibited any "noisome or injurious Smells or Vapours" and also regulated hog sties and hog keeping. The Home Office did not challenge the hog-keeping law but rejected the "Smells and Vapours" law, because it "might interfere with some trades now carried on."[110] The Devonport council responded by drafting a fresh bylaw that dealt specifically with decaying biological material and required it to be a "Nuisance to the public" before it could be removed.[111]

In addition to these concerns about scope, in other cases the Home Office prohibited bylaws that were based on unusual mechanisms. Droitwich, for example, adopted Worcester's inspection inquest into sanitary nuisances (described above), yet in Droitwich's case the Home Office deleted the bylaw.[112] Tewkesbury, too, was very enthusiastic about the Worcester mechanism—the council noted that Worcester's inspection inquest bylaw was of "great importance"—and believed that the adoption of this bylaw itself more than compensated local residents for the delay the council experienced in framing bylaws. Yet the Home Office deleted the bylaw when the Tewkesbury council submitted it.[113] In these two cases, the Office's objection may not have concerned the process, because Worcester's inspection inquest survived even though the Home Office forced it to tighten its list of nuisances.

Finally, the Home Office may have objected to the conditions that made nuisances dangerous, the third component of local nuisance bylaws. Great Yarmouth's proposed sanitary nuisance bylaw declared that if any one of several situations was "offensive to any person," it was to be deemed a nuisance and subject to removal.[114] The copy of the Great Yarmouth bylaws in the Home Office has this provision completely crossed out. S. M. Phillipps wrote to the town clerk, informing him that this bylaw should be omitted altogether.[115] The council prepared a fresh, and acceptable, bylaw that omitted the "offensive" provision and controlled several of the same substances but only if they were a "common nuisance."[116] Hull's nuisance bylaw was similarly edited, at least at the Home Office. Hull's bylaw initially listed a range of things and required only that they be "offensive" to any person. An undated, stand-alone copy of this bylaw found in the Home Office records struck out the "offensive" passage and stipulated instead that they had to be a common nuisance. Given contemporary understanding of the term, a common nuisance, requiring the judgment of magistrates, was a potentially much higher bar than an offense to an individual. In any event, the unidentified Home Office author clearly believed that this distinction mattered.[117]

The Home Office's revisions of corporation health-nuisance bylaws from 1835 to 1840 thus continued, even if inconsistently, the pattern it had established in the 1831–32 cholera epidemic, when local authorities wanted summary power and central authorities did not want to give it. Parliamentary ambivalence emerged again in the 1839 Metropolitan Police Act. The Home Office promoted the act primarily for purposes unconnected to the control of sanitary nuisances, but the act's one sanitary nuisance section suggests that the Office was concerned with limiting the ability to police things and situations increasingly identified as sanitary nuisances.[118]

Central thinking on the matter was finally consolidated in 1846, when Parliament wrestled with the feared reappearance of cholera and the failure of any public health legislation to reach the statute book. The 1846 Nuisances Removal Act cut through many of the controversies around danger, democracy, and property that had swirled in towns during the 1830s.[119] The variety of offending objects was explicitly listed. The conditions that made them so were also made explicit: they had to be a danger to health or a nuisance. The final piece of the puzzle was process. The Home Office could not ignore the manifest desire of local authorities for summary nuisance power, but it needed an appropriate mechanism, and the various models that the councils proposed evidently did not provide one. Rejecting the lay focus and even the democratic character of these examples, the Home Office squared the circle of speed and control by enrolling physicians in the process. Identified items could be removed only if certified as a nuisance by two medical men, notwithstanding the fact that few if any councils relied on this mechanism.

The 1846 statutory health hazard clearly resembles the hazards identified by the central government during the 1832 cholera epidemic. But to suggest that precedent as the only or even the most important influence in its making seems, to me, one sided. Nor should we see medical involvement simply as a tribute to official appreciation of the need for professional judgment and qualification in matters of health.[120] Parliament would shortly pass a Public Health Act that allowed "unqualified" nuisance inspectors to perform this work.[121] Equally important as an influence, it seems to me, were the bylaws that the councils produced. Since late 1837, the Home Office had waged an ongoing tug-of-war with municipal corporations, revising and rejecting their attempted definitions of a health hazard. It is highly unlikely that this work did not influence the form of nuisance control in 1846.

ಶ ಶ ಶ

I have examined statutory and bylaw nuisance provisions through the lens of sanitary reform, but these provisions were part of a broader project of regulation. The control of private property had as its obverse the establishment and reordering of public spaces. Indeed, local acts before 1835 and bylaws after that date often contained a vast, catch-all code of behavioral regulation.[122] These codes have themselves been seen as complementary to voluntary projects of moral reform, which likewise entailed substantial redefinition of public space. A host of people engaged in newly prohibited behaviors were harassed, and a host of activities were driven out of public spaces into private or commercial areas.[123] Historians of local law (and law enforcement) have noted that this remaking of public space was never wholly successful.[124]

I have not examined the enforcement of nuisance laws, although historians have noted that the regulation of sanitary nuisances was uneven.[125] This inconsistency was in part a function of changing definitions of what counted as a hazard to health, and in part a function of a changing context of application.[126] The category itself, though, remained in the statute book. The 1846 Nuisances Removal Act, initially temporary but soon made permanent, became the model for statutory nuisance law throughout the nineteenth century. Even such an enthusiastic champion of the common law as Joshua Toulmin Smith believed that an act more calculated to do good had "seldom been passed" and he "earnestly" hoped that it would be made permanent.[127] Nuisance law after 1846 evolved to include an increasing array of potentially dangerous things, especially industrial nuisances and housing. Parliament developed different definitions of danger and the means to control it, but the mold was now set.[128]

In the next chapter, I turn to another attempted redefinition of property: liability for healthy drainage. Parliament was unable to pass comprehensive public health legislation before 1848, notwithstanding Chadwick's *Report on the Sanitary Condition* and the Royal Commission on the State of Large Towns and Populous Districts. Local authorities, ranging from sewer commissioners, first appointed under Tudor legislation; to improvement commissioners, acting under local laws; to private companies increasingly led the development of these services. These bodies were as conceptually innovative as the corporations elected after 1835. They too responded to epidemics by adopting miasmatic arguments in order to redefine drainage as a public good. The challenge to property that they promoted, however, was as unpalatable to national elites as that promoted by corporations, though in this case the courts led the fight against them.

Chapter Two

Private Benefit and Public Service

Paying for Sewers before 1848

In the first half of the nineteenth century, utilities such as bridges, water supplies, and gas undertakings could all be privately owned; by mid-century about 90 percent of gas undertakings were privately owned, and only 10 out of 190 municipal corporations possessed their own water supply.[1] Over the second half of the century, these services, at different times and to different degrees, were municipalized. Though it was by no means first in the field, the Birmingham council's takeover of its gas and water supplies in the 1870s caught the attention of contemporaries and historians, particularly once it became part of the narrative of the municipal gospel associated with Joseph Chamberlain's mayoralty.[2] However, one utility that is usually absent from analyses of municipalization is the lowly sewer. In part, this absence makes sense. As far back as the sixteenth century, sewers were controlled by public bodies such as sewers commissions. By the end of the eighteenth century, there were approximately one hundred provincial sewers commissions across the country.[3] Because of their public status, these commissions did not have to be municipalized, even though their constitutions and powers changed over time.

Yet the failure of sewers to find a place in the discussion of municipalization has, I suggest, led to a neglect of important problems and questions related to the provision and even the nature of this particular public good. The public provision of sewers is sometimes taken for granted in the literature on municipal provision.[4] Private provision was, however, a real albeit infrequently chosen option for nineteenth-century towns.[5] An analysis of why some towns first chose and then rejected it may tell us something about the nature of municipal provision.

Public sewer commissions also changed significantly over time. One of the most important of these changes involved rating. According to the Tudor Law of Sewers, parties could be forced to pay for sewers only if their property benefited from or avoided damage as a result of them.[6] This law was still in force at the start of the nineteenth century, and sewer commissioners spent much time and energy attempting to avoid its consequences. A related but distinct change involved drainage areas. Public sewer commissions (and local improvement commissions) increasingly wrestled with the geographic and hence the social scope of this public service and its burdens, especially in response to population increase, disease, and suburbanization.

The widespread existence of public commissions and public control at the start of the nineteenth century is thus only one part, and not the most interesting part, of the story of the growth of sewers as a municipal service. An exploration of changes in rating and areas provides us, I believe, with a fresh perspective on the politics of drainage. In older histories of public health, drainage per se was seen as an empirical and apolitical solution to urban health problems. The politics of drainage, where one was even thought to exist,[7] was presumed to come in at the implementation stage. But even here the question often asked about drainage—Why did it take so long?—presupposed an answer and led to accounts oriented around clean versus dirty, or progressive versus reactionary, proponents and opponents.[8] More recently, scholars from a variety of disciplines have identified a rich and complex politics surrounding the nature, function, and timing of urban drainage.[9] In this chapter, I use sewer financing and drainage areas in order to explore the establishment of urban drainage as a public good, financed with a rate on all property.[10] This outcome was only partially achieved by 1848 but was the result of a protracted legal and political struggle; as Daunton noted, drains raised important issues of political and philosophical principle.[11]

In the first part of the chapter, I examine two different private sewer ventures in Taunton and Cheltenham in the 1820s and the early 1830s. I draw particular attention to the ideological considerations that underlay their creation, but I stress that the private turn in these two towns was not solely or even primarily a function of local ideological commitment to market-based provision. Taunton and Cheltenham both adopted private provision not as their first choice but after other experiments with sewer building failed. In this experimentation, we can see local elites oscillating between conceiving of sewers as public or private goods. As they moved from one conception to the other and sometimes back again, local elites highlighted the difficult issues, such as the boundary between individual and collective benefit and the nature of taxation necessary to finance it, that dominated debates over financing until mid-century.

Private sewer building in both Taunton and Cheltenham did not, in the end, satisfy local residents, but in the second section of this chapter, I show that the problem with the provision of drainage was not only that private enterprise delivered an inferior product, because areas with public provision were similarly dissatisfied.[12] The problem was the nature of the service itself. The principal statute under which public sewer commissions were organized in the Tudor period was 23 Hen. 8, c. 5.[13] This statute was mainly intended to facilitate the protection of land from inundations from the sea or from overflowing rivers and streams. Because sewers were initially conceived as protecting lands at risk from water, the liability to contribute to them was calculated differently from other local public charges, such as the poor rates, county rates, church rates, and highway rates, whereby, with particular exceptions, all real property within the district was rateable. The language of the statute suggested that all who derived benefit (or avoided damage) from the works of commissioners were liable.[14] The decision about who benefited and who did not was made by a jury.[15] In time of need, the commissioners of sewers summoned, through the sheriff, a jury of men who, in theory, examined the matter and reported back to the commissioners with their recommendations. This "presentment" of the jurymen became the foundation for the rate that the commissioners levied when the Court of Sewers, as it was called, issued its decree.[16]

The importance of this law in nineteenth-century London resulted from the fact that even though some metropolitan sewers commissions operated under new updated legislation, these new local acts did not necessarily repeal the old statutes, especially in regards to rating. Several commissions (Poplar Marsh, Tower Hamlets, and Greenwich) still worked under the Tudor statute.[17] The idea that the sewers tax could be levied only on those receiving benefit or avoiding damage was thus well entrenched. The mid-nineteenth-century legal and political commentator Joshua Toulmin Smith clearly drew on this tradition when he wrote that "the sewer rate is the most just and equitable tax that was ever imposed; and the principle of its imposition is perfect; namely, that no man can be compelled to pay it unless it can be proved that he derives a benefit from the sewers themselves."[18]

In this section, relying on records of the Westminster Commission of Sewers, I show that the traditional benefit requirement, and the courts' interpretation of it, seriously affected the commissioners' ability to raise revenue and even to build new works. In response, the commissioners attempted to undermine the power of traditional benefit as a guiding principle of rating for sewers, shifting the benefit from property onto people and redistributing the costs among people presumed to benefit, by identifying health as one of the indirect benefits of good sewerage.

This effort, initiated in 1817, was a radical rethinking of liability for rating. This agenda did not emerge fully formed in 1817, and the evolution of the commissioners' thought was promoted and punctuated by successive epidemics and threats of epidemics. The commissioners began, as typhus swept though London in 1817–22, by arguing only that all individuals occupying property in the neighborhood of sewers benefited from them by avoiding disease and should help pay for them. By the time of the first cholera epidemic in 1831, the commissioners saw their mission in part as the prevention of disease. They privately acknowledged the need not only to tax people hitherto unrated but to build sewers in areas hitherto unprovided with them. In the course of this effort, the commissioners realized that some new way to finance sewers was needed. In the late 1840s, as cholera again loomed, they promoted a bill that would have allowed them to redistribute significantly the costs of sewerage in the jurisdiction. This long-standing effort, operating at times in advance and independently of the much better-known public health movement, was only partially successful by the time the commission was abolished in 1847, in part because Parliament did not share the commissioners' enthusiasm for redistributive taxation.

In the third section of this chapter, I explore the conflict between parliamentary and governmental priorities and local preferences from 1845 to 1848, a crucial moment in the evolution of the early English public health movement. I argue that both Parliament and the central government adhered to a largely traditional notion of the benefits and burdens of urban improvement. Benefit was still the principle that underlay liability. Various central actors, including parliamentarians and officials, carefully controlled schemes that spread the burden of urban improvement beyond tightly drawn limits. This control occasionally created conflict with local urban elites, especially in terms of areas for drainage, and Parliament changed local bills in order to bring them into conformity with central preoccupations.[19] Provincial and metropolitan elites often had very different visions of urban improvement from Parliament's. These contrasting visions exposed and expressed the increasingly contested terrain on which drainage, health, and suburbanization intersected, linking sewers with the broader debate over the costs and benefits of urban life in nineteenth-century Britain.

Private Provision: Taunton and Cheltenham, 1822–33

As we saw in chapter 1, the period leading up to the first cholera epidemic witnessed a flourishing of local laws. From 1,177 local laws in the 1760s, the number rose to around 2,000 per decade in the first half of the nineteenth century.[20] One of the standard powers of these improvement commissioners was provision of drainage and sewerage.[21] Yet not all towns embraced public delivery of this service, and both Taunton and Cheltenham experimented with private, for-profit sewer ventures, one informal, the other statutory. These private ventures were, I stress, experiments in reconciling the delivery of a good increasingly seen to be public with its historically and ideologically private financial basis. They were more experiments in financing than in delivering this service.[22]

In both towns, the local statutory and political environment powerfully influenced but did not determine the private turn. In Taunton, the structure of local administration exerted a particularly noticeable effect.[23] Insofar as there was a local government in the town, it was the Market Trustees.[24] The trustees were called into being in the late eighteenth century, largely to establish a market but also to discharge other basic municipal functions, such as street cleansing and nuisance removal. Unlike other improvement commissions, however, Taunton's Market Trustees did not have the power to rate property, and all of their income came from market tolls. Initially, their powers were somewhat limited, but in 1817 the trustees obtained a new act, authorizing, among other things, the construction of street drains. Nonetheless, the Trustees still were unable to rate the town.[25]

That the trustees obtained power to build sewers in 1817 suggests that they were alive to the need for them. In 1821 they began to discuss providing the town with them. In 1822, when the trustees finally decided that the town should be drained, they informed the public that they would build some deep drains and that property owners could connect to them for a fee, based on their property's rateable value, in order to offset (partially) the capital costs. The trustees stressed that the project required a significant advance buy-in from the townspeople, like some kind of modern condominium development.[26]

This 1822 proposal embodied an interesting politics of urban improvement. First of all, the drainage was to be publicly built and maintained. The financing of it was, in addition, unusual for the time. The Market Trustees could have built the sewers and paid for them solely out of the only revenue they controlled: market fees. This kind of indirect taxation was not uncommonly used for municipal purposes.[27] At the national level, indirect taxation dominated revenue generation after the 1816 abolition of the income tax. Yet taxes on consumption, such as market duties, were comparatively regressive and controversial, especially in the aftermath of the Napoleonic Wars and the political battle over the national debt.[28] The trustees elected not to build the sewers solely with this revenue. Instead, they opted to raise revenue by effectively taxing property. The trustees did not, however, have statutory authority to tax property, and the scheme was voluntary.[29] Drainage was a hybrid public-private good for Taunton's trustees; individuals chose to contribute or not, but drainage was publicly provided, and indirect taxes partially underwrote the costs of construction.

The trustees' 1822 proposal apparently ended up with few subscribers.[30] The trustees must have been relieved when a private individual stepped in and offered to build the system. They entered into an agreement with James Lackington Rice, who would build the sewers, charge customers a market rate for connecting with them, and turn them over to the trustees only once he recovered his costs plus a suitable return (defined as interest).[31] The trustees thereby seemingly accepted the idea that sewers were analogous to goods often provided entirely through the market, such as gas and water.[32] Yet the decision did not reflect a particular ideological commitment to private provision. Entering into a private agreement was not the trustees' first choice, and they only did so when the preferred option failed. The assumption that the trustees would take over maintenance once the capital costs were paid also suggested some kind of hybrid public-private good.[33]

The trustees' decision to rely on private provision did not, however, satisfy the desire for town drainage. Mr. Rice built some sewers, but given a low demand for the service, or perhaps given his monopoly power, he charged a very high rate for people to connect, thereby further driving down the demand.[34] As a result, the sewerage was very incomplete. The trustees returned to the matter of drainage in the center of the town during the cholera scare of 1831. Recognizing that consumer demand (and capitalist supply) were unreliable, and that a purely voluntary public scheme would likely fail, the trustees offered to pay most of the costs. Nevertheless, the trustees could not emancipate themselves from the notion that drainage was simultaneously a private good, and they also insisted on a voluntary contribution from the properties in the very limited part of town for which the scheme was intended.[35]

This new 1831 model embodied another politics of benefit and liability. First, the trustees decided that they would use their own revenues to finance most of the project. They provided no rationale for what was in effect an outrageous subsidy given to property owners in the affected street. Market failure may have eased their consciences about relying on indirect taxes, but it is also possible that the decision to use their own revenues suggests that the trustees envisioned the benefit from sewers in a new way. Both 1822 models, for example, assumed that owners were consumers and charged only those who wanted to connect. The 1831 model, in contrast, required a contribution from certain properties whether they connected or not. Owners and occupiers in 1831 were not merely consumers. The benefit was general for the affected properties; thus, a contribution could be, in a sense, required.[36]

The trustees' 1831 proposal was one step away from compulsory municipal taxation, yet even at one remove the challenges of municipalized rating immediately appeared and frustrated the trustees' intentions. They had to decide how to apportion the contribution on which they insisted. The sum Taunton's trustees required was apportioned among local owners according to their frontage (instead of the rateable value of their property), and apparently all but one of the fronting owners agreed to their contributions. The one holdout claimed he would have been faced with about half the cost [of the voluntary contribution] and that another one hundred houses in the neighborhood that happened to drain in another direction would effectively pay a trifle.[37] Deprived of one of the key contributions, the project collapsed. This new hybrid model was as unsatisfactory in terms of outcome as the private scheme it was intended to supersede, and Taunton remained badly drained in the 1850s.[38]

These vignettes in Taunton illustrate the difficulties local authorities sometimes faced as they contemplated even the smallest of drainage projects. In the span of nine years, the Market Trustees tried to finance sewers in three different ways—assessed value, market price, market duties/frontage fees—each of which embodied some model of benefit and liability. But each of these models generated a different kind of difficulty, and in each case the difficulty was insurmountable.[39] The difficulties Taunton experienced in financing sewerage surely explain why the Market Trustees made no attempt to provide any further for the construction of sewers and drains when they obtained a new local Act in 1833, although they had prepared another plan for draining the town that year.[40] And the refusal of one property owner to make a voluntary contribution in 1831 highlighted the critical contemporary question: How does one measure, and assess, benefit?[41] For this one owner, in contrast to the trustees, drainage was a public good from which all parties in the locale drew a benefit, and to which all should thus contribute. Frontage, implying as it did a relatively restricted sphere of benefit, was for him an inappropriate metric.[42]

Attitudes not unlike those of Taunton's trustees shaped the contours of the drainage debate in Cheltenham. According to one of its historians, drainage proposals circulated widely in Cheltenham in the 1820s.[43] Cheltenham's Improvement Commission was permitted to make drains and sewers, but the statute under which they worked was inadequate to the scale of the project, probably as a result of its inability to take on sufficient debt.[44] A common response to cases of statutory inadequacy was to obtain a fresh grant of power in an amending act, but Cheltenham's Improvement Commission chose not to do so for political reasons, opting instead to support a private solution. An 1833 act created a new private corporation, the Cheltenham Sewers Company, and empowered it to build sewers and charge customers for draining into them within Cheltenham.[45] It is clear that the Improvement Commission was not opposed to this new corporate venture, because in various sections the act spoke of the interaction between the two bodies. It is highly unlikely that the act would have been passed had there been significant local elite opposition.[46]

The formal private provision model embodied in the 1833 Cheltenham Sewer Company Act is not entirely surprising, given the devotion to market-based provision so characteristic of the time.[47] Cheltenham already had a private water-works company, and Cheltenham's elites and Parliament apparently believed that there was no *a priori* reason that sewers could not be made to pay on the same basis.[48] Yet as was the case at Taunton, the contemporary appeal of market-based provision does not fully account for the decision to support private provision. Local drainage promoters in Cheltenham saw the benefit from sewerage as a private good, and they were opposed to paying for a service from which they claimed in general to derive no benefit. The parish vestry, a political rival[49] of the unelected commissioners, initially approached the commissioners in 1831 about the need for improved drainage. However, the vestry clearly envisioned a limited scheme applying to one part of the town only, and they approached residents in that area who expressed themselves willing to underwrite the costs of constructing the sewers. The vestry stressed that it wanted to avoid a situation in which any residents "should be taxed for the Sewer who do not partake of the accommodation it is intended to afford."[50] The commissioners, in contrast, wanted a more comprehensive scheme financed by property-based taxation, but conflict associated with the political reform of local institutions doomed this project.[51] The vestry's view of drainage as a private good forestalled the adoption of a general system of drainage financed by rates on property.

As was the case at Taunton, the drainage of Cheltenham by the private venture was not, in the end, satisfactory to local inhabitants. By the late 1840s, fifteen years after the company was created, only one ninth of Cheltenham's houses drained into the company's sewers, and only half of the houses that could connect to the company did so. The drainage was almost entirely absent in the most densely populated and poorest part of town.[52] Capitalist provision, based on the assumption of consumer choice of private goods, again failed to deliver, though as at Taunton, it was not the commissioners' first option.

In both Taunton and Cheltenham, local elites lost faith in private solutions in the late 1840s.[53] A variety of problems were associated with private provision. Private providers could not force people to connect to their service, they charged a tariff that priced many people out of the market, and they did not even attempt to service low-income areas. These issues were hardly unique to sewers; the same was true of other private utilities, such as water supply.[54] But the failure to provide proper sewerage in these two towns reflected a deeper ideological problem. The issue was not the delivery, public or private, of this service, but rather the nature of it. At the root of the difficulty was the conception of the service itself. As long as drainage was conceived as a private good, it would be difficult to provide on a large scale, because it would be difficult to pay for in the absence of a rate on all property. Taunton's trustees resolved to obtain permission to rate the town four times between 1833 and 1840, though they never did.[55] Drainage was not the only reason they applied for permission, but it was certainly one of the important reasons. Cheltenham built a sewer system in the 1850s only by levying just such a rate.[56] But taxing all property in the city for this particular service necessitated a revolution in the philosophy of local taxation, redefining sewerage as a public rather than a private good, and relocating the benefit from property to people, even if property continued to be the instrument through which most local taxes were raised. This decision, however, to charge all property with the cost of the main drainage was, as Cheltenham's experience in the 1850s showed, not without controversy and came up repeatedly in parliamentary hearings in 1852 on Cheltenham's improvement bill.[57]

Taunton and Cheltenham illustrate the value of following a road less traveled. Private provision of this service was probably infrequent, though there is some evidence that it may have been more common than we suspect.[58] Although we are not sufficiently informed about the extent to which small towns passed through phases of private provision, the fundamental issue raised in Taunton and Cheltenham was common, and a similar story can be told for London and towns across the country, even though many of them had public providers.

Health and the Public Good: The Westminster Commissioners, 1817–47

The rating difficulties Taunton and Cheltenham faced had their statutory counterpart in the Tudor Law of Sewers, which, as we have seen, permitted rating but only on those properties receiving benefit or avoiding damage. This law, formulated in a different time and for quite different circumstances, increasingly generated conflict when it was applied in early nineteenth-century urban contexts. Flood defenses were still crucial for certain metropolitan commissions of sewers, but for some and even for parts of all, sewers were also used for surface drainage. In addition, after 1815, sewers began to be used for the drainage of household wastewater and even for sanitary waste as water closets spread in the city.[59]

The legal doctrine of benefit was ill suited to these new purposes. This doctrine had two major consequences for metropolitan authorities such as the Westminster Commissioners of Sewers (WCS). The most obvious consequence was that commissioners could not automatically rate all parties within their district and were thus deprived of potentially much-needed revenue. When demand for sewers escalated during the period after the Napoleonic Wars— whether as a result of population growth and associated land development, increased demand for the amenity (itself possibly the result of increased water supply), or disease—the financial stress on the commissioners could be severe.[60] A related yet distinct financial consequence was the barrier that benefit posed to the construction of new works, quite apart from the revenue that needed to be raised for them. The traditional notion implied that a sewer was like any other home improvement for which benefit was both easily identified and individualized. Once the benefit was paid for in one area, it was unfair to call on that area to pay for the improvement of other areas. This attitude clearly created difficulties for the commissioners, particularly in draining older (and impoverished) districts.[61]

In the remainder of this section, relying in the first instance on a casebook maintained by the commissioners, I describe the Westminster Commissioners of Sewers' attempt to deal with these consequences.[62] The casebook is overwhelmingly a record of legal opinion, some of which concerned ongoing or imminent litigation and some of which concerned new initiatives whose possible legal consequences worried the commissioners. These last cases, in particular, were policy departures by the commissioners and are a valuable supplement to the decision-making record normally left by minutes. Of particular interest are cases involving rating, several of which ended up before the courts. On the basis of these cases and legal opinions, I argue that the commissioners engaged in a thirty-year-long attempt to redefine the benefit and redistribute the costs of sewerage. They increasingly identified health and the prevention of disease as the goal and justification for this redefinition.

The commissioners' earliest attempt at redefining benefit in the casebook came in 1817.[63] The issue arose as a result of some repairs the commissioners made to an outlet for a sewer that passed through Paddington on its way to the Thames. Believing that the part of the parish within the boundaries of the Ranelagh level, or drainage area, benefited, the commissioners rated that entire part.[64] The parishioners, stressing that the work done by the commissioners at the outlet was more than two miles away from the parish, and never before having been rated for the sewers, challenged the rate.[65] In a careful analysis, parishioners divided the parish into four parts, specifying the different benefits, usually negligible, that accrued to each part from sewers the commissioners maintained. Counsel retained by the parishioners agreed that only a small part of the parish benefited under the law.[66]

In response to the parishioners' claim, the commissioners naturally sought their own legal opinion and developed a carefully reasoned account of the nature of benefit as they understood it.[67] The most significant obstacle in the way of rating, the commissioners believed, was the fact that the laws of sewers were "so imperfectly understood." Parties believed they were not liable to the rate if they were not connected to the sewers. The commissioners acknowledged that there might be streets on which none of the houses were connected to a sewer that ran down it. Yet somebody had to pay for its repair, and the commissioners' practice was to rate all land and houses adjoining public ways that drained into sewers and watercourses that they maintained. The commissioners' rationale for this liability was twofold. First, removal of the waters ensured that the streets were passable and all parts of the district thus remained accessible. Second, if the sewers and watercourses were not properly repaired and maintained, the water would stagnate and become a common nuisance.[68]

The cautious and unenthusiastic opinions the commissioners received on their case can hardly have reassured them, although, to be fair, their legal advisers probably were apprehensive about the commissioners' case as a result of *Masters v. Scroggs*, a similar 1815 case in which Masters' house was ruled to be so far above the Holborn and Finsbury commissioners' sewers that he could not derive any benefit from them.[69] John Richardson of Middle Temple seemingly agreed with counsel for the parishioners when he stated that the commissioners were on solid ground only in a small part of the parish, but in other parts the liability was "questionable."[70] Robert Gifford, the solicitor general, agreed with the parishioners that benefit still determined liability but tentatively claimed he "cannot help thinking" that the commissioners' reasoning on this were "more correct" even though the benefit might be "remote."[71]

Nonetheless, after hearing both opinions, the commissioners decided that the Ranelagh parishioners were "generally rateable" and proceeded with the rate.[72] As it turned out, the commissioners ended up in front of the courts for the Ranelagh rate, even though the case originated with a resident of another parish, Ann Stafford.[73] When forced to defend at trial their claim that the property in question benefited, the commissioners proposed a two-pronged strategy. They claimed first of all that water from the property drained, albeit rarely, into sewers they maintained, which satisfied, they argued, the test for rateability. They also argued that Stafford received benefit in the form of convenience and health. Internal documents were even more specific, linking badly drained areas to typhus.[74]

The commissioners' claim that health was a benefit was a particularly interesting part of their argument. Even the rationale that the commissioners developed in their 1817 case—that stagnant water could become a common nuisance—was not this explicit. The concern with health appears to have been a new one for them. In a slightly earlier and unrelated correspondence with the Dean and Chapter of Westminster concerning some property owned by them, the commissioners noted that their primary interest was with the drainage of public ways, and they made no mention of health or disease.[75] The idea that filth was somehow associated with disease was embodied, as we saw in chapter 1, in a number of contemporaneous local acts, and in general terms this was not a new idea.[76] The commissioners' claim that defective or improperly maintained sewers could engender typhus fever and other diseases was, however, both much more specific and more medically and legally contentious. The commissioners' typhus claim clearly reflected the increased prevalence of typhus in London during the postwar period.[77] It also reflected what historians have identified as an increasingly common though controversial medical claim about an environmental etiology of this fearsome disease.[78]

The genesis of the commissioners' environmental position in this developing controversy is unclear and, some might say, unremarkable. One might ask,

What else would the Westminster Commissioners of *Sewers* say if not that sewers were partly to blame? In practice, furthermore, official responses to epidemics typically included measures of environmental sanitation in addition to isolation and other medical and social measures.[79] Yet it seems to me that this was distinct from the commissioners' acceptance of their particular responsibility. The commissioners might just as easily have said, Typhus isn't *our* problem. There was no consensus that they were part of the problem; the 1818 Select Committee on Contagious Fever in London made no reference to drains or sewers and interviewed virtually only medical witnesses, all of their recommendations being directed toward hospital provision.[80] The Westminster commissioners certainly knew of "medical gentlemen" on whom they could rely to defend their position and who possibly inspired them. But it appears that some such environmental belief was increasingly common, even in the WCS papers.[81] The commissioners noted that the typhus claim was suggested in a letter from a Mr. Wilberforce and other residents of the neighborhood.[82] Ultimately, the extent to which medical debates inspired the commissioners is unclear.[83]

The inspiration for this belief is, in any event, unimportant, because the commissioners were not interested in developing a theory of disease but rather a theory of liability; health was the occasion and the instrument. The fact that sewers under the commissioners' control could prevent airborne disease necessitated the change in the nature of sewer financing. This financial change, though important, was limited at that time. For example, the Commissioners did not argue and would not have argued that sewer financing should be on a commissionwide basis, let alone a metropolitan-wide one. At this point they argued only that certain people in the level should contribute. Stafford and her neighbors benefited, and they should pay for the service provided to them.[84] They did not suggest any course of action that would have redistributed costs or benefits among areas or residents. Further, nothing suggests that they believed they needed to embark on a program of sewer building in particular neighborhoods. This was improvement by and for the middle classes.[85]

Even if the commissioners' ideas were limited at this time, they clearly were uncertain of this new position. They mainly framed their defense in terms of the actual drainage of the plaintiff's property, and the claim about typhus appeared only in a single paragraph at the end of the six-page document. Their caution was not unwarranted, because their counsel was uninterested in the health argument. The commissioners specifically asked counsel if the evidence for drainage was good enough, or if counsel thought they should in addition have "medical gentlemen of talents" testify on the health effects of bad drainage at the trial.[86] Mr. Serjeant Taddy declined to recruit medical witnesses, because he believed there was little they could say that was not well known already, and the trial itself showed that the commissioners' legal team had little interest in medical input or evidence.[87] No medical witnesses were called, though the commissioners' counsel did refer to the wholesome quality of the properly drained neighborhood.[88]

In 1822, the case finally was closed when a jury returned a verdict in favor of the commissioners, though we do not know the reason for their unanimous decision. They may have been persuaded by the argument that Stafford directly benefited, even if minimally, from the commissioners' sewers. But they also may have been persuaded by the more general claim that the commissioners advanced about the sound and wholesome state of the neighborhood surrounding Stafford's property and the requirement that she pay for this general benefit.[89] Interestingly, Hullock, the counsel appearing for Stafford, made no mention of this more general benefit that the commissioners posited, suggesting that it was a ground on which he chose not to contest their claim. If the general benefit claim was *prima facie* ridiculous, it is a virtual certainty that he would have pointed it out, with relish.[90]

The victory in Stafford's case was locally crucial for the Westminster Commissioners of Sewers, and their clerk, John Houseman, claimed that they subsequently collected many rates from Stafford's neighborhood.[91] The commissioners' victory did not pass unnoticed. In the 1823 Select Committee on the Metropolitan Commissioners of Sewers, Houseman came under particular scrutiny over Stafford's case. He stressed that everybody in the metropolis benefited from surface drainage of the streets, though he did not stipulate the nature of the benefit.[92] Houseman's reticence in front of the select committee has, I think, obscured the nature of the project in which the commissioners were engaged. By declining to speak explicitly of health benefits, Houseman downplayed what was by that time five years of reflection and argument among the commissioners and between them and their legal advisers over the benefits of drainage. Although there is evidence that other commissions in the metropolis adhered to the Westminster Commissioners' health view, as a jury finding on a matter of fact *Stafford v. Hamston* set no precedent.[93] *Masters v. Scroggs*, with its traditional interpretation of benefit, continued to shape metropolitan sewer law.

The effects of this traditional notion of benefit extended beyond restricting the commissioners' ability to raise revenue in their district and also compromised their ability to build new sewers, as is clear from the casebook.[94] The matter came to a head during the cholera outbreak from November 1831 to January 1832.[95] The commissioners already subscribed to the notion that bad drainage caused disease.[96] So, it seems, did a number of parishioners within the district, at least on the basis of correspondence with the commissioners at the start of the epidemic.[97] The commissioners could do little in most of these cases of defective drainage (see below), but they did pledge to do all they could "for the Health and general Benefit of the Inhabitants," reiterating their newly conceived twin benefits of drainage.[98]

The commissioners' sense of helplessness had strong legal foundations. As a result of fears of an outbreak in one area, the commissioners obtained four different legal opinions on their ability to build sewers in existing neighborhoods unprovided with them and, just as important, on their ability to pay for them. Thomas Andrews, part of the legal team in the *Stafford* case, advised them to build the sewers and pay for them out of an assessment raised on the owners of property to be benefited. Yet Andrews was less clear on who those parties might be, and he stressed that the commissioners could not pick out particular parties within the district and require them to pay for the work.[99]

Sensing that Andrews was perhaps unfamiliar with the exact nature of the circumstances and desiring further clarification, the commissioners immediately sent him a fresh version of the case, making clear that the street in question was Long Acre and the sewer was primarily intended to benefit private houses. The public, as it were, did not require any particular drainage of the street, because it was on the ridge of a hill and water naturally drained off it. The problem was that the houses and courts on the street had nowhere to dispose of their wastewater.[100] In his second opinion, one of the longest in the casebook, Andrews argued that it was "morally and physically impossible to ascertain with exact precision" the limits of benefit, and he suggested that the commissioners identify some larger district than the street itself that could be presumed to benefit and rate it.[101] His convoluted answer highlighted the fact that the difficulty in which the commissioners were placed with respect to existing, unsewered streets was due as much to rates as to legal power to build.

The commissioners were unwilling to rely on a single opinion in this matter, so they also sent versions of the case to John Campbell, the future Lord Chief Justice of the Queen's Bench, and to Attorney General Thomas Denman and Solicitor General William Horne for their opinions. Campbell told them that he could see no way for the commissioners to build sewers in existing streets unless they paid for the cost entirely out of public funds, essentially meaning that the entire district would pay for the street. Although Campbell "very anxiously" studied the statute and believed that the commissioners "unquestionably" had this power, he did not suggest that they actually should use it. Instead, he suggested (in a postscript) that the commissioners apply to Parliament for a new act, especially given the danger "now existing to the public health."[102] Denman and Horne expressed themselves even more strongly against the commissioners, stating that the commissioners had neither the power to build new sewers nor the power to pay for them if they did. "The Law," Denman and Horne intoned in early 1832, "appears to us not to have provided for the present case."[103]

The various opinions obtained in 1831–32 put the commissioners in a difficult situation. It must not have appeared prudent, particularly given the opinions received by the Law Officers of the Crown in 1832, to proceed with the building of new sewers. According to the law, the commissioners could only repair existing sewers; they could not make new ones. Yet the status quo in fact provided the commissioners with a partial way out of their dilemma by claiming that old ones were being repaired.[104] The commissioners appear to have operated this way even during the 1832 cholera epidemic.[105] And the chairman, Thomas L. Donaldson, suggested this as their strategy in an 1836 Select Committee hearing.[106] In August 1838, the commissioners instructed the surveyor to prepare a report on the drainage requirements of areas densely inhabited by the poorer orders, consistent with these powers and practices of the commission.[107] Pushing the limits of the commissioners' repair mandate by "repairing" old sewers so as effectively to make them new, the surveyor prepared a list of thirty projects costing more than £12,000.[108] If the 1839 estimates were correct, the completion of sixteen of these projects in the next three years cost something on the order of £6,000. This may seem like a trifling sum, but it was almost double what the commissioners spent annually, on average, for all purposes from 1800 to 1806.[109]

The period from 1831 to 1838 thus marks a new phase in the commissioners' thinking about health and property, in several senses. In 1817, the commissioners' objective was limited: to capture some hitherto exempt property. In the course of this initiative, the commissioners tentatively deployed a new understanding of the health benefits of drainage and the corresponding liability of property. During the 1831–32 epidemic, in contrast, the commissioners sought not to capture new rates but to build new sewers. This initiative makes sense only if we assume the commissioners believed that part of their mission was to preserve health.[110] Yet the commissioners also focused their attention on poor areas and their residents, another difference from their agenda in 1817–22. This redirection was again apparent in 1838. The instruction to the surveyor reflected not just a completely conventional belief that areas densely inhabited by the poorer orders were more susceptible to disease but also an entirely nonstatutory belief that these areas were thus an important responsibility of the commissioners.

This shift in the social concern of the commissioners is striking. It of course paralleled the intensification of the national government's concern with the health of the poor and their environments.[111] It also anticipated later central bureaucratic concern with drainage. As was the case for the first phase discussed above, the shift in social concern can be linked to local demand. Complaints to the commissioners from ad hoc voluntary parochial bodies at the very outset of the cholera epidemic drew attention to class-based differential access to infrastructure in a way that was not apparent in 1817–18.[112] To some extent this was unsurprising: the connection between victims of cholera and poverty, usually formulated in terms of behavior, was a staple of the first epidemic.[113] The parochial committees shared that attitude, but their reaction to cholera was more nuanced. If all they wanted to do was blame the poor, there was no reason to write to the commissioners. Parishes wrote to the commissioners because they believed that the commissioners could, or should, do something and that they were to some extent responsible.[114]

Just as they had in 1817, the commissioners responded to local demands.[115] Yet even as they added the role of "conservator of the public health" to their long-standing role as protectors of private property, their understanding of the liability of private property evolved more slowly.[116] This second phase of the commissioners' thinking about sewers did not, for example, involve significant redistribution of costs among property owners in their jurisdiction. In his opinion to the commissioners in 1832, Campbell acknowledged that they could distribute the costs of draining Long Acre onto the level as a whole, but the commissioners themselves appeared ambivalent about this possibility. In the margin of their instruction to the Law Officers of the Crown, sent after Campbell's opinion was received, the commissioners stressed that this did "not seem equitable," because property would be improved, with other property underwriting the expense.[117]

This marginal comment reflected the incompletely reconciled tension between their roles as conservators of public health and protectors of private property, and between the burdens that these two goals implied.[118] Miasmatism may well have implied that everyone was liable to the disease, but it implied nothing about liability to taxation; fear of disease may have opened philanthropic purses, but it did not change the law of rating.

The threatened return of cholera in late 1846 triggered a fresh round of conceptual innovation by the commissioners. If poorer areas were going to be sewered, they realized, other areas had to pay for it. In late 1846, probably frustrated that Parliament had not passed a new sewers act for all metropolitan commissions, the WCS obtained a new local act.[119] In the bill, and to a lesser extent the act, we can see the commissioners' commitment to redefining the benefits and redistributing the costs of urban improvement in the name of health. The act marked the first time the Westminster Commission statutorily relied on health.[120] At first glance, the act appears timid. It did not, for example, explicitly redefine general liability for the rates or repeal the rating provisions of 23 Hen. 8, c. 5 (1531).[121] Nor did the commissioners attempt to broaden the categories of property rated, a process on which they had been engaged for nearly a decade.[122] This apparent failure of nerve made sense, however: the commissioners must have known that the latter attempt would be vehemently contested, as would perhaps the former, seriously jeopardizing passage of the bill. Pragmatism trumped principle, hardly surprising as the commissioners prepared for a fresh onslaught of cholera.

The commissioners' strategic decision not to redefine explicitly general liability must also be weighed against the act's multiple redistributive possibilities. The commissioners were worried primarily about the building of sewers and drains in existing streets and houses in already established neighborhoods.[123] A major issue, since the act made clear that the commissioners could build and order new drains and sewers to be built, was cost: who would pay for the improvement of these streets and properties? The bill required frontagers to pay but permitted the commissioners to throw the expense onto such levels or districts as they thought derived a benefit if the sewer was larger than strictly necessary for the street in question.[124] Given that the commissioners were, willy-nilly, constructing a system of drainage, most sewers were probably going to be larger than strictly necessary for the street in question, and the commissioners clearly intended by this section to spread the cost of drainage as widely as possible.[125] Although the commissioners indeed decided to avoid a full-scale conflict over rates, they circumvented the problem that individualized benefit created by other means.

The promise and peril of redistribution posed by the act was apparent in the reaction of the commissioners' solicitors to it. The solicitors drew particular attention to the sections permitting the commissioners to throw part of the costs of new works onto the public as a whole, noting that the commissioners "will require carefully to consider how the provisions . . . can be carried out in the most satisfactory manner." The solicitors also appended to their report a legal opinion on these sections and these sections only. Charles Hall stressed that the commissioners could make sewers a public charge only under limited circumstances.[126]

The sections allowing the commissioners to throw part of the costs onto the district were quickly tested in Long Acre, a thorn in the commissioners' sides dating back to the 1831 cholera epidemic.[127] In response to the commissioners' query about how to execute and pay for Long Acre's drainage, the solicitors, noting that it was likely to become a precedent, responded with a lengthy opinion, seconded by the solicitor who had drawn up the bill. They noted that the act left the commissioners with two options, the difference essentially being the amount of expense that would be borne by the public. The solicitors stressed that the choice between these options was not a matter of law but of policy, yet they twice drew attention to the fact that the act allowed the Commissioners to charge individuals as opposed to the public and cautioned, or warned, that their decision to relieve individuals "needs to be based on strong grounds of advantage to the public."[128] It was the job of legal advisers to give cautious advice to clients, yet one cannot but be struck by the consistently narrow advice that their solicitors and other counsel gave to the Commissioners from 1815 onward.

As it turned out, the abolition of the Westminster Commission in late 1847 along with all the other commissioners in London brought the saga of Long Acre to a temporary stop. But it did not abolish the problems with which these urban improvement authorities wrestled. A deeply ideological vision of the benefit worked by sewers and drains—confined to property rather than people, sanctioned by Parliament, enforced by courts, and endorsed by large sections of the legal profession—constrained the ability of metropolitan commissioners to do their work. The Westminster Commissioners countered by adopting a rival ideological vision founded on collective health, but by 1847 they had made only limited gains. Sewers, in Westminster, were still incompletely municipalized.

Parliament, Public Health, and Public Works, 1842–48

By the late 1840s, it seemed clear to virtually all interested observers that Parliament was going to pass some kind of law dealing with public health. The government's determination to legislate in public health had multiple roots: the approach of a fresh cholera epidemic, ongoing problems with metropolitan commissioners of sewers, an avalanche of local legislation, and, last but not least, the growth in the early 1840s of a diverse movement directed toward improving the public health. Among its leaders was Edwin Chadwick, Secretary of the Poor Law Commission. The first phase of his work culminated in his 1842 *Report on the Sanitary Condition*, in which he argued that much surplus death and disease in the community and especially among the poor was caused by the presence of decaying animal and vegetable matter.[129] As a result of the impetus Chadwick and other interested parties gave to issues of urban improvement, the government created the Royal Commission on the State of Large Towns and Populous

Districts (hereafter Health of Towns Commission, or HOTC) in order to flesh out the argument and recommend the next steps necessary.[130]

The Health of Towns Commission sat for over two years and issued two typically stout reports. The commission ranged over a large number of topics—water supply, building regulations, nuisance provisions, and drainage, among others—each of which required some sort of investigation and recommendation. Given the amount of litigation that rating produced and the challenges it raised, the Health of Towns Commission might have been expected to give it serious attention and offer serious recommendations. Yet the commission's treatment of this subject was cursory at best. After a brief review of rating provisions in local acts, the commission made only two recommendations (out of thirty) directly related to rating for drainage—one primarily about rating poor tenements, the other primarily about paying for private improvements. The Health of Towns Commission tossed out the suggestion that main and branch drains should be paid for by the owners of properties benefited, without any further discussion of the difficulties involved. For the great financial battles that the metropolitan commissioners of sewers were fighting, the Health of Towns Commission offered little of value or interest. Even provincial elites would have found little to guide them in the exceptionally difficult matter, for example, of exemptions from rating for urban improvement.[131] The Health of Towns Commission noted that a variety of exemptions existed but did not directly address the justice of them, unhelpfully pleading only for uniformity.

The Health of Towns Commission's reticence on rates was matched by its reticence on areas for drainage, which did not yield a concrete boundary recommendation. This would depend on local conditions, but the commission stressed that natural drainage or watershed considerations should prevail.[132] Depending on the case, that could have meant less land in whatever was conceived as the local urban area, but it often likely would have meant more. The commissioners also recognized that suburban areas posed a particular problem. On the one hand, they should not be taxed for purposes unconnected with rural life, but on the other, they too needed works done, and excluding them from urban improvement areas meant they often had no provision.[133]

Further guidance for localities soon emerged, however, in the form of Lord Lincoln's 1845 Health of Towns Bill.[134] Lincoln's bill provided for a wide range of powers, including sewerage, paving, and general purposes. Each could be paid for with a separate rate, and Lincoln carefully defined and policed the benefit and burdens of each. Under the bill, the inspector appointed by the central government to visit boroughs seeking to adopt its provisions was empowered not only to recommend the district's boundaries but also to recommend that a district be subdivided for the purposes of drainage and sewerage. Once a district was divided, the local commissioners were required, not merely empowered, to rate it separately and to ensure that each subdistrict as near as possible paid only for its own works.[135] Whatever the rating district chosen, all property was meant to be rated, although land used for purposes such as pasture or market gardens was rated at one quarter net annual value.[136]

It is worth pausing for a moment to consider the assumptions that underlay Lord Lincoln's bill and the message it sent to local elites. This bill circulated widely among provincial towns, and several of the inquiries in 1847 (see below) made reference to it.[137] Acknowledging a long-standing demand of metropolitan commissioners, the bill proposed that all premises within districts should be rated. But by allowing the central inspector to divide the district for sewerage purposes, the bill encouraged local elites to see sewerage not as a municipal service but rather as a localized amenity for which localized pockets of property should pay. Local desire for sewerage, furthermore, required central oversight in order to protect land from being plundered by town dwellers. The division of the district, left to the judgment of the inspector, did not evidently provide enough protection, and the bill guaranteed further protection in the form of rate reductions. The fact that certain lands were rated at one quarter value only reinforced the notion that sewers were still rated on some sort of differential benefit scale. Although all property within the district was rated, sewers in this bill were not municipalized.

Lincoln's bill did not pass. In the short term, legislative progress came through the local act procedure, revamped by Parliament. The 1846 Preliminary Inquiries Act mandated that local acts had to have an on-site preliminary inquiry, overseen by the Office of Woods and Forests.[138] The last few weeks of 1846 and the first few of 1847 were a flurry of activity, with Woods and Forests having to recruit suitable surveying officers, as they came to be called, and formulate the procedures by which the preliminary inquiry would be held. Because evidence was going to be given, Woods and Forests believed that barristers should take it, but given the nature of the work the bills would likely propose, engineers or architects with extensive practical experience were soon drafted as the second group of official members of the local inquiry.[139]

Staffing the inquiries was only the first part of Woods and Forests' problem. If a local inquiry was going to be held, promoters of local acts needed to be told what they were expected to tell the inquiry. Woods and Forests accordingly sent local promoters tables of questions, which the surveying officers used for gathering evidence.[140] Woods and Forests drafted the tables but based them on suggestions from other parties with particular experience in the field, including, in the case of drainage works, Henry de la Beche, Thomas Page, and Lewis Hertslet.[141] With his service at the Westminster Commission of Sewers, Hertslet, who apparently recruited Page and de la Beche, was the most experienced voice in matters pertaining to administration, including rating and extent of jurisdiction. He specifically suggested asking promoters if all parties in the district would be rated, and if not why not, implying that it was the absence rather than the presence of a rate that required justification in the urban setting.[142] He made no explicit reference to benefit, and neither did de la Beche, although Page raised the issue.[143] Given Hertslet's position, this omission is startling and suggests something of the discontent with which metropolitan commissioners viewed this concept. However, the final tables repeatedly linked sewers to benefit and thus assumed something that Hertslet denied and de la Beche ignored: benefit was still a salient variable.[144]

The preliminary inquiry procedure was only one of the initiatives Parliament developed to assist local act promoters.[145] The other was a series of model clause acts that could be incorporated without fear of controversy into local acts, the clauses already having passed parliamentary scrutiny.[146] One such model act, the 1847 Towns Improvement Clauses Act, included sections on drainage. Given the content of the questions for the preliminary inquiry, it is hardly surprising that local commissioners were empowered (with central approval) to divide their districts for the purposes of drainage works and required to ensure that money was collected and spent in the separate districts.[147] In addition, the Towns Improvement Clauses Act rated land used for agricultural and other purposes at one third annual value.[148] It was, in many ways, analogous to Lincoln's bill, although in rating land at a higher value, even if the difference was modest, the Towns Improvement Clauses Act signaled the controversy over the respective burdens that land and houses should bear in the Tory and Whig political imagination.

Local improvement bills promoted in the 1847 and 1847–48 parliamentary sessions were thus subject to a number of potential official influences. The 1847 bills were first prepared in late 1846, when the only government guide the promoters had was Lincoln's bill.[149] They were examined in early 1847 under the procedures of the Preliminary Inquiries Act, and they passed through Parliament at the same time as the Towns Improvement Clauses Act, which some of them incorporated into their own local acts. These government bills and procedures sent a consistent message to local elites that benefit was still the principle, and subdivision the preferred method, of rating for drainage.[150] The extent to which the message was shared (or at least heard) is apparent from the local acts that passed during these sessions, but the 1847 and, to a lesser extent, 1847–48 preliminary inquiries[151] give us a different look at the local bill-making process and in particular at local elite understanding of the benefits and burdens of drainage and the appropriate framework for its provision.[152]

The least controversial aspect of local acts concerned the framework for provision of drainage. In the past, Parliament had supported private provision, and the preliminary inquiries guide assumed at least the possibility of private provision, but almost all bills saw drainage as a service to be provided by public bodies.[153] Almost all provincial bills also abandoned the various attempts to restrict the rate to properties explicitly deemed to benefit; henceforth, echoing Hertslet's view, the bills rated all property within the district.[154] The promoters of the Bingley Bill, for example, made no distinction between properties benefited and not benefited by their proposed works. According to William Barr, appearing for the promoters, "Premises are intended to be benefited by the sewers, and all to pay the rates."[155] At Rochdale, local promoters openly acknowledged that many people who currently paid their "paving and sewering" rate derived "no direct advantage," and they would continue to pay in the future.[156]

At Colchester, Surveying Officer Nathan Wetherell noted that the proposed bill rated the whole town "with regard to good sewerage or not."[157]

In an important sense, then, the original debate over municipalization was over for many local elites. Not only was drainage publicly controlled but all property was to be compulsorily rated whether it directly benefited or not. This open disregard of the traditional benefit principle of liability was remarkable, particularly given the struggles to get around it in London. It is not clear if local promoters believed that benefit was simply irrelevant or if they believed that a new kind of benefit demanded a new kind of rating. Promoters did not, unfortunately, make their underlying principles clear. It is noteworthy that promoters did not frame the need for drainage in terms of personal convenience, as they might well have, or in terms of the protection of property per se, as had been the case for more than three hundred years under the Tudor Statute of Sewers. It is possible, although there is no direct proof, that in the minds of the promoters, health legitimated the significant departure from the Law of Sewers that their rating provisions made. It is hard to imagine what other principle legitimated rating property owners or occupiers "good sewerage or not."

Although health was thus potentially a crucial concept for local promoters, both promoting drainage and altering its property relations, the significance of physicians for this development was again somewhat uneven. Physicians, sometimes more than one, testified at most, but not all, preliminary inquiries, even those at the smallest of places.[158] Given the increased prominence the public health movement gave to medicalized drainage, this may seem unremarkable. Nevertheless, the drainage section of the guide to the inquiries did not make any request for local mortality tables or morbidity records, in contrast to the detailed plans demanded for the works themselves. There is no evidence in Woods and Forests' records that physicians were consulted over the preliminary inquiries procedures, nor did Woods and Forests' guide instruct the surveying officers to examine local physicians. The few questions with medical content were scattered throughout the document.[159]

The presence of medical personnel at local inquiries thus reflected local decisions alone.[160] Although it may be the case that promoters believed that medical evidence helped convince local inhabitants and the surveying officers of the need for legislation, the testimony by local medics was not always wholly reliable from the perspective of promoters. They usually, but not exclusively, wanted medics to testify in support of the medical need for drainage works.[161] Yet medics were not always on side on the issue. John Leigh at Saint Ives, for example, saw "close air and want of ventilation" as of equal, if not more, importance than drainage.[162] Thomas Dugdale, surgeon at Blackburn, gave his self-described "somewhat singular" opinion that improved drainage would, "perhaps," make the town healthier but implied that perhaps it might not. He could not name any special cases of ill effects from bad drainage, though he weakly agreed that bad drainage "has its influence."[163]

Even in cases where medics delivered the goods promoters wanted—and in cases such as Taunton they definitely did—it is not clear that their evidence was needed or appreciated.[164] At Taunton, bad drainage was clearly the lever whereby local promoters hoped to overturn the local governing body. They trotted out three practitioners, the first bearing a petition signed by all the physicians and virtually all the medics in the town. But after the first medical witness had testified, opponents of the bill objected to the examination of another, and the surveying officer agreed that the need for improved drainage was already clear.[165] On considering other locations, one wonders if even the first witness was necessary. After Henry Houghton, a surgeon at Lytham, was sworn, he was asked just four questions, one of which confirmed his occupation.[166] At the Surrey and Kent Commission of Sewers hearing, which spread over six days, two surgeons very briefly testified.[167] At Rochdale, no medical witness appeared. If, as Christopher Hamlin argued about inquiries carried out under the 1848 Public Health Act, these hearings were a piece of local political theater, physicians were bit players.[168]

Notwithstanding the relatively uniform acceptance of the need for better drainage and smooth passage of local general rating clauses, the controversy over paying for urban improvement was not over. The debate in the provinces no longer concerned the propriety of rating within the district but rather involved the proper extent of the district and the proper distribution of charges among different kinds of property within it.[169] These issues already had been dealt with in various central initiatives in 1845–47, yet the drive for drainage at the local level forced local elites to confront them in a way they had not before. There was, for example, no consensus on the exemption from rating that should be given to certain kinds of land (primarily agricultural land, parkland, and market gardens).[170] Some promoters rated at the 1845 Health of Towns Bill level, some at the 1847 Towns Improvement Clauses Act level, and some higher.[171] The issue of agricultural exemptions would be controversial for the remainder of the century.

A related but distinct issue concerned boundaries and official and parliamentary enthusiasm for subdivision, an even more controversial matter for local drainage authorities. To be sure, parliamentary adherence to subdivision clearly reflected provincial opinion in some places. Leeds, to take one example, obtained a major local act in 1842 that gave power to the town council on an impressive scale.[172] Early in the process of planning for a drainage system, the Leeds Town Council decided that only the three central townships (out of eleven) would be drained.[173] This strategy eliminated the local political difficulty of rating outlying townships, such as the relatively wealthy Headingley, for work carried on in the central areas.[174] Because there was no provision in Leeds's 1842 local act for subdivision, the Leeds Town Council was forced to seek a new act authorizing it in 1847–48.[175] The council's decision to create what was, in effect, a special drainage district within the borough was legally unproblematic, because the Towns Improvement Clauses Act envisioned exactly that scenario. This feature of Leeds' 1847–48 bill was supported by the surveying officers Joseph Burnley Hume and William Tite at the preliminary inquiry. The exclusion of outlying areas attracted no comment in the parliamentary hearings.[176]

In other cases, however, local elites did not share the official fondness for subdivision. The 1847–48 Huddersfield improvement bill apparently proposed to levy one single general rate on all property within twelve hundred yards of the town center. At the preliminary inquiry, the surveying officers Henry Horn and Ambrose Poynter openly intervened, suggesting to the promoters that "hardships" would likely result from this. The principal benefit of the works might be conferred on one portion of the district only. The surveying officers suggested that the promoters avail themselves of the section in the Towns Improvement Clauses Act that permitted them to divide their district. This was necessary, they added, even though under the Towns Improvement Clauses Act, land was to be rated at one third only and was thus already protected.[177] The 1847 preliminary inquiry at Taunton unfolded the same way.[178] Taunton's ultimately unsuccessful bill proposed to take the parliamentary borough as its boundary, encompassing land outside the ancient municipal borough. Landowners in areas within the parliamentary borough but outside the town naturally protested, and the surveying officers John Maurice Herbert and Thomas Page pushed Orlando Reeves, solicitor for the promoters, to exempt land. Reeves believed that this decision should be a matter for public discussion, but after a valiant attempt at resistance, he relented.[179] At both Huddersfield and Taunton, the surveying officers exerted a critical influence on the boundaries of the local public service.[180]

The most vigorous local debate over the proper extent of a district and the proper distribution of costs within it for drainage came in a bill promoted by the Surrey and Kent Commission of Sewers in London.[181] This commission encompassed a huge range of land on the south side of the Thames, from the Ravensbourne River (dividing Deptford from Greenwich) in the east all the way to East Moulsey (as it was called in the bill), opposite Hampton Court, in the west. Its southern border was not precisely established but included lands draining into the Thames from highland areas through sewers under the commission's control. The effective jurisdiction of the commission, however, extended over only part of this territory, the lowlands adjacent to the river. The bill's preamble stated that significant new building had taken place within the commission's purview but outside its effective jurisdiction.[182] This building necessitated the construction of new sewers and the repair of old sewers in the proposed new district. But it also supercharged sewers in the lowland portion of the district controlled by the commissioners, and thus required new and improved and repaired sewers there as well. The bill accordingly extended the effective jurisdiction of the commission and unambiguously allowed it to build new works and to repair old works. It also allowed the commission to rate at half value every property in the new district more than two hundred yards away from any sewer or drain.[183]

The universal rating provision (even if at half value) was perhaps the most daring feature of the Surrey and Kent bill, linking it with the ongoing provincial disagreement over the proper distribution of local burdens and benefits. The Surrey and Kent Commission's attempt to overturn the existing order needed a compelling rationale, and the commission partly justified its desire to increase its jurisdiction through a pragmatic and equitable analysis of the local watershed. The commissioners admitted that water from the highlands naturally flowed down to the lowland area, yet they also saw that that water was carried away by sewers in the low-lying areas. Without those sewers, the lowlands would be a swamp, and people would not be able to travel across the lowlands to get to the highlands.[184] The Surrey and Kent Commission and some local residents of the low-lying areas saw the old and new parts of the district as an interconnected whole, with the proper drainage of each being necessary to the proper functioning of the whole. These equitable considerations legitimated rating all parties, including those more than two hundred yards away from any existing works, even if they got a reduced rate.[185]

The Surrey and Kent commissioners and their servants relied, however, on more than equitable considerations alone. These commissioners, like the Westminster commissioners, used health as a lever with which to move opinion. There was an immense amount of discussion about health, very little of it by medics. The Surrey and Kent commissioners' advocates and witnesses argued, for example, that new works covering over open sewers, many of which would be in the new district, were needed almost exclusively for medical reasons, and a number of witnesses testified to the ill effects of open sewers. Reflecting a consensus long identified by historians, virtually all parties agreed that open sewers were unhealthy, that unsewered areas were unhealthy, and that this bill was about health, that it was a sanatory act.[186] Very few physicians testified at this lengthy hearing, but the commissioners knew that their battle-tested professional staff had testified repeatedly at parliamentary hearings and would do a better job of defending the commissioners' objectives.[187] Indeed, it is clear from their testimony and from the questions they asked that the commissioners' servants and other interested parties from the district had devoted a considerable amount of thought to the nature of their local environment and the medical and equitable principles that should govern its workings.

This medical and equitable practical political philosophy adumbrated by supporters of the Surrey and Kent bill was, however, summarily dismissed by the barrister Henry Horn (the same barrister who conducted the preliminary inquiry at Huddersfield discussed above) and the engineer James Walker. They were opposed to some of the critical rating provisions and disagreed openly with the equitable principles developed at the local level. The surveyors did not think that in law or in fact the highlands derived a benefit from lowland sewers. So hostile to the objectives of the bill were they that they even questioned the manifest support for expansion from the outlying new district, attributing the absence of opposition to the local farmers' ignorance.[188] The surveying officers argued that anyone farther away than two hundred yards should be exempt. When the bill subsequently came before a parliamentary select committee, that committee agreed that property more than two hundred yards away should not be rated. Parliament's decision to exempt such property from the rates effectively subdivided the Surrey and Kent commissioners' district.

The boundary outcomes of these four bills, which were promoted in 1847 and 1847–48, were similar. In Huddersfield and Taunton, the surveying officers cajoled promoters into excluding outlying land. Parliament acquiesced in these semicoerced exclusions in Huddersfield and Taunton and again in the voluntary one in Leeds, and it forced subdivision on the Surrey and Kent Commission of Sewers. It is important to recognize the political nature of these decisions. In each case the dispute was spatially organized and in Surrey and Kent revolved around simple distance, but distance, like all spatial differentiation, was socially and functionally structured. In the Surrey and Kent Commission of Sewers, properties more than two hundred yards away from the commissioners' works in the new district were more likely to belong to gentry or farmers. In 1847, including such property, even at the reduced rate, meant politicizing drainage in particularly volatile ways.[189]

It would be a mistake, however, to think that this urban-rural conflict in the Surrey and Kent Commission exhausted the politics of drainage. The conflicts traced in this chapter were both complex and variable, and middle-class divisions along religious, political, economic, and residential lines make the interpretation of continuity, change, and conflict in these towns similarly complex and variable.[190] The debate over the Surrey and Kent bill, the most thorough of the 1847 hearings here considered, illustrates this. There was no local consensus on areas and rating in this bill; whether one lived in the old riverfront district or the new upland district did not necessarily predict one's position.[191] Some parties in the high ground rejected the Surrey and Kent Commission's expansionist argument, noting that their water found its level and they had nothing further to do with it, and they feared they would be rated for works they did not require. But not all of the opposition to the expansion was from the highlands. In fact, as the surveying officers noted, most of the evidence from the highlands, including that of landowners, supported the extension of the commission's effective jurisdiction.[192] Some of the most vociferous opponents of extension were from riverside parishes. Much still needed to be done in the old district, and they believed that adding new areas would only dilute the energies of the commission. In addition, they argued that the rates they would be forced to pay would be used to construct works in the highlands from which they would not benefit, and they believed that they had already paid rates from which they did not benefit.[193] Some parties in the old district stressed that "aristocratic" property would derive an unfair advantage under the proposed bill and had derived an advantage under the existing bill.[194] But not all opponents of the bill from the old district were opposed in principle to incorporating the new district; for some, everything depended on the terms. A Mr. Elkington, appearing on behalf of Bermondsey, a riverfront parish, summed this position up: "We, at present in the low lands, are in a species of partnership; the high lands are to be brought into that partnership, and the question is, on what conditions they should join us." Elkington suggested that the highlands, "the more wealthy firm, so to speak," should pay the same or even a higher rate.[195] The politics of drainage cut across a number of conventional political markers.

In their powerful analysis of the dynamics of metropolitan growth, Dyos and Reeder link slum and suburb together as manifestations of the relatively unrestrained movement of capital in the metropolis. In their view, the movement toward municipal socialism at the end of the century arose, in part, from a desire to redistribute the financial burden of metropolitan life, caused by this freedom of capital, among poor and wealthy parishes.[196] We can, I believe, see a similar process at work when, in the first half of the century, the Westminster Commissioners of Sewers and the Surrey and Kent Commissioners of Sewers struggled to municipalize their sewers. In both cases, the commissioners also responded to some manifestation of spatial differentiation in their local environment, be it residential segregation or recent suburbanization.[197] The developments traced in this chapter chart a concerted effort to redefine the burden attached to property.

The impetus for this redefinition came not from socialist ideas, however, but from a socialized notion of health. From the 1810s through the 1840s, in parliamentary committee rooms and courts of law, various sewer authorities fought to alter the established law of sewers so as to permit districtwide rating. Commissioners believed that the subdistrict rating, whether based on parishes or levels, was, in the first instance, impractical, because it was effectively impossible in certain situations to confine benefit to one level or parish alone. But commissioners and their officers went beyond pragmatic considerations and challenged the very benefit principle that underwrote level financing. One of the most common rhetorical strategies the commissioners deployed to support districtwide rating was to claim that the benefits the sewers provided were indirect or general. Calling a benefit indirect or general, however, conveyed little positive meaning and seemed only to distinguish this new kind of benefit from the standard direct benefit (i.e., land was drained) while still trying to bring the benefit within ideologically acceptable limits.

In order to give indirect and general benefit more precise meaning, commissioners sometimes compared the benefit from the sewers with other presumably equally indirect benefits, such as paving and highways.[198] Increasingly frequently and successfully, though, some commissioners, such as the Westminster Commissioners of Sewers, claimed that the sewers produced generally better health for all, including ratepayers not directly connected to them but living in the area. This shift from an analogical to a mechanistic argument was a key move. The commissioners justified sewers not on the basis of an analogy but on the basis of a causal mechanism. Thus did miasmatism haltingly become a doctrine of liability, not of disease transmission.

The first two chapters of this book have demonstrated the conceptual innovations that various local actors developed, among them town councilors, improvement commissioners, and sewer commissioners. These chapters also have demonstrated that the principal means by which these local actors responded to their local environment was a creative interpretation and application of miasmatism. The miasmatic theories they deployed had a family resemblance, to be sure, but they were not identical, and their differences were driven less by medical ideas than by the need to protect property. The power of miasmatism in the hands of local actors is clear, yet so were the limits, which emerged most clearly in the case of property's liability. The Westminster Commissioners of Sewers used miasmatism to make important changes in the law of rating, but they could not and would not use it to sanction significant redistribution within their districts. The Surrey and Kent Commissioners of Sewers likewise imposed their own limits in rating properties more than two hundred yards away at half value. This may have been strategic, but when Parliament eliminated even that qualification it showed miasmatism's limits very clearly; the local authorities discussed in this chapter did not use miasmatism to significantly redistribute rates. If a large district was going to be rated to provide infrastructure for a restricted part of it, some new justification was required. In the next chapter, we will see that local authorities and the judges who ruled on their actions provided just that.

Chapter Three

The Boundaries of Health, 1848–70

The previous chapter showed that the physical boundaries of drainage were increasingly controversial in both London and the provinces. In this chapter, I analyze boundary-making processes under the 1848 Public Health Act (PHA). I demonstrate that boundaries, for both opponents and supporters of the PHA, were not simply physical or administrative. They were simultaneously political, ideological, and financial, defining not only membership but responsibility and, more important, liability. In the course of boundary making, local PHA promoters and local boards of health developed a view of public health that amounted to a new view of community, integrating spatially, socially, and functionally distinct kinds of property into a common political and financial regime. In legal terms, this was controversial, but in contrast to the situation under the Tudor Law of Sewers, local promoters successfully persuaded the courts to expand the circle of liability. In this case, as in the creation of the statutory health hazard, public health activists changed the law of property's liability.

The PHA was one of several laws enacted in the first half of the nineteenth century that had significant boundary-making implications.[1] The 1832 Reform Act, the 1834 New Poor Law, and the 1835 Municipal Reform Act also demanded spatial reorganization. These acts required some kind of physical boundary, often a novel one, for parliamentary constituencies, poor law unions, or municipal corporations. Boundary making was hardly the primary purpose of these acts, but it was inextricably linked to all of them. Parliament clearly recognized the importance and sensitivity of the matter, devoting significant parliamentary time to the discussion of boundaries and insisting for the 1832 and 1835 acts that it alone could establish or change them.[2] As a result of these boundary-making exercises, spatial and hence political and financial relationships among the country's rural, urban, and suburban populations changed in highly significant ways.

It was, perhaps, predictable that boundaries emerged as a topic of parliamentary interest during the 1830s merely as a result of the growth of cities. Yet urban areas had experienced significant population growth for decades, and Parliament previously had discussed boundaries only infrequently.[3] Rather, politics and especially parliamentary reform in 1832 drove the increasing parliamentary concern with boundaries. Given that some partisans regarded the enfranchisement of new boroughs as an alteration in the balance between the manufacturing and agricultural interests, attempts to create boundaries for parliamentary boroughs invariably uncovered and perhaps generated conflict between rural/agricultural and urban/industrial interests.[4] Henceforward, boundaries were an increasing if irregular part of parliamentary concern, the cartographic manifestation of structural change.[5]

It is understandable that the physical boundary-making exercises of the 1832 Reform Act and the 1835 MRA have attracted less historical attention than have their constitutional and political consequences.[6] Yet the debates around boundaries in 1831–32 and again in 1835–38 are interesting, because they articulated contemporary notions of municipality at the time.[7] Two main models circulated. When debating particular parliamentary borough boundaries in 1831–32, ministers stressed that they strove to construct communities of interest. The idea that a community was an undifferentiated whole with a well-defined consensual and collective interest was, of course, a fiction. Rather, the enfranchisement of new boroughs and the establishment of their boundaries was influenced by various political compromises and realities.[8] Nonetheless, the ideal reflected what scholars have identified as the traditional view of parliamentary representation of specific interests and industries, such as shipping, the cloth trade, and manufacturing, as opposed to "mere numbers."[9]

A different model dominated the discussion of municipal boundaries, which also were controversial. Both the Commons and the Lords debated appropriate boundaries and the constitutional means for forming them.[10] The government believed that neither parliamentary nor historic municipal boundaries were ideal for municipal purposes, the former frequently being too large and the latter frequently too small.[11] Although Parliament rejected the Whig proposal to have boundaries for some boroughs determined in the first instance by an appointed boundary commission, the commission was already engaged in its work by the time the 1835 act passed, and the Whigs presumably believed that Parliament would agree with some of the recommendations it came up with.[12] The instructions issued to the Whig-appointed boundary commissioners provide interesting insights into the conceptualization of municipalities at the time. Municipality, for the boundary commissioners, was not about some hypothetical community of interest but rather very concrete service provision. It implied two things: jurisdiction and police.[13] Those two functions rested on different foundations, but my main concern is with the police, which implied not merely law enforcement but rather a wider, eighteenth-century notion of municipal governance that included paving and lighting as well as watching.[14] What seemed to unite these communities were the shared burdens and benefits of municipal taxation. Indeed, the commissioners' recommendations often involved collapsing parliamentary boundaries in order to liberate adjoining land from municipal burdens.[15] According to the 1835 commissioners and their Whig masters, municipal boundaries reflected less communal interest than self-interest.[16]

The 1830s ideas of municipality are important for this study because the boundaries struck under the 1832 and 1835 acts often became the boundaries used for local board of health (LBH) districts. Boundary making under the 1848 Public Health Act is relatively understudied.[17] However, as was the case with parliamentary and municipal boundaries, it was often highly controversial, in part because the idea of community constructed by some local boards of health did not mesh seamlessly with preexisting ideas. Indeed, tension surrounding conceptions of community implicit in these three statutes provided the dynamic for some LBH activity. Communities, for some local boards of health, were united not by direct benefit but by indirect benefit, especially health and the need to provide the means of obtaining it.

In the first section of this chapter, I trace the initial formation of physical boundaries for LBH, the contests it generated, and the efforts of newly created local boards of health to change those outcomes in the early PHA period. Although it may seem that efforts to modify proposed LBH boundaries amounted to little more than a contest between expansionist desires to increase the pool of ratepayers or contractionist desires to circumscribe the limits of liability, the character of change that expansionist local activists sought belied this cynical motive. In some cases, expansionist local promoters tried to use the PHA to force hitherto exempt urban property, suburban houses, regional industry, speculative developments, and agricultural land to bear a greater share of the cost of urban improvement. In order to achieve these objectives, the promoters developed an explicit ideological justification for their expanded notion of liability. In so doing they redefined the benefits and therefore the burdens of urban improvement.

This section also examines the role of the General Board of Health (GBH), comparing and contrasting it with the activist role that many local promoters played. Although the GBH's superintending inspectors—the central government officers responsible for suggesting local board of health boundaries—emerge as sympathetic allies of the expansionist group among local promoters of the PHA, local attempts at boundary extension often, though by no means always, failed. One of the main reasons was that the administrative and political leadership of the GBH undercut local wishes and often their own local inspectors. Local boards of health were not always deterred by these initial failures, and they sometimes tried again once the district was formed. The Eton LBH, for example, spent five years trying to extend its district boundaries on three different occasions. These efforts were unsuccessful, and the GBH was a conservative force, delaying and denying in turn. The attempt to increase the amount of land within LBH boundaries was frequently no more successful than local act attempts to capture outlying land before 1848.

The establishment of a local board of health physical boundary did not settle disputes over boundaries. In the second part of the chapter, I argue that in the long term, physical boundary making was less important than financial boundary making. Once a physical boundary was set, the LBH still had to make difficult decisions about distributing the costs of sanitary improvement within it. The PHA left decisions about rating to the discretion of local boards of health, and I show that their rating decisions consistently pushed the financial boundaries of health, rating much property hitherto exempt from these charges, notwithstanding GBH suggestions to the contrary. Although the GBH could not prohibit these decisions, the courts could, and LBH initiatives often were challenged in court. The outcomes of these challenges were highly significant, making law and thus influencing policy well beyond the borders of the particular LBH districts in which the challenges were launched. For example, after a long legal struggle, the Epsom LBH successfully convinced the Queen's Bench, Parliament, and even the GBH of the justice of its highly redistributive program of sewer building, establishing in law the importance of indirect benefits in rating for urban infrastructure.

Epsom's victory, I would suggest, brought about the most fundamental revision of the law of sewers in two hundred fifty years. In the third section of this chapter, I consider the significance of this ruling for the General Board of Health and for other local boards of health. Apparently the GBH did not aggressively promote the court's decision in Epsom's case, but it immediately began responding to local boards of health in light of the decision, drawing attention to it and tacitly consenting to projects that distributed costs over larger districts than those that benefited directly. Some local boards of health were fortified by this information, redistributing costs locally in ways that might have seemed impossible before the decision, and in the process forging new communities of health.

The Physical Boundaries of Health

The process of physical boundary making under the Public Health Act was structured by the mechanism that Parliament created for adopting this permissive act.[18] When a locality petitioned to adopt the Public Health Act, the General Board of Health directed a superintending inspector to conduct a preliminary inquiry in the district, reporting on the state of the area, recommending district boundaries, and suggesting remedial works. Boundaries of local boards of health were intended to be determined on the basis of watershed considerations.[19] The mechanism for putting the act in force, however, assumed that at least some of the time the act would be applied to places with already defined boundaries, such as a parish, corporate borough, or parliamentary borough. It was highly unlikely that those boundaries, formed as they were for ecclesiastical or political purposes, would coincide with watersheds, and the legislature thus recognized the limits to the scientific and engineering logic that underlay the Public Health Act. Given that many of these already existing boundaries encompassed large areas with, in some cases, highly dispersed populations, the process of boundary making under the PHA was highly controversial.[20]

Eton illustrates the controversial character of boundaries and some of the moral, ideological, and political meanings of making them. Eton was (and is) the location of an elite public school, and around it was a town of some thirty-five hundred. In the early 1840s, in consequence of the publication of Edwin Chadwick's *Report on the Sanitary Condition*, Eton College spent several thousand pounds perfecting its own internal drainage arrangements.[21] Eton town, in contrast, remained unimproved yet apparently not uninterested in improvement; it was one of the earliest places to petition to adopt the PHA.[22] The application of the act, however, generated opposition, one of the principal concerns being Superintending Inspector Edward Cresy's proposed boundary. Cresy's draft report suggested that the college and its precincts "might be very advantageously included" in the proposed LBH district. However, Cresy's boundary recommendation was corrected by a reader at the GBH, and the final report recommended that the College "should be" included in the district.[23]

Cresy's rationale for his recommended boundary is not entirely clear. Eton College was in the heart of the district, so it did not merely happen to get captured because of the way Cresy envisioned the outer limits of the local watershed. Nor was the college itself included because it needed significant improving; it needed at the most a small amount of additional work. Cresy's report indicated that the college should be included for unity of administration; keeping the college out, he appeared to believe, would lead to clashes of interest. This would be believable in a district of unequally improved, publicly accessible areas, such as those towns administered by multiple paving or improvement commissioners. However, because the college recently had constructed its own sanitary arrangements and because it was a private establishment, administrative unity was not a serious consideration. Given the strength of feeling subsequently shown by the local board of health in the matter, Cresy's recommendation possibly reflected his sympathy with the position of those about to be elected to the LBH. The GBH at this time evidently felt even more strongly about the matter than Cresy did.

Regardless of the GBH's reasoning, the college immediately swung into action and argued that it should not have to pay for the town's drainage, having recently completed its own.[24] The town's self-appointed committee on sanitary reform seemingly accepted this rationale,[25] and the GBH left the college out of the proposed district. The elected members of the LBH apparently did not agree, because they almost immediately asked the GBH about expanding the district. The GBH rebuffed them, and the LBH temporarily gave up and began to construct a drainage scheme for its own district.[26] Once the town's sewerage scheme was underway, however, the ostensible reason for keeping the college out of the district disappeared, because the college would no longer have to pay for drainage of the town. The LBH accordingly again petitioned the GBH to alter the district, expanding it to include the college and cottage property nearby.[27] Cresy again presided over a three-day inquiry, extensively reported in the local press, and in his second report produced an even more forceful statement in favor of uniting the college with the town in a single district.[28] The college memorialized the GBH against the proposed extension, which triggered a countermemorial and a deputation from the LBH.[29]

The debates around extending the district—at the inquiry, in the memorials, and at the deputation—reveal some of the diversity of issues at stake in boundary making, at least at Eton. The newspaper report of Cresy's second public inquiry focused almost exclusively on the Eton LBH's claim that because it was excluded, the college largely escaped paying highway rates.[30] This was an important if predictable objection; disputes about highway rates would be a recurring cause of conflict in setting boundaries for various local government districts for the next several decades.[31] Yet it is not clear that the college or the local board of health saw this as the only issue or even the most important one. It is perhaps unsurprising that the college did not mention highway rates in its memorial against the proposed extension. For the college, extension was a political issue, and the possibility that an elected LBH would have power over them filled the college's officers with "dread."[32]

The fact that the college's officers were as worried about this as they evidently were invests this town-and-gown conflict with a particular political meaning. The Public Health Act, like the New Poor Law, used a property-weighted voting scale that awarded owner-occupiers up to twelve votes.[33] In Eton, this ensured that individuals such as the Provost and Fellows of the college had multiple votes. Of the forty-five properties rated at more than £50 in the parish, the Fellows and Provost occupied thirty-one.[34] In addition, the PHA empowered the General Board of Health to set property qualifications for local board of health members. In Eton's case, Cresy recommended that LBH members be possessed of property worth £25.[35] In the face of a local board of health so stacked in favor of property, the college's resistance to LBH supervision suggests a profound anxiety about participation in democratic fora and about democratic control in the Age of Reform.

For its part, the LBH petition in favor of expansion noted the desirability of unity of administration, as had Cresy's Preliminary Inquiry. The LBH also prominently mentioned the highway rates but framed the issue beyond pence in the pound. The LBH developed three additional arguments. First, students frequented particular locales in the town that Cresy had highlighted in his Preliminary Inquiry as particularly insalubrious; one of them was now drained at the expense of the LBH. Yet the college did not participate in this burden, though the LBH believed that it derived the benefit.[36] A second argument relied on notions of the responsibility of property. If sanitary reform in part benefited the poor, or was represented as so doing, the college should help pay for it.[37]

These two LBH rationales in favor of extension were in some ways conservative, appealing as they seemingly did to traditional notions of benefit and the responsibility of property.[38] Yet the LBH simultaneously challenged the usual conception of the benefits and burdens and thus the boundaries of health. Just as did the metropolitan commissioners of sewers before 1848, the LBH promoted an alternative and expanded notion of benefit that widened the circle of parties presumed to benefit and thus were liable to pay. The LBH laid a particular claim on the nonresident regular users of the LBH district, such as the Fellows and students of Eton College, arguing that they should pay for that privilege.[39] This argument, under different circumstances than those that prevailed at Eton, could lead to rural and suburban incorporation with urban areas, forcing those who relied on the city to pay for it, even if they had escaped it.

The LBH's third and most radical argument for extension relied on the injustice of the fact that the college, the wealthiest part of the Eton Local Board of

Health District, entirely escaped taxation.[40] This was neither a reiteration of the LBH's claim about the responsibility of property nor a simple-minded fairness argument; the LBH was not arguing that "we're paying and they aren't." The LBH wanted to effect "an equitable adjustment of local taxation."[41] To be sure, the LBH developed this argument in part because it needed to avoid being seen as simply plundering valuable property, as the college implied; that would have been a fatal weakness in the LBH's case.[42] But the LBH's concern went beyond the politically expedient. Its decision to shine a light on the inequitable incidence of taxation among rich and poor ratepayers linked its concerns with long-standing radical arguments about class legislation.[43] The LBH, in a later document, referred to the need to effect an "equalisation" of taxes in the district, linking its quest with highly controversial movements to reform the Poor Law.[44]

The LBH's petition to extend its district was quashed in 1851 at the deputation that the LBH members had with the GBH, ostensibly because of the lateness of the parliamentary session. The LBH accordingly renewed the struggle for a third time in early 1852, and the Eton LBH files among the GBH papers record an extended correspondence.[45] The LBH did not win this long-running battle for extension. It is almost surprising that the board even tried, given the college's political power. In fact, the boundaries of the Eton LBH District were not changed until 1868, and then only at the college's request, the LBH paying for the privilege. The college must have been surprised at its good luck, except that it was hardly luck and the college quite likely was unsurprised.[46]

I have dwelt at some length on Eton's struggle, because it highlights the ideological character of boundary making. At Eton, the controversy was dominated neither by the complexity of the engineering nor by the cost of the works; instead, issues of democracy, equity, and morality were uppermost. The political struggle at Eton also highlighted the central government's ongoing reluctance to make certain kinds of local property pay the costs of urban improvement. The GBH abandoned its own original boundary recommendation, then initially refused to entertain an application for extension. When it did institute a second inquiry, it again neglected its own inspector's 1851 recommendation.[47] Another application for extension in 1852 met with delay until an outbreak of disease in the town gave the GBH an excuse for a third inquiry, whose disputed results provided it with further occasion for delay and, ultimately, refusal.[48] The GBH occupied an ambivalent position, alternately promoting and impeding sanitary reform.[49]

The Eton LBH was hardly the only one to attempt this kind of boundary expansion. Some other campaigns to extend them were more successful. At Swansea, the petition to adopt the Public Health Act came from the "Town and Franchise" (comprising the old town plus some suburban and agricultural land) of Swansea, an area much smaller in size than the boundaries of the corporate borough.[50] In the report on his preliminary inquiry, George Thomas Clark noted that his investigation "necessarily" led him to explore parts of the corporate borough not included in the petitioning area, particularly groups of population clustered about copper and other works on the riverbank, quite some distance from the town itself.[51] This somewhat extraordinary mode of proceeding led Clark to suggest applying the act to the entire corporate borough, by his reckoning an area more than twenty times larger than the town of Swansea. Clark would not have decided spontaneously to go further afield than the petition required; he presumably responded to the wishes of some local promoters. It is clear from newspaper reports that parties living outside the town proper were concerned about being rated for town improvements; Clark repeatedly stressed that the future local board could levy rates on only those districts benefited.[52] This must have smoothed over the difficulties, because during the second inquiry necessitated by this recommendation, Clark asserted that there was very little opposition to his proposed boundary, and it accordingly passed.[53]

At Bangor, as well, the LBH aggressively promoted local boundary extension. In Bangor's case, the original petition came from the parliamentary borough, which comprised a portion of Bangor parish and a small amount of land in another parish.[54] The LBH almost immediately requested an extension, and just as quickly retracted that request, because it had decided on an even greater extension. The Bangor LBH proposed to capture, in the words of one of its members, all land reasonably expected to be built on in the neighborhood. The proposed new boundary also captured railroad property that was rated to the poor and apparently also was drawn for the purpose of capturing a hotel at the outermost tip of the new district.[55] The railroad and other ratepayers protested against the boundary extension at the local inquiry and to the GBH. One ratepayer's complaint nearly exactly foreshadowed the case that would be made against the Epsom LBH in 1855. The fall of this ratepayer's land lay in another direction from Bangor, and he would derive no advantage from the drainage.[56] Superintending Inspector T. W. Rammell blandly asserted that the ratepayer in question would derive "a full share of advantage from any improvements in the sanitary arrangements of the district."[57] Rammell backed LBH requests for early extensions, and the GBH also backed him.

At both Swansea and Bangor, PHA promoters and local boards of health successfully expanded the boundaries of health. The GBH did not obstruct these expansions, but unlike in Eton, in these cases the local opposition was either blunted (Swansea) or not politically powerful enough (Bangor).[58] The documents for Swansea and Bangor do not permit the kind of analysis possible for Eton, yet in both we see expansionists capturing industrial works, agricultural land, building land, or suburbs to pay for urban improvement, and PHA promoters and local boards of health aggressively redefining the boundaries and burdens of health. Undoubtedly numerous other examples are waiting to be found, but further examples are not critical, as getting this property inside the boundary was only the first step. Getting it to pay was the next and more important one.

The Financial Boundaries of Health

In the remainder of this chapter, I want to explore the way in which local boards of health pushed the boundaries of health once their districts had been formed. They did so not only by extending the districts physically but also by extending them financially. The 1848 Public Health Act opened up this possibility for local boards of health. In the first place, it created potential new categories of property to rate, removing some exemptions even as it preserved others. Local boards of health were quick to capture them. In a second and more controversial step, it opened up new ways of distributing costs. The boundaries of LBH districts often were quite extensive, being composed of different types of settlements, often improved to quite different degrees and requiring quite different degrees of further improvement. The politics of improvement in this sort of situation varied from place to place depending on the circumstances but obviously were complicated. Places already improved, or believing themselves not in need of improvement, or far down the LBH list of candidates for improvement clearly were going to be unenthusiastic about paying for the improvement of some other part of the district. The PHA, however, gave local boards of health discretion about distributing costs over a whole district or only over parts of it. Some local boards of health used this discretionary power to redistribute the costs of urban improvement and further redefine the boundaries of health.

The possibility of capturing new property was a strategy that was eagerly if largely unsuccessfully pursued by the Westminster Commission of Sewers during the 1840s.[59] The members of the vast majority of local boards of health probably would have been unaware of those cases; if they were, they probably would have been discouraged. The PHA did not, in addition, hold out much hope to those keen to rate new kinds of property, because one of its provisions guaranteed exemption from rating of any property that had been exempt under any local act in force when the PHA was adopted.[60] The earliest cases brought under the PHA to the superior courts showed the willingness of local boards of health to test these new powers.

The first case was brought by the Chelmsford Board of Guardians against the Chelmsford LBH. One section of one of the local acts under which the town of Chelmsford was governed exempted from rating any property outside a fixed distance from the parish church of Chelmsford. The workhouse of the Guardians of Chelmsford Union was outside these limits (but was within the parochial boundaries) and was thus unrated for the purposes of the local act.[61] The Public Health Act, however, applied to the entire parish, not just the town. The LBH assessed the workhouse in a general district rate made in 1851; the Guardians appealed the decision. In a special case, the court ruled that the rate was good. The local act granted two sorts of exemptions: one based on the kind of property that might be rated (houses, hop gardens and so forth), and another on a property's location relative to the town (within a certain distance from the church). The kind of property exempted in the local act did not include the workhouse. The judges unanimously decided that if it had been within the distance prescribed by the local act, it would have been rated under that act. Because the PHA extended over the entire parish, the workhouse was thus eligible for rating.[62]

A local board of health also was the respondent in a somewhat more contentious case that involved rating dwelling houses within the cathedral precincts of the city of Carlisle. The city was governed under a local act, and according to counsel for the appellant, the property within the cathedral precincts was exempt from rating. The PHA applied to the whole city, and the LBH accordingly levied a rate on dwelling houses within the cathedral precincts. In their reasoning on this case, the judges again relied on a careful reading of the relevant statutes. In this case, they disputed that the local act created an exemption for property within the precinct, and they held the rate good.[63]

The last early rating case arose out of the Swansea LBH's decision to rate railroad property within its district.[64] This case differed from the previous two in the sense that the PHA, irrespective of any local act, itself created exemptions from rating. The eighty-eighth section specifically directed that "the occupier of any land used . . . as a railway" should be assessed at one quarter the net annual value. The South Wales Railway Company owned and occupied a substantial amount of property in Swansea, including not only the tracks and embankments but stations, platforms, warehouses, sheds, offices, and other potentially rateable, and valuable, property. For the purposes of a general district rate, the LBH assessed the actual rail line at one quarter but all other property at the full net annual value. When the case appeared before the court, the judges clawed back some of the property that the LBH wanted to rate fully into the one quarter annual value category, but allowed a substantial amount of property to be rated at the full net annual value.

These early rating decisions illustrate the importance of local boards of health in the ongoing construction of financial liability for the costs of the PHA. For example, although local boards of health had a duty to rate all property required to be rated and could be legally challenged if they did not, that does not mean that all local authorities rated all legally liable property.[65] Carlisle's improvement commissioners clearly misinterpreted their own local act in not rating the cathedral precincts. There must have been other local authorities who negotiated with ratepayers, especially corporate ones, and arrived at some informal understanding of liability that may or may not have withstood challenge, as may well have been the case at Newport. LBH legal responsibility to rate all property legally liable also did not mean that a local board of health had to bring all rating cases to Queen's Bench. As we shall see, the Epsom LBH backed off two rates after it was defeated at quarter sessions, including a rate that the Queen's Bench validated when it was levied again four years later. Few ratepayers would fault a local board of health for abandoning a case it lost at quarter sessions. The fact that these local boards of health took these cases to Queen's Bench makes clear their role in the establishment of rating law.

These early cases also reveal the extent to which judges participated in the evolution of rating law. In their rulings, the judges not only articulated their understanding of the meaning of the statutes in question but simultaneously developed an equitable justification and framed their holding in those terms. Lord Chief Justice John Campbell, consulted by the Westminster Commissioners of Sewers in an 1831 case discussed in chapter 2, observed in Chelmsford that the court's reading "works justice," and that it was "fit that the benefit and burthen should be coterminous."[66] Justice William Erle noted that the Carlisle cathedral precinct "is the very kind of property which ought to be rated."[67] In the same case, Justice Charles Crompton claimed that even if the LBH did not, for example, light the cathedral precincts, the properties would be benefited by the rest of the city's being lit. In the Swansea case, the judges likewise gave the general district rate an equitable justification.[68] Chief Justice Campbell argued that it was a "fair interpretation" of the language of the statute to rate fully much of the property in question, because it was only "just" that these properties, which derived a benefit "in perhaps a greater degree than any other species of property," should be fully rated.[69] In all three cases, the judges relied on benefit, thereby linking these decisions with a very long line of rating decisions, although in none of these cases did they make clear the nature of the benefit they believed these properties received.

The most important case of LBH financial boundary making came at Epsom and revolved around the rating principle adopted in sewer bills and legislation since 1833 (and in law for centuries before that): property was not required to pay for any works from which it did not derive a benefit. As we have seen, in practical terms the benefit principle was realized by subdividing sewer districts into smaller areas so as to make assessments of benefit more meaningful. In the usual language of the time, separate districts were to be identified, and as near as possible each district was to pay for its own expenses. The 1848 Public Health Act, in contrast, provided no explicit direction requiring local boards of health to divide their districts into separate drainage areas (or levels). The act permitted local boards to divide their districts and rate areas separately, but it did not require them to do so.[70] Even more important, the 1848 Public Health Act did not impose on local boards of health a duty to ensure that each such district should, as near as may be, bear its own expenses. The PHA thereby neglected a provision found repeatedly in local bills and acts of the period.[71] The 1848 Public Health Act thus permitted local boards to construct drainage works for a district encompassing several hitherto distinct subdistricts and to rate all of the ratepayers of the district for the work, instead of throwing the cost on the most densely populated and sometimes poorest part of a district.

Although the Public Health Act permitted districtwide, equal, and uniform rating, the General Board of Health, the central agency responsible for overseeing the operation of the PHA, seemed as ambivalent about these redistributive or equalizing provisions as it was about boundary extension. In its advice to local boards of health, the GBH stressed that benefit should be the criterion governing rateability. This issue attracted the GBH's attention with increasing frequency in 1851 as local boards established their operations and began levying rates for various purposes. Although the official minutes of the GBH do not record the receipt of every letter from a local board or a local resident or the contents of every reply for those they do, it is revealing that the board repeatedly recorded its opinion that local boards could divide their districts for rating purposes. This was obviously an issue about which they felt some anxiety.[72] In his 1852 edition of the PHA, Cuthbert Johnson claimed that in the GBH's opinion local boards did not have any discretion about rating parts of their district not benefited by works.[73] In correspondence about rating with the Gainsborough local board of health in 1852, the GBH suggested dividing the district for rating purposes and stressed that "no part of the Special District rates . . . can be fairly charged upon any but those parts of a District which are directly benefitted by such works."[74] The General Board of Health reiterated this when the Newport local board of health appealed to the GBH for advice regarding rating its district in late 1853. After a longer delay than normal, the GBH noted that it had "very carefully considered" the question submitted by the LBH, and it appears to have recommended that the LBH divide the district for rating purposes, because "the principle of the Public Health Act is adapting burden to benefit wherever practicable."[75] Consistent with this advice, the GBH's instructions to the superintending inspectors, responsible for suggesting local board of health boundaries, stressed that "every district will be protected by the General Board of Health from contributing more than its fair share of rates, proportioned as nearly as may be practicable to its share of the advantages which . . . will be derived."[76] In response to the GBH's wishes and formal instructions, the superintending inspectors emphasized in their reports that local boards were to charge districts according to the benefit they received.[77]

It is clear that some local boards of health shared the GBH's ambivalence about uniform and equal rating. Bristol was a large city and county composed of several different parishes.[78] One of the most pressing tasks facing the LBH was the imperfect sewerage of Bristol. According to David Large, the LBH planned its work methodically, dividing the city into six separate drainage districts that were progressively sewered over the next twenty years.[79] The LBH began by quickly approving a scheme for the Clifton High Level sewer in 1853, and as was their practice the LBH assessed the district benefited with a special district rate. Having once decided to do that, the LBH was more or less forced to do so for the next extension of the system.[80] The completion of these two projects left much of the city still undrained. The LBH returned to the subject in 1857 and agreed to drain three more districts, with each separate district bearing its own costs, "by which means the practical difficulties of providing the cost of constructing works. . . will be obviated."[81] Districts benefited by the works paid for them.[82]

The General Board of Health's caution in interpreting the Public Health Act's redistributive provisions thus resonated with at least some local boards of health. But the GBH was not entirely of one mind on this matter. The inspectors and the General Board of Health regularly drew boundaries, particularly for market towns, that included areas that they surely knew would not benefit directly from any drainage works. The GBH, furthermore, did not always support appeals for formal separation.[83] In addition, the GBH sanctioned works that clearly did not benefit outlying districts in any direct manner. The General Board of Health's ambivalence about the equalizing provision of the act reflects contemporary unease with the politics of redistribution. Indeed, the redistributive potential of the PHA was established not by the central government but, more important, by local boards and by the judges who ruled on their actions.

The importance of local boards of health for determining the limits and significance of the statute is clear in the case of Epsom's local board. This small board spent the first four years of its life engaged in repeated struggles to define the justice of rating and responsibility, winning two victories at Queen's Bench. The district of this local board comprised the entire parish, including the town of Epsom (about one seventh of the parish) and much surrounding agricultural and other land. It was apparent from the start that the Epsom LBH intended to test the limits of rating to the fullest.[84] The first legal threat the LBH encountered came as a result of the very first rate it tried to raise for highways. Highway rates would become a sore point under the PHA, and Parliament was quickly forced to return to the subject. Although the confusion may have arisen from statutory ambiguity, the dispute about rating for highways was fundamentally political in nature. Under the 1835 Highway Act, all houses and land within a parish were rated equally. Under the 1848 Public Health Act, however, land of various sorts was rated at only one quarter its annual value, in contrast to houses, which were rated at full net annual value. The decision for local boards of health was whether they would raise highway rates under the 1835 act or the 1848 act. The difference mattered, because landowners would pay a substantially lower bill under the 1848 act than the 1835 act. The Epsom LBH decided to rate under the 1835 act. Landowners, believing that the LBH had to rate under the PHA, immediately appealed the rate. Perhaps as a gesture of goodwill and out of a desire to save costs, the LBH dropped the rate.[85]

The LBH's legal difficulties over rating reappeared in an 1851 rate for several purposes, including lighting and general administration. Prior to the passage of the Public Health Act, Epsom Parish was lit under the General Lighting and Watching Act. In Epsom, only part of the parish had gas lamps and, consistent with the Lighting Act, only part of the parish was assessed to pay for them.[86] The principle that only those who had gas lamps paid for them seemed completely straightforward to most contemporaries. The statute governing parochial lighting explicitly recognized this principle; indeed, the draft bill for the statute proposed that individual streets could adopt the act.[87] That provision did not survive parliamentary passage, presumably because of feasibility concerns, yet its mere inclusion at any point indicates the extent to which individual benefit regulated the financing of public services.

Members of the Epsom Local Board of Health apparently did not subscribe to this interpretation. In 1851 the local board repeatedly sought the opinion of the General Board of Health about its desire to rate the entire parish for lighting, even though only a small portion had lamps.[88] The General Board of Health repeatedly noted that the local board could basically do what it wanted but suggested that the lighting rate be confined to places that actually were lit.[89] Unsatisfied with this response, the chair of the local board, Sir Richard Digby Neave, personally solicited Edwin Chadwick's opinion.[90] In reply, the GBH claimed that the local board had to pay for lighting with a rate levied on the entire district, even if only part was lit.[91] The GBH's rationale for this decision was that the Public Health Act recognized that all parties within a district had a beneficial interest in lighting any portion of the district.[92] Notwithstanding the GBH's breezy assumption of communal benefit, several ratepayers within the Epsom district protested the rate raised for lighting and other purposes and argued that the local board should rate for lighting only that part of the parish which was lit.[93] The rate was contested at the Surrey Quarter Sessions in 1852, and both the LBH and the appellant agreed to quash it. The Epsom local board decided that it would divide its district for the purposes of lighting and rate the separate divisions accordingly.[94]

The third and most important Epsom local board rating conflict came with the sewerage and waterworks. The LBH decided to embark on a scheme of main drainage and water supply for the town.[95] The scheme was estimated to cost approximately £14,000.[96] This posed a problem for the local board: according to the 1848 Public Health Act, local boards were allowed to borrow no more in any given year than the annual estimated rental. The town site in Epsom Parish (one seventh of the total) had an estimated annual rental of £12,000. The Public Health Act thus imposed on the Epsom local board a duty either to raise more money than the town site provided or to alter its scheme so as to lower the cost. The board opted for the former. In order to pay for this drainage scheme, the board proposed raising the money through a special district rate on the entire parish, valued at approximately £20,000 for poor rate purposes, even though the drainage works pertained almost exclusively to the town. The General Board of Health sanctioned the various loans.[97]

We can infer the Epsom local board's rationale for this decision only from documents produced after the fact.[98] The board members appear to have relied on considerations of both law and equity.[99] In the first place, they argued, the 1848 Public Health Act gave them sole discretion to determine whether the district should be divided for rating purposes. Their second argument did not rely on any specific provision in the statute but relied instead on the act's implicit redefinition of the benefit criterion against which individuals' liability to the sewers rate was determined. Because the act did not impose on local boards a duty to ensure that each part of each district paid only for its own benefits, and because it permitted the union of different parishes and parts of parishes for the purpose of drainage works, the Public Health Act implicitly redefined the nature of the benefit that an individual was meant to receive in order to be taxed for drainage works. If one was to pay for works carried out in another part of one's district, then at the very least the nature of the benefit one received was indirect. And thus the Epsom local board argued. According to newspaper accounts, Epsom's legal counsel claimed that the benefit "was not a direct, but indirect and general good."[100]

The local board's claim that the benefit was indirect rather than direct echoed the argument it had made about lighting and reflected a consistent policy of attempting to force suburban householders and landowners to pay for their share of the benefits provided by town dwellers.[101] The local board must have known that ratepayers previously exempt from paying rates would not accept this. Ratepayer challenges had already led the Epsom local board to abandon its districtwide highway and lighting rates. Nonetheless, in late 1853, the LBH levied a special district rate for drainage purposes on the entire parish. Several ratepayers not directly benefited by the works immediately filed notice of their intention to contest the rate. At a quarter session in Guildford in July 1854, the justices quashed the rate. The chairman of the session agreed that the appellants in that case "derived no benefit" from the works.[102]

One might imagine that at this point, the Epsom local board would have admitted that its project of financing drainage with a tax on the entire district was a failure. Indeed, the board was dismayed; shortly after the decision all the board members appear to have considered resigning.[103] At a loss as to how to proceed, the local board instructed its clerk to prepare a case for the opinion of the Solicitor General and of their own counsel.[104] A deputation from the board met with Sir Benjamin Hall, the president of the General Board of Health. The local board's clerk had several meetings with the solicitor general, who was of the opinion that the case was important enough that the opinion of the Law Officers of the Crown should be sought.[105] After receiving the Law Officers' opinion, which supported the Epsom Local Board of Health, the newly fortified board decided again to raise a rate on the entire district to pay for the works, although several members of the board clearly had lost their nerve.[106] Predictably, appeals against the rate followed.

The Epsom local board again appeared at the Surrey Quarter Sessions. Although the trial turned on a technicality and went against the board, it was clear that the chairman of the sessions, James W. Freshfield, was sympathetic to the board.[107] He noted that there might be an improvement to an entire district that justified a rate, and he was not in any case prepared to affirm the dictum of no individual benefit, no rate.[108] After further legal maneuvering, the parties agreed to send the case to Queen's Bench for a definitive ruling. At the hearing in June 1855, the Epsom Local Board of Health again relied on its two arguments about local board discretion and indirect benefit. The justices recognized that the "question raised in this case"—whether the occupier of a residence can be rated for the sewers where the residence derives no direct and immediate benefit from them—"is one of very general application and great importance."[109] In their questions, the judges initially seemed skeptical of the board's attempted redefinition of benefit. Pressed that the entire district should benefit, the board's legal counsel agreed that the property of the appellant (Henry Dorling) lay far from the town site and that the appellant would not derive any immediate benefit from the system of sewerage. Yet the board's counsel claimed that he would derive indirect benefit in the form of reduced poor rates.[110]

All the evidence suggests that the LBH made the same basic argument as its counsel. Three months earlier, the Epsom LBH had appeared in front of the House of Commons Select Committee on the Public Health Act.[111] As was usually the case in such situations, the select committee heard testimony from various parties interested in the measure, including William Everest, an Epsom solicitor acting on behalf of the parties appealing the special district rate levied over the entire district.[112] Everest indignantly told the story of local landowners, paternalists all, who were being forced to contribute to the drainage of the town of Epsom, all because the LBH unjustly and perhaps illegally refused to confine the special district rate to the town. In Everest's view, properties should only be rated if they benefited. Although he did not define benefit, he seemed to believe that connection to the works was the principal criterion.[113]

Everest's argument apparently was satisfactory to the Select Committee, which decided that local boards of health should be forced to divide their districts for rating purposes and charge only those areas benefiting. The Epsom LBH presumably heard Everest's testimony and sensed the direction of the select committee's thoughts on the matter, because the LBH clerk, George White, appeared in front of the select committee on the same day as Everest's second appearance.[114] White was faced with the task of justifying a decision still before the courts in front of a hostile committee. "It has been suggested to the Committee," Sir Benjamin Hall informed him, that rates for works benefiting a particular part of the district should not be charged to the whole district, "and they agree very much in the suggestion."[115] Having already pointed out how little land itself actually contributed to the rateable value of the LBH district, White answered that individuals might not be directly benefited, but that medical testimony would prove indirect benefit accrued.[116] He did not elaborate, and in what must have been a humiliating reminder of the value attached to medical testimony, the committee did not even call the medical officer to testify, although he was present, and White again referred to him in a subsequent question.[117]

We do not know if the Epsom LBH's counsel based his argument on indirect medical benefits, but it would be odd if the LBH advanced one argument in front of the House of Commons and another one at the hearing three months later.[118] In any event, the justices of the Queen's Bench sided with the Epsom Local Board on both points. They agreed with the board that the appellant would derive benefit from the works and that the decision to divide the district was at the discretion of the board.[119] Although Justice John Coleridge insisted on strict statutory interpretation, he began with a digression on the nature of benefit and the justice of rating parties for other than direct benefits. The appellant claimed that his property could not possibly receive a benefit from the Epsom local board's drainage works. Yet that all depended on how benefit was defined, and the statute was silent on the nature of benefit required. In a remarkable display of statutory interpretation, Coleridge claimed that Dorling, whose property was nearly a mile away and on the other side of a hill from the nearest sewer, derived, "undoubtedly, not only benefit, but benefit precisely of that kind which it must be considered the Legislature had in view for the population of all classes when it passed a public health Act."[120] In *Dorling v. Epsom*, Coleridge's imaginary outlying landowners and occupying farmers benefited because the value of their land appreciated, their visits to the town to sell their products were more pleasant, and they paid lower poor rates because the town's poor were healthier.[121]

Coleridge's analysis of indirect benefit is noteworthy for a number of distinct but related reasons. To begin with, none of the benefits he identified were part of the 1848 Public Health Act; indeed, the very notion of indirect benefit was entirely nonstatutory.[122] In addition, the one indirect benefit that Coleridge's agricultural ratepayer did not get was health. In other words, individuals paying rates for an act intended to promote the public health did not necessarily get their own health promoted. Some people did, however, and even if they did not directly pay rates, they were apparently entitled to have someone pay the bill for them. Better health for some was thus premised on higher rates for others. That was an astonishing admission of the necessity of redistribution, but as Coleridge's indirect benefit argument showed, the court (and the LBH) appeared ambivalent about the ideological rationale for redistribution—framing it in part in terms of reduced poor rates—even as they accepted the need for it.

The Epsom Local Board of Health's successful decision to finance drainage works by rating the whole parish illustrates the dynamics of sanitary reform in one small town. At least three different sets of actors were involved in the outcome of this decision. Clearly, the framers of the Public Health Act were crucial.[123] Parliament passed a statute that abandoned the benefit principle formulation that had appeared in sewers laws for the previous fifteen years. We have no reason to assume that this was other than deliberate, particularly because the principle did not reappear in the failed Public Health Act amendment bill of 1855.[124] Statutes were crafted carefully, and the 1848 Public Health Act reflected a deliberate balancing of interests between agricultural and house property,[125] between owners and occupiers,[126] and between present and future generations in its rating provisions.[127]

We have evidence, then, that the 1848 Public Health Act was a carefully crafted document, and that the outcome of the *Dorling v. Epsom* case thus reflected parliamentary intentions. But those intentions had to be interpreted by the judiciary, the second group critically involved in the outcome of the case. The role of the judiciary in forming English law is well known in the case of contract law, for example, but Albert Venn Dicey observed nearly a century ago that even some sections of statutes "derive nearly all their real significance from the sense put upon them by the Courts."[128] In this case, the justices were confronted with a new statute, and they would have claimed that all they did was discover the meaning of the statute.[129] It seems unlikely, however, that the meaning of the statute could have been as crystal clear as the unanimous judgment of the Court implied; at least two quarter sessions cases had not seen it that way, and one of them had quashed the rate. The Solicitor General was uncertain enough about its meaning that he advised formal consultation with the Law Officers of the Crown. The statute had to be interpreted, and the Queen's Bench overturned at least one previous judgment in doing so. Justice Coleridge himself argued that the final decision was grounded in both the construction of the statute and on general considerations of benefit, suggesting that even the judges recognized that strict statutory interpretation itself was not enough.[130]

The license that Coleridge took in defining benefit shows us that the redistribution promoted by the 1848 Public Health Act owed as much to friendly judicial interpretation as to clear-minded drafting. The role of the judiciary in the evolution of public health clearly varies across issue areas, times, and jurisdictions, as the work of several historians has shown. Brenner and Dingle argued that the common law was a poor instrument for resolving industrial nuisances, in part as a result of judicial rulings, and we know that local magistrates were often unreliable in the case of sanitary nuisances.[131] In the Epsom case, however, judges facilitated rather than obstructed local action.

Yet the Epsom local board was the most important actor in bringing about the outcome for at least three reasons. First, the LBH had to decide to rate this way in the first place; the statute was permissive in its rating clauses. In correspondence with other local boards facing similar decisions about dividing their districts for the purposes of paying for works, the General Board of Health stressed that the principle of the Public Health Act was the adaptation of burden to benefit wherever practicable, and this usually meant dividing districts wherever practicable.[132] It clearly would have been practicable to divide the Epsom LBH district, and it is difficult to imagine the circumstances under which such a decision could have been so much as challenged, let alone reversed. Second, the LBH had to stick to its guns. Although it was perhaps inevitable that some local board of health would bring a case such as this forward, the circumstances under which the Epsom case reached the bench are noteworthy, because the Epsom LBH persevered through two different rejections at the lower court level. Third, the Epsom LBH advanced an argument about indirect benefit that the judges, on balance, found compelling, even though it was not part of the statute and even though the judges might have interpreted indirect benefit in their own way.

The Epsom LBH was not yet finished testing the justice of taxation. Flush with its victory in the *Dorling* case, the board decided to test the law of rating one last time in 1855. The topic this time was highway rating, the first rating experience that the LBH had had and from which they backed down in 1851. In late 1855, the LBH imposed a highway rate under the powers of the 1835 Highway Act, thereby taxing outlying land at full annual value.[133] Appeals were launched, including one by a board member named Samuel Hanson, and the parties agreed to submit a special case to Queen's Bench, which upheld the rate.[134] The Epsom LBH's second major rate victory in under six months did not set a precedent in quite the same way as did the *Dorling* decision, but the lack of long-term success in Hanson's case does not detract from the political commitment of the LBH.[135]

The *Dorling* Decision after 1855

The Epsom Local Board of Health does not typically figure in histories of English and Welsh public health. When smaller towns such as Epsom do appear, the point generally is not to highlight their importance. But following the legal history of public health gives a political agency and significance to small-town residents that we do not normally see. In this case, the effects of the *Dorling* decision reverberated well beyond Epsom. The GBH, which had paid for a shorthand writer for the case, framed its advice to local boards of health about the justice of rating quite differently.[136]

As we saw earlier in this chapter, the local board district of Swansea was a sprawling area coextensive with the municipal boundary.[137] It included the town of Swansea, suburban land, agricultural land, and industrial sites with their associated housing. Some of the industrial sites were three miles away from the town. Incorporating such disparate and dispersed populations within a single district was bound to pose problems. In blunting opposition to the boundary at his inquiries around adopting the Public Health Act, Superintending Inspector G. T. Clark had repeatedly noted that the LBH would be able to rate districts according only to the benefit they received.[138] Yet Clark also challenged local notions that only districts directly benefited by works should pay. Clark noted that Parliament rated land at one fourth its annual value and claimed, "The legislature assumed that houses and lands in the vicinity of a town were, to some extent, benefitted by their proximity to town, that the occupiers often frequented the town, and that they decidedly derived some advantages from the improvement in town."[139] He did not resolve these two potentially conflicting views, leaving that to the Swansea local board.

The board got its chance in the mid-1850s. The Swansea LBH was an active promoter of sanitary reform. In 1854, the board received GBH sanction to borrow £30,250 to purchase a private waterworks built in and serving the lowlying part of town. In 1856 the LBH started to make arrangements to pay off the loan.[140] The LBH had every intention of extending the water supply to the whole district, and Robert Rawlinson was at that moment in the town working out a plan, which the LBH believed would eventually be implemented. In the meantime, the loan to buy the works had to be paid off, and the LBH wondered over what district the rate should be levied. The clerk noted to the General Board of Health that it was hardly fair to rate properties unable to obtain water, yet it was also unfair to rate only those deriving the immediate benefit, because they would be paying the capital costs for a plant that would subsequently be used by all the town. The GBH recommended that the LBH should rate the entire district to be benefited eventually.[141]

The GBH's view no doubt appeared reasonable when the issue was seen from Gwydyr House (the London headquarters of the General Board of Health), but at the local level this was profoundly difficult. As part of a hoped-for settlement of rating controversies in Swansea, in 1854 the local board of health created a new town district to be rated for the cost of improvements from which the remainder of the LBH district derived no benefit.[142] Notwithstanding this attempted resolution, questions of equitable local taxation continued to disturb the LBH, coming to a head in late 1856. The LBH received a report on Rawlinson's drainage plan for the Mynydd district of Swansea Town. Replaying the debate over the water rate, a member suggested that the interest on the loan for the works should be paid only by the recently created town district. Another member pointed out that the inhabitants of the town were very poor, and some members wanted the rate extended over the entire LBH district.[143] No decision was taken, and after a further inconclusive LBH meeting, the clerk sought the GBH's opinion. In reply, the GBH carefully noted that the decision was the local board's, but that it could levy the rate on any district deriving "direct or indirect benefit" from the works. The GBH explicitly drew attention to the *Dorling* case.[144] The GBH's view did not apparently help the LBH; multiple motions were defeated at the board's January 1857 meeting.[145]

The members of the Swansea LBH were clearly at a loss as to what to do, much as the members of the Epsom LBH had been in the summer of 1854. The Joint Finance and Works Committee was established and sought legal opinion on the matter. The Swansea LBH clerk consulted one of the junior members of the Epsom team, who told the Swansea board what the judgment in *Dorling* had said: that the decision was the LBH's. In what obviously was a contentious meeting, the joint committee voted to rate the entire LBH district, with the chair casting the deciding vote. At the full LBH meeting, a renewed attempt was made to restrict the rate to the recently created town district, but the motion lost. In the end, the LBH voted to rate the entire district, abandoning its recently adopted scheme for distributing local burdens between two districts.[146] This decision triggered much dissatisfaction and within a few years generated a petition to split the district.[147]

It is easy to assume that these debates are without general interest, reflecting nothing more than a desire to shift the burden of local taxation onto other parties. Certainly residents from outside the core area believed that board members associated with Swansea Town had snookered them, as did the editor of the *Swansea Herald*, but supporters of the extended rate do not appear to have been so cynically motivated.[148] On occasion, as when one member supporting the extended rate appealed to opponents as members of one common family, the debate was cringeworthy, but most speakers honestly wrestled with the difficulty of deciding who should pay. Of course, opponents of the districtwide rate spoke the language of benefit narrowly defined, and even some of the supporters worried that the town district as defined in 1854 still required many parties to pay who would derive no benefit. Other members realized the implications of that claim and pointed out that they either had to rate the entire borough or rate strictly according to benefit. In the latter case, they would need a separate rate not just for each district but "for every street and every house."[149] This was not the *reductio ad absurdum* it appears, and Justice Colin Blackburn of the Queen's Bench made the exact same argument in an important case in London several years later.[150]

Thus, the debate at the Swansea LBH was exactly the debate that metropolitan commissioners of sewers had been having for fifty years and that the Queen's Bench had addressed in the *Dorling* case. Indirect benefit apparently provided the key.[151] One of the major proponents of the districtwide rate noted that residents, even poor residents, in the outlying districts got many kinds of benefits from living in association with the town, although an opposed member protested that outlying areas derived no more indirect benefit than any casual visitor to the town. The *Swansea and Glamorgan Herald*, too, was deeply skeptical, calling the benefits to outlying areas "metaphysical."[152] On balance, though, *Dorling*'s promotion of indirect benefit gave enough Swansea LBH members the discursive resources they needed to make sense of their decision to rate the entire district for works that would directly benefit only a part of it. As was the case in Epsom, the decision by some Swansea members to adopt whole-district rating apparently was an amalgam of equity and law. The effect was to distribute the costs of Swansea's improvement over a wider circle of parties, including proprietors of large works.

The General Board of Health's promotion of the *Dorling* case at Cheltenham highlighted the redistributive potential of the Public Health Act in a different way. Social differentiation at Cheltenham was pronounced, with so-called private estates, full of valuable housing, surrounding the town site but within the parochial boundaries.[153] Cheltenham is interesting as well because of the presence of the private sewer company. (The conditions that led to the 1833 creation of the company were discussed in chapter 2.) Until the early 1850s, the company seemed not to generate any "outward and visible hostility" from residents.[154] However, the drainage of the district was not satisfactory to local inhabitants; thus, Cheltenham was one of the early petitioners to adopt the PHA.[155] Although Edward Cresy recommended the application of the PHA to Cheltenham, for a variety of reasons Cheltenham's elites decided to obtain a fresh local act.[156] After an 1851 attempt failed, Cheltenham succeeded in 1852.[157]

One of the principal purposes of the new act was to enable the new commissioners to build a main sewer system. As was the case at Epsom and Swansea, distributing the costs of these works was not a simple matter. Residents in the private estates had long been paying their landlord for such drainage as they had via a rent charge. Customers of the sewer company had likewise been paying a rental charge for their drainage for many years. To some residents, it seemed unfair to tax people twice for the same service.[158] The new local act incorporated provisions of the PHA, and the local commissioners had the option to pay for the works with a special district rate levied only on the part deemed to benefit. The town committee, however, decided to insert a special clause stipulating that the "arterial" (or main) drains should be paid for with a districtwide rate.[159]

Given the reluctance of Cheltenham's vestry to rate property not benefited by sewers in 1833, the decision in 1850 to charge all property was a remarkable turnaround. Once again, miasmatism was the key. Removal of the nuisance associated with the three brooks was deemed to benefit all; hence all should pay. This decision to charge all property with the cost of the main drainage was not without controversy and came up repeatedly in the select committee hearings on the 1852 bill, though neither the Commons nor the Lords struck it.[160] The new Cheltenham improvement commissioners quickly completed the arterial drainage scheme and embarked on a plan to build the branch drains that would be necessary to complete the system.[161] Once again, the issue of rating came up. The commissioners expected that they would be doing a great deal of work on the branch drainage in general but that some areas would require less work than others. The commissioners preferred to rate the district as a whole, but they asked the GBH if they were obliged to rate parts of their district separately. The GBH minute stressed that the decision was the commissioners', but GBH Secretary Tom Taylor noted that "the benefit from improved sewerage may extend far beyond the particular district sewered. There are some important remarks of Mr. Justice Coleridge bearing on the subject" in the *Dorling* case.[162]

Cheltenham's desire to rate the entire district for its works highlights another aspect of the PHA. Throughout the hearings on Cheltenham's bills, witnesses testified that drainage was almost entirely absent in the most densely populated and poorest part of town.[163] These places thus needed the most work. In contrast, witnesses testified that the company had sewered the best part of the town; the private estates, which had their own drainage, were filled with first-class houses. When Cheltenham's local act promoters decided to rate the entire borough for the main drainage works, and when the commissioners wanted to rate it again for the branch drains, they were at the very least implicitly redistributing costs associated with drainage from poor parties onto rich parties. There is no reason to assume any particular benevolence here; they may have been entirely self-interested. Yet their decision nonetheless highlights the redistributive potential of the PHA.

Even in cases where we have no evidence of GBH intervention, local boards of health themselves apparently relied on *Dorling*. The Woolwich LBH, for example, comprised land on both sides of the Thames. Districts such as Woolwich cried out for division; indeed, in an 1829 Tower Hamlets sewer case, Chief Justice Charles Abbott remarked on the absurdity of having parishes on one side of the Thames pay for works on the other side.[164] Yet that was exactly what the PHA permitted the Woolwich local board to do, and that was exactly what it did in 1859. One aggrieved ratepayer in North Woolwich contested the rate at the Kent Quarter Sessions, and the bench quashed the rate. Frustrated by the quarter sessions decision, the members of the LBH wanted to move the case to Queen's Bench.[165] At a subsequent meeting, after hearing that the decision to divide the district was at the LBH's discretion and that property on the north side of the river benefited "indirectly," the LBH decided to remake the rate.[166] It is, of course, possible that Woolwich LBH independently arrived at the same conclusion as the Epsom LBH, but they probably took their cue from the ruling in the *Dorling* case.[167]

The full impact of the *Dorling* decision will be difficult to determine, because the extent to which other local boards of health acted on its principle can be determined only through a laborious review of local records.[168] Yet in one sense *Dorling*'s impact was limited. Although the GBH recommended the *Dorling* holding to several local boards of health, official support for this principle did not translate into legislative endorsement. When Parliament passed the Local Government Act in 1858, it did not attempt to enshrine the principle of indirect benefit in law. Parliamentary ambivalence about this development surfaced again in the 1860s, when Parliament struggled to introduce suitable local government into parts of the country where it was lacking. The resulting statutes permitted precisely the kind of subdivision against which the local authorities described in this chapter struggled.[169] The Royal Sanitary Commission, in addition, did not endorse the principle in *Dorling*, notwithstanding hearing testimony on that very point.[170] On the other hand, the fact that Parliament did not enshrine the principle of indirect benefit in statute law did not mean that it had no impact. Parliament also did not prohibit the kind of decision that Epsom and other local boards of health had made, leaving the decisions to elected local officials.

❧ ❧ ❧

In late 1870, the Abersychan local board contacted the Local Government Act Office (LGAO, the successor to the GBH) about rating its district. The district was large in extent, comprising about seven thousand acres of farm- and pastureland under which were found extensive coal and iron deposits, and three thousand acres containing settlements of workers employed in the mines. The local board resolved to sewer the settled portions of the district, whereupon landowners in the unsettled seven thousand acres objected to being rated for drainage purposes when their land would not benefit. The board believed that it had "absolute discretion" over the area to be rated for the sewerage works and intended to rate the entire district. The LGAO, in reply, noted that the board's absolute discretion had to be guided by justice and good reason. In this case, however, the LGAO implied that the district not directly drained by the sewerage works should contribute to "the cost of the sewerage which would not be necessary but for the requirements of the population they have been the means of collecting."[171] Although the LGAO did not make any reference to the *Dorling* decision, its tacit consent to the project reflected the extent to which indirect benefit had become part of the landscape. It is difficult to imagine that Abersychan could have taken this decision before *Dorling*; if it had, the case would be known under Abersychan's name instead of Epsom's. It is perhaps fortunate that Abersychan did not: there is no guarantee the outcome would have been the same.

❧ ❧ ❧

The decisions taken by the various local boards cited in this chapter illustrate the way in which new properties and new kinds of properties were made liable for local public health rates. Although rates were collected from individual properties, they were based on areas. These rates accordingly helped define new communities—what we might call communities of health. These communities of health were neither constructed according to a particular logic of health or disease, nor, as Briggs suggested for London, were they stitched together by underground drainage pipes. The infrastructure for which property was rated often did not extend to all of the places within the area; there was no particular medical or technological determinism at work here.[172] These communities were instead based on preexisting boundaries formed for very different purposes.[173] Epsom and other local authorities took existing boundaries and reenvisioned them in terms of equalized financial liability for health. This was a revolution in liability, significantly redefining benefit by making all property potentially liable.

The flip side of this community of ratepayers was the community of beneficiaries. The members of this community were not a homogenous population. If a local board decided to build a drainage system, some members of the community were entitled to the indirect benefit of health, whereas others had to pay for it. Those who got the indirect benefit, furthermore, were not a random sample of the population. It is clear from Cheltenham and Swansea at the very least that the local boards undertook the expenditure in part for the benefit of poorer residents. This kind of redistributive taxation was unusual at the time. The closest model to which local public health rates approached was the Poor Law, whereby resources were explicitly distributed from ratepayer to pauper. The chief difference between poor relief and public health lay in the fact that there was no workhouse test required to receive the benefit of health and no civil disability or stigma that resulted from its receipt.[174] This was a straight redistribution of the cost and benefits of health. Historians have recently described this sense that the incidence of disease fostered a new communality as cholera citizenship or sanitary citizenship.[175] Ideals of citizenship at the time typically implied duties, such as payment of rates, although they were less assertive about correlative rights.[176] Sanitary citizenship implied, even if a right to health was discretionary and qualified, a right to health, a right that legitimated the redistribution of rates from one area to another.

Chapter Four

The Benefits of Health

London, 1848–65

In order to build healthy infrastructure, Epsom's local board of health had to persevere through two defeats at quarter sessions, a hostile parliamentary select committee, and a hearing at Queen's Bench. Similar efforts in London were even more difficult. Aspects of this struggle, including the immense engineering and technical difficulties, are well known, and I do not intend to revisit them.[1] My focus here is on the struggle to pay for them. I do not mean the political struggle of getting elected bodies to vote taxes; I mean the prior and in some ways more fundamental struggle to obtain the legal power to levy rates for metropolitan purposes or even for purposes beyond those benefiting individual properties. In the course of the effort to establish this power, various levels of London's government faced mass civil disobedience, powerful corporate adversaries, hostile metropolitan and parliamentary opinion, and skeptical judges.

Part of the problem in London was that there was no "London" on a map, apart from the City, and no administrative entity with oversight over the whole of it. There was no agreement even about where it ended. In 1840 the largest border belonged to the Metropolitan Police District, supervised by the Home Office, which spread out roughly fifteen miles from Charing Cross.[2] In 1851, the Registrar General developed the much more compact metropolitan census district, but it was a statistical, not an administrative, entity.[3] Even the metropolitan census district comprised parts of three counties (Middlesex, Kent, and Surrey), the City of London, forty-two Poor Law authorities, and more than sixty parishes, precincts, liberties, and extraparochial places. Within each of these boundaries, a wide variety of what the Webbs called statutory authorities for special purposes carried out a host of activities.[4] From the perspective of this book, the most important statutory authorities were the ancient separate commissioners of sewers, sprawling over an ill-defined but large area of potential jurisdiction.[5] But they made up only a fraction of the total; as Briggs notes, two hundred fifty local acts of Parliament controlled ten thousand commissioners of one or another kind in London.[6]

This profusion of authorities, often exercising overlapping functions, was only partially reformed by the Whigs in the 1830s.[7] The Royal Commission on

Municipal Reform did not include the City of London, the only corporate entity in the metropolitan area, and the results of a Royal Commission on it in 1837 yielded nothing.[8] The next major opportunity for the reform of London's local government came during the era of public health legislation. Yet London, as is well known, fitted uneasily into this movement, if at all. Lord Lincoln's 1845 Health of Towns Bill did not include London, and although the initial draft of Morpeth's 1847 Health of Towns Bill did, opposition quickly forced him to drop it.[9] In the spring of 1847, the prospects for significant administrative change in London were slim.

The approach of cholera in 1847, however, created fresh opportunities to pursue the remodeling of London's government.[10] Yet another Royal Commission was appointed, this one on the Health of the Metropolis. On the basis of its recommendation, late that year the government abolished the separate commissions of sewers and created a unified Metropolitan Commission of Sewers (MCS).[11] The history of this little-lamented body has yet to be written, perhaps because the Metropolitan Commission of Sewers built few new works and was paralyzed by internal dissension and external attack.[12] In the space of little more than eight years, six separate commissions were appointed (and in one case partly elected), their predecessors having resigned or been replaced.[13] The commissioners had serious plans available but no ability to conclude them.

Responsible parliamentarians, including the metropolitan MP Benjamin Hall, president since 1853 of the GBH, knew that something had to be done to reform London's governance, especially in light of the return of cholera in the early 1850s. Hall's decision making was structured by a widely shared and deeply entrenched antipathy not just to Chadwickian centralization but to any nonlocal control—which meant, in the metropolitan context, nonparochial control.[14] Hall thus relied on London's parishes, notwithstanding their widely differing topographies, sizes, populations, economies, and wealth. It was obvious that a main drainage system for London could not be constructed by parishes operating individually, yet an appointed body to coordinate parishes and oversee the metropolitan component (the Metropolitan Commission of Sewers) had been tried and by 1855 was manifestly a failure, even when leavened with an elected component. An 1854 Royal Commission on the Corporation of London provided a way out. It argued that the metropolis's diversity precluded a single, undivided authority and recommended instead a federal structure with a Metropolitan Board of Works populated with delegates from elected vestries of large parishes and groups of vestries of smaller ones.[15] In 1855 Hall set up just such a two-tiered structure for the government of London in the Metropolis Local Management Act (MMA).[16] All parochial ratepayers elected vestries. Larger parish vestries selected representatives from among their members to sit on the upper-tier Metropolitan Board of Works (MBW). Smaller parishes were pooled into District Boards of Works. They also sent some of their members to the upper tier, which thus was indirectly elected.[17]

An important task of the MBW was the construction of a main drainage system for London. It did so in collaboration with either the local vestry (V) or district board of works (DBW), depending on the area. (These V/DBW also had numerous other functions.) The MBW constructed the intercepting and main drainage; the V/DBW constructed the branch and household drains.[18] In fashioning new drainage authorities for London in 1848 and 1855, Parliament had perforce to decide how their operations would be financed but, as we saw in chapter 2, there was no consensus on how to pay for sewers in London. For nearly thirty years, the separate commissions of sewers in London had pushed the boundaries of sewers funding, but their efforts were often thwarted by the courts and not supported by Parliament or perhaps even public opinion. In 1848 and again in 1855, Parliament took only tentative steps along the trail the commissioners had blazed; neither the MCS nor the MBW could levy a metropolitan-wide rate for drainage.

In this chapter, I focus on the struggles of the MBW and its second-tier partners to overcome this powerful limitation. The MBW, the vestries, and the district boards of works pressed the agenda, testing the limits of the 1855 legislation at both the metropolitan and submetropolitan levels. As they tried to pay off the debts of the Metropolitan Commission of Sewers and raise revenue for their future work, the MBW and V/DBW pursued rating policies that quickly created a little-studied crisis in the financing of metropolitan health and improvement.[19] Various parties went to court to challenge the taxing powers of both the MBW and the V/DBW. The courts again thwarted the boards' efforts to raise the necessary revenue, triggering a vigorous response by the MBW.

I will reconstruct the history of these rates and legal debates in some detail, because I believe that it reveals the way in which, as Martin Daunton observed, mundane matters such as drains involved issues of political and philosophical principle.[20] Indeed, in response to this crisis, the MBW and its second-tier partners aggressively and ultimately successfully promoted what the former Attorney General and soon to be Chief Baron of the Court of Exchequer Sir Fitzroy Kelly, MP called in 1860 "a total revolution" in metropolitan taxation, redistributing the burden of taxation in ways that would have seemed impossible to their predecessors.[21]

The legal conflicts generated by the metropolitan authorities' policies were largely resolved in favor of the MBW and V/DBW during the 1860s. Thereafter, neither level of metropolitan government was restrained in law from raising revenue for drainage and redistributing its costs locally as seemed to it just, at least not in the same way as before the 1860s. In one sense, the outcome of these contests in London was similar to those under the Public Health Act in which liability was redefined and discretionary rating reaffirmed. Yet the situation in London was different; the stakes were significantly higher, the opposition more numerous and powerful, the parochialism more entrenched, and the battles more frequent and intense. The resolution of these conflicts, furthermore, both reflected and reinforced other controversial metropolitan political movements. The recognition that health required new principles of liability particularly challenged the parochial basis of improvement work, and thus it was part of a broader trend described by John Davis and David Green toward equalizing various rates between parishes in London.[22]

The first part of this chapter analyzes the influence of the courts on the MBW and V/DBW. It introduces the section (s. 170) governing the MBW's rating powers and that (s. 159) governing the allocation of expenses by V/DBW, the two sections of the 1855 Metropolis Local Management Act around which the chapter is organized. In decisions and dicta delivered in 1857 and 1858, the Queen's Bench made clear that it regarded a narrow reading of benefit as the unchanged criterion of liability for health and improvement. In the second part, I explore the MBW's response. The MBW tried to amend the 1855 Metropolis Local Management Act six times between 1858 and 1862, with important parliamentary successes in 1858 and 1862.[23] Rating, and especially section 170, was a central feature of this process. In the course of these attempts, the MBW established in law the ability to levy metropolitan-wide rates for healthy purposes, undermining the commitment to traditional benefit. The third part of this chapter explores the operation of section 159, particularly in Whitechapel, and demonstrates that debates and cases fought over it were permeated by contemporaneous debate over poor rate equalization. The MBW linked the two issues in its internal correspondence, as did some vestries and district boards. Opponents of the MBW's legislative agenda explicitly drew parallels between the two issues. The period from 1855 to 1867 was a critical time in the history of metropolitan health and poverty, and I show that the political economy of metropolitan poverty intersected with concerns about metropolitan health in multiple ways.[24] In the final section, I return to the courts to illustrate, with a new collection of decisions from 1860 to 1865, the acceptance by justices of the arguments of the MBW and its associated bodies.

The MMA Goes to Court, 1856–58

As would be expected, given the scope and complexity of the MMA, the MBW and its second-tier partners spent much time in their early years in court. Cases against rates were, not surprisingly, among the earliest that the MBW and its associated bodies encountered. Two broad sorts of challenge appeared in the early years, one contesting the liability of property for the debts of the old Metropolitan Commission of Sewers, the other contesting the liability for future improvements. Within each of these categories, the MBW, the vestries, and the district boards fought battles over the kind of property that could be rated, the principle that should govern its liability, and the justice of distributing costs at the local level. By the end of 1857, as a result of legal decisions, the MBW knew that the rating provisions of the MMA had to be amended; future cases only reinforced this view.

The first rating case heard at Queen's Bench involving the MBW concerned some property belonging to the Vauxhall Bridge Company.[25] That the first appellant against rates was a company was predictable. As we have seen, pre-1848 Commissioners of Sewers attempted to extend their rating powers to the maximum possible, and the MBW's decision to try to rate corporate property was consistent with that objective.[26] The MBW's decision, however, came up against the benefit principle. Under the old law of sewers, only property benefited paid, and the company claimed that its property did not benefit. The MBW did not contest or even address the company's liability under the old system, arguing instead that the benefit criterion applied under the Tudor Law of Sewers was inapplicable to sewers as they were understood at least since 1848. The MBW particularly noted that sewers now served sanitary purposes, which implied a different kind of liability.[27]

The company lost the case because it had not appealed against the sewers rate within the statutory time limit, but the parties to the *Vauxhall Bridge* case considered that the question at the heart of the matter—the liability of property—had not been answered. Both parties asked the court for guidance. Though the ruling did not require it, the court believed it appropriate to give an opinion on this "great question."[28] Stressing that he was speaking extrajudicially and in a nonbinding way, Lord Chief Justice John Campbell suggested that the burden of proof was on those who argued that the ancient law of sewers had been changed. They could see no evidence in the statute that the ancient law was changed; on the contrary, the statute carefully preserved the ancient principle of rating: if there was no benefit, there could be no rate. During oral arguments, Justice Charles Crompton even suggested that the statute was drafted so as to make clear that the law had not been altered.[29] Campbell specifically rejected the MBW's contention that health demanded a different liability, noting that "although it might be considered fair to distribute equally over the district all expences incurred with a view to the general health of the district," he could see no statutory justification for it.[30]

The Court's extrajudicial opinion in this case must have surprised the MBW and its legal team. The Court, for this hearing, consisted of John Campbell, William Erle, John Coleridge, and Charles Crompton. The latter two had decided *Dorling v. Epsom* in 1855, with Coleridge delivering the Court's opinion in that case. In *Dorling*, discussed at length in the previous chapter, the Court ruled that any assessment of benefit must include "indirect" benefits, and Coleridge engaged in a remarkable display of statutory interpretation in justifying them. Yet in this case, albeit explicating a different statute, Coleridge and Crompton were silent on the nature of benefit. It is not clear why the Court believed that a different set of principles should govern sewers law in the provinces than in the metropolis, given that the circumstances in the provinces were generally much stronger for the ancient principle. That the Court volunteered this opinion suggests a particular attachment to the benefit principle in the metropolis and a particularly interventionist approach to its maintenance.

Less than a month after issuing its extrajudicial ruling in the *Vauxhall* case, the Court again expressed its opinion on another challenge to the law of rating under the 1855 MMA. This case, argued three days after the *Vauxhall* case, involved a paving rate levied by the Vestry of St. George in the East on property belonging to the London Dock Company.[31] The company based its case on the 159th section of the MMA, which authorized vestries to exempt parts of parishes from rates if they were made for purposes not equally benefiting all parts of the parish. The company argued that the rates in question were for purposes from which not all their property could possibly derive a benefit. The vestry was, they argued, required to exempt such properties. The case turned on the meaning on the 159th section, but it of course made no sense apart from a belief that the old principle of no benefit, no rate still held. The vestry board members, relying on the plain meaning of the statute, argued that the decision to divide the parish was theirs and theirs alone.

The Court accepted the London Dock Company's argument and ruled that the company had to be relieved of part of the rate. The vestry must have been shocked, because the act clearly did not require the vestry to so apportion the rate; even the counsel for the London Dock Company, Sir Fitzroy Kelly, admitted that the statute said "may" but claimed that it should be read as saying "must."[32] The Court accepted that argument because of its conviction that the old principle of rating continued to apply to the MMA; under the Act, "the duty is cast on the vestry . . . to apportion the burden according to the benefit."[33] The Court argued that "the general purview of the statute is directed more to a change in the power of administration than to a change in the liability of property to be rated." Indeed, the ruling implied that there should be not only benefit but "equality of benefit."[34]

Between them, the *Vauxhall Bridge Company* case and the *London Dock Company* case must have sent a chill into the MBW and its second-tier partners. Although *Vauxhall* was extrajudicial and Lord Chief Justice Campbell stressed that the Court's opinion was not binding, the case was routinely cited as having made the point that the old principle of rating still held.[35]

In these two cases, decided within a month of each other, the Court thwarted attempts to broaden the basis of paying for health, in one case stretching the limits of statutory interpretation. To be sure, the courts did not invariably rule in favor of companies. The Wandsworth District Board successfully rated some West Middlesex Waterworks Company property, and Paddington Vestry successfully defended a rate levied on the Great Western Railway Company in early July 1858.[36] Yet the courts also continued to express the opinion that benefit was still the ruling principle. In a complex series of cases argued over eight months in 1857–58, for example, the Court ruled that some particular exemptions to rating for sewers were sound, being grounded both in practice and principle, "namely, that of actual benefit received by the property rated."[37]

As we shall see in the next section, these legal decisions convinced the MBW that the rating provisions of the MMA needed significant amendment. But the Queen's Bench rulings in these rate cases did not exhaust the new authorities' rating problems, and benefit loomed large in judicial consideration of the MBW's other legal rating problem, the liquidation of the debts of the old Metropolitan Commission of Sewers. By the time it was superseded by the MBW on January 1, 1856, the Metropolitan Commission of Sewers had contracted several hundred thousand pounds of debt in anticipation of building major metropolitan works, and the discharge of that debt triggered a major controversy over the cost of metropolitan improvement.[38] Deciding who should pay for what drain involved the MBW in difficult discussions about the relative financial responsibility of different kinds of property, from agricultural and building land to houses, and thus the responsibility of different groups of people for metropolitan improvement. But in keeping with the Metropolitan Commission of Sewers' practice, the debts were ultimately discharged on the basis of the rateable value of the parishes within the commission.[39]

These rates could hardly have been expected to be other than highly controversial. Allocating expenses among fifty or more metropolitan parishes, each of which wanted to pay as little as possible and get as much as possible, was a thankless task. It was extremely unlikely that any method of apportioning the debt would have been satisfactory to all the parishes. Yet the decision to allocate on the basis of rateable value was particularly calculated to rile parochial ratepayers, and within weeks, memorials protesting the assessment began arriving at the MBW.[40] As we have seen, the traditional law of sewers, dating back to the Tudor period, allocated charges for sewers only to those properties deriving a benefit from them, and some parishes argued that the costs should be apportioned on the basis of the relative benefit a parish derived. Parishes, furthermore, tended to equate benefit with expenditure; whatever was spent actually building sewers in the parish was the limit of liability.[41] They were unwilling or unable to see the interconnected nature of the works being constructed.

Greenwich is an example.[42] Greenwich, like many parishes, believed that little of the work for which it would pay actually benefited it.[43] The Greenwich representative to the MBW unsuccessfully tried to delay the issuing of the precepts, the instruments that ordered parochial overseers to collect rates on behalf of the MBW.[44] Even after this failure, the issue continued to be agitated in the district, and the MBW was forced to demand payment from individuals in the rate book rather than from the parish's overseers.[45] The exact number of individuals to which the rate applied is not clear, but the MBW requested nearly five hundred summonses for nonpayment in what was a striking instance of civil disobedience.[46]

Other parishes decided to protest the rates in front of Queen's Bench, hoping to secure relief from the courts.[47] In November 1858, for example, the St. Marylebone Vestry contested its portion of the cost of the Victoria Street sewer. The Court declined to hear the vestry's argument about the assessment, but a comment from the Bench invited further litigation. Justice William Erle noted that in *Vauxhall* the Court had given an extrajudicial opinion that the MBW should be guided by considerations of benefit, and in the St. Marylebone case he suggested that it "is very fit that the matter should be brought before us in the form of a special case."[48] St. Marylebone immediately notified the MBW of the decision.[49]

Coming as it did after the *Vauxhall* case, in which the Court had decided to give an opinion on a matter not required for the case at hand, this open invitation to litigation must have seemed extraordinary to the MBW. Twice within eighteen months, the Court appeared to be itching for a fight, and the MBW clearly was paying attention. The MBW, relying on the judgment of its clerk, Edmund Humphrey Woolrych, late clerk to the Metropolitan Commission of Sewers, had, with one exception, steadfastly resisted revising the initial apportionment of the old Metropolitan Commission of Sewers' debt. In early 1858, the MBW strongly reiterated its opposition to any reapportionment and prepared a bill amending the 1855 MMA that recommended none.[50]

The MBW was, however, having trouble collecting the rates due to it.[51] In the face of this popular resistance, and taking account of the signals the Court was sending about the legality of these rates, the MBW must have believed a reapportionment according to benefit was necessary to protect the Board's financial position. In late 1858, less than a month after the *St. Marylebone* ruling, the Finance Committee recommended that the debt be reapportioned accordingly.[52] Given the strength of the MBW's previous opposition to reapportionment of these debts, it is difficult not to conclude that this course of action was forced on them.

The reapportionment of the old debts of the Metropolitan Commission of Sewers consumed a significant amount of the time of the Works and General Purposes Committee and the servants of the MBW.[53] The question was, How does one measure the benefit of drainage? The MBW considered several different metrics, including the physical area of a parish benefited by the works and the rateable value of that area. These two methods resulted in different winners and losers in the reapportionment. Depending on the circumstances, adopting the physical area benefited as the metric instead of that area's rateable value could significantly redistribute the cost of work among land and houses. The rateable value of any given area was in part a function of the value and density of the houses on it. Two equal-sized areas, one covered with houses and the other only agricultural land, paid very different rates based on rateable value, with the built-up portion paying much more.[54] If, however, the calculation was based merely on physical area, the Works Committee ignored the rateable value of the land and houses, forcing agricultural land and urban land covered with houses to pay a proportionate share.

The process by which the MBW apportioned the debt thus brought the politics of improvement into relief. As the Works Committee struggled with the justice of the reapportionment, it prepared at one time or another tables showing the cost of particular works calculated according to four different criteria. Each of these methods involved a different politics of liability.[55] In general, the outcome of the MBW's reapportionment exercise was a move away from the comparatively progressive Metropolitan Commission of Sewers' apportioning.[56] Yet to lay the blame for the resulting inequities at the door of the MBW is to ignore both the role of the court in driving this reapportionment and the way in which the ideological construct "benefit" systematically disadvantaged certain areas and, therefore, certain people in London. As we shall see in the next section, the benefit principle that the courts insisted on was inconsistent with the MBW's broader agenda.

Constructing, Deconstructing, and
Reconstructing Benefit: 1855–62

The legislative history of the Metropolitan Local Management Act was short, although the act itself was long and permitted the MBW and V/DBW to carry out an enormous range of actions.[57] With an act of this size and scope, problems were inevitable. As early as 1856, Parliament passed an amending act to clarify some of its provisions.[58] In early 1858, the MBW drafted its own amending bill.[59] Although the MBW bill contained upward of fifty clauses, more than a quarter of the accompanying report focused on just three clauses dealing with rates. In an extended and carefully reasoned fashion, the MBW recommended repealing the rating section (s. 170), its grandfathered exemptions (s. 164), and the qualified rating section for extraparochial places (s. 175).[60] Given the importance of benefit to all three sections, the repeal of section 170, the general rating clause, was crucial.

The history of section 170 of the MMA was somewhat mysterious. As originally presented, the Metropolis Local Management Bill proposed that in raising revenue to pay for its works, the MBW should have regard "to the benefit derived from the expenditure by the several parts of the metropolis, and the annual value of the property in such respective parts."[61] Early in the bill's journey through Parliament, that clause was amended, dividing up the board's work into drainage and nondrainage works. Hall stressed in Parliament that if the rate was split up, poorer tenants would better be able to pay the smaller sums.[62] The drainage works were to be paid for on the basis of the benefit derived from the works. All other works were to be paid for on the basis of the rateable value of property, irrespective of whether it derived benefit or not.[63] In the Commons, Sir Benjamin Hall, the bill's sponsor, defended the idea that the MBW should assess benefit as a means of sparing districts from having to pay if nothing had been spent on them.[64]

Thus, the MMA upheld the benefit principle on which the Metropolitan Commission of Sewers and the provincial sewers commissions operated. Yet the MBW believed that the reference to benefit defeated the original intention of the bill.[65] A solicitor involved in preparing the original bill claimed further that the reference to benefit was meant to be excised, but was left in inadvertently.[66] Regardless of the section's provenance, the MBW noted that the decision to make only some of its operations dependent on benefit did not rest on any defensible principle. It led, the MBW further claimed, to absurdity. A few parishes would bear the whole cost of a main sewer, designed to be part of a metropolitan-wide system, but all parishes would be forced to contribute to the establishment of Finsbury Park, in all likelihood a purely local amenity. Similarly, a main sewer line would be rated according to a different principle than a main thoroughfare. Aligning all of the MBW's operations with one uniform principle of rating not only made more sense, they argued, but it respected what they believed was the original intention of the 1855 Metropolis Local Management Act. The MBW stressed that the project in which it was engaged was a metropolitan one; provincial sewer commission standards, based as they were on benefit, could not apply.[67]

Although the MBW's strategy would have led to its being able to rate uniformly over the metropolis, the board did not stress that. The experience of its predecessors showed that a uniform, metropolitan-wide rate was politically controversial. In early 1853, the Chair of the Metropolitan Commission of Sewers, Richard Jebb, received a request from the Home Secretary, Lord Palmerston, for suggested amendments to the law governing the commission's powers. In his reply, Jebb stressed that the division of the metropolis into thirty or so separate and financially distinct drainage districts was counterproductive and needed to be changed.[68] One of the particular problems that resulted from this division was the variability in rate income in the different districts. Property on the north side of the river yielded about three times as much as property south of it, and this meant that comparable expenditure required much higher rates in the much poorer southern districts. Jebb tossed out the suggestion that perhaps the MCS should be allowed to raise a rate levied on the whole metropolis, but recognizing the futility of that suggested instead dividing the metropolis into two districts only, separated by the river, and levying equal rates on parishes within each district.[69] Even that proposal was ambitious.

Jebb was hardly the only one who recognized the obstacle that financially separate districts created, particularly south of the river. Sir Robert Stephenson, MP, who served on the MCS, also believed that there had to be some adjustment of rates between rich and poor districts, though he rejected fully equalized rating.[70] The MBW's Chair, John Thwaites, was probably aware of these discussions because he served on the MCS, but he was also no doubt aware that the bill floated in late 1853 to remake the MCS made no such provision for equalizing rates.[71] Thus, in 1858, the MBW did not argue that rate reform was needed in order to ensure rate equalization among the many separate districts in the metropolis, even though that was what its bill effectively promoted.[72] This silence probably was not accidental.

Whether the rate-reform strategy that the MBW pursued would have been successful is unknown. As it turned out, the MBW in part obtained its object independent of this amending bill. Because of a series of problems in the original act with respect to even designing a system of main drainage and having borrowing power to finance it, the MBW had not made much progress in building the system.[73] In mid-1858, in the midst of the Great Stink, and after extensive negotiations among the MBW's Chair, John Thwaites, and several ministers, the government agreed to introduce a bill dealing with the main drainage alone.[74] This bill authorized the raising of a new rate levied on rateable property in the metropolis. It made no reference to differential benefit; indeed, the bill contained a separate clause stipulating that all parts of the metropolis "shall be deemed to be equally benefited by the Expenditure under this Act."[75] Considering the MBW's forceful denunciation of the benefit criterion two months earlier, Thwaites almost certainly seized the opportunity of the government-sponsored amending act to obtain this clause, which effectively neutered the traditional benefit principle. The act's preamble also explicitly linked the MBW's work to "the Health of the Metropolis." It is again hard to believe that this phrase was not inserted by Thwaites (and his advisers) in response to the court's assertion that "although it might be considered fair to distribute equally over the district all expences incurred with a view to the general health of the district," there was no statutory justification for it.[76] There was now.

It is worth pausing for a moment to consider how far opinion on this matter had traveled. As we saw in chapter 2, in 1817 the Westminster Commissioners of Sewers wanted only to make parties in the vicinity of a sewer pay for it because the sewers helped them avoid disease. In 1831, they wanted to build sewers in poor neighborhoods in order to prevent disease, but they could not legally or ideologically justify providing a subsidy to do so. Even their 1847 act did not permit districtwide rating for new works. In 1858, the MBW obtained power to rate the entire metropolis in order to sewer the whole city, because the health of its residents demanded it. This was not just about the protection of property; it was about the protection of health. The imperative to provide a disease-free environment, with the right to freedom from epidemic disease it implied, justified this extraordinary redistribution of rates. If sewers were merely about the protection of property, it is difficult to imagine that Parliament would have forced one group of ratepayers to subsidize another. This development, furthermore, helped create a new imagined local community.[77] The metropolis was not simply a collection of parishes cooperating, for technological reasons, in the completion of an engineering task. The MBW's action defined a new metropolitan community, united by a shared liability, even as champions of anticentralization crowed about the vindication of parochialism.[78]

The passage of the rating clause in the 1858 amending act was a major accomplishment for the Metropolitan Board of Works, one often overshadowed by the vigorous contemporary debate over debt ceilings and ministerial control of the main drainage project.[79] Had the MBW promoted this change on its own, the cost and trouble of defending it would have been significant (as would be seen in 1860). We do not know the basis on which John Thwaites convinced the government to go along with the MBW on the equalized main drainage rate, but the board was right to offer Thwaites its thanks.[80] The passage of the 1858 act was also extremely fortunate for the MBW, whose own amending act plans were derailed by the legal rulings discussed above. These rulings convinced the MBW that it had to reapportion the Metropolitan Commission of Sewers debt. Because the board believed that reapportionment required statutory sanction, delays meant that the MBW could not seriously submit an amending Act until mid-1859. The 1859 bill was introduced too late for passage, and as a result the MBW again ordered an amending act prepared for the 1860 session.[81]

The MBW's 1860 amending bill was the culmination of three years' debate and discussion at the board. The MBW's report on the this bill again made clear that rating principles were critical; the internal justification for the two sections dealing with rating (clauses 8 and 19) were the longest in the report.[82] As in 1858, the MBW defended its proposals in equitable terms, quoting large sections of the justification it had prepared in 1858. But the MBW added considerable new material to this justification, highlighting health and sanitary concerns five different times. The MBW drove home the point that sewer rates under the 1855 MMA served wholly different purposes from those under the old statutes; they accordingly required a new principle of contribution.[83] Sewers per se were not responsible for new rating; sewers had been around for a long time. It was the goal of the expenditure—the public's health—that required new property relations.

The MBW's 1860 bill attracted serious opposition and thus serious parliamentary attention, including a select committee that met for more than two weeks. More than eighty petitions against various clauses in the bill arrived.[84] The select committee spent ten days (out of fourteen) dealing with the rating and MCS debt provisions; the battle against the 1860 bill was, once again, joined around benefit. Notwithstanding this vigorous opposition, the select committee accepted the MBW's rejection of the benefit principle explicitly in its support for the repeal of the benefit section (s. 170).[85] Vindicating the MBW's original position, the select committee also struck the clause reapportioning the debts of the MCS (the so-called Rock Loan).[86] The failure of the reapportionment surely delighted the parishes onto which the costs of the work had been thrown and also probably pleased the MBW, which had taken the task only as a result of legal fears. Although the MBW did not get all it wanted, its determination to reframe the liability for rating the metropolis was largely successful.[87]

The select committee did not provide a rationale for its decision to accept the repeal of the benefit principle, a principle that the House of Commons explicitly had endorsed when it passed the original act five years earlier.[88] In part, the select committee may have been convinced that benefit could not be apportioned precisely. The MBW had always argued that it was not possible to do so, but even the witness called by opposition counsel—presumably to testify that it was not difficult to apportion benefit—was not convincing on the stand. Thomas Hawksley, who had been one of the board's consulting engineers, claimed that there was no real difficulty in dividing districts so as to apportion benefit.[89] Counsel for the MBW pointed out to Hawksley that six different parishes contributed to the cost of one sewer in central London and forced Hawksley to admit that he could not apportion the benefit precisely, but he claimed he certainly could avoid "doing violent injustice."[90] The select committee must have wondered if this sufficiently answered the MBW's argument that benefit could not be apportioned. The "absence of violent injustice" (to paraphrase Hawkesley) would have been an odd standard on which to ground taxing power and a fruitful, and frightful, source of litigation.

Indeed, the whole notion of benefit as determined by engineers and surveyors must have seemed increasingly meaningless to the select committee. Under repeated questioning, Joseph Bazalgette, the chief engineer of the MBW, stuck to the party line that "all districts in the metropolis derive a benefit from an improvement of the drainage of the metropolis."[91] Asked about the benefit a parish on the north side of the river derived from main drainage works carried out on the south side, Bazalgette finally admitted that main drainage works carried out in, say, Rotherhithe would not directly benefit St. George's Hanover-square, but there was a general, though unexplained, benefit.[92] Hawksley, too, admitted that he supported the principle of the 1858 Amendment Act, whereby intercepting sewers were paid for on the assumption that all people within the metropolis benefited equally. Yet when asked how they all benefited, he admitted that it was "very difficult to say."[93] Clearly, neither Bazalgette nor Hawksley had a firm idea of the meaning of benefit from an engineering standpoint, and neither wanted to advance a medical argument.[94] The MBW, we know, believed that health determined liability. Under questioning even Hawksley admitted that the benefit provided by the intercepting and main sewers was the "general health they promoted."[95] The select committee may well have accepted that argument.

In contrast to its usual practice for what was essentially a local act, the Commons seriously debated the clauses that the select committee had already approved. This unusual proceeding was presumably a result of the significance of the bill; according to Sir Fitzroy Kelly, the bill "effected a total revolution in the entire system of taxation of the Metropolis." Notwithstanding this total revolution, the House overwhelmingly supported the select committee's decisions during the critical debate in early August.[96] The Commons' 1860 debate showed, however, that there were multiple objections to the redefinition of benefit proposed by the bill. Some MPs clearly recognized the implications of this bill, with its new rating clauses, for the contemporary debate over the equalization of poor rates.

The Politics of Equalization: Section 159

In important ways the history of financing healthy infrastructure traced in this book is part of the long, contested history of local rate equalization. Equalization was increasingly important to the central government and to various political actors beginning in the 1830s, although the term meant different things to different groups and individuals at different times. According to an 1834 parliamentary report on county taxation, equalization usually meant some kind of equitable adjustment between the taxation of agricultural and nonagricultural property,[97] but it also meant equity among parishes within a county.[98] Counties raised a levy on their parishes relative to the total parochial assessed value, so if a parish was undervalued relative to others in the county, it paid proportionately less than other parishes. This last concern with equalization reflected a conviction that the counties raised rates for the good of all the inhabitants and thus all parishes should pay a fair share, not one artificially depressed by an unrealistically low property assessment.[99]

Debates over rate equalization also arose frequently around the Poor Law, the costs for which were very unequally distributed among parishes across the country.[100] In part this was a result of the law of settlement.[101] Since the seventeenth century, the right to relief was determined by one's parish of settlement, often but by no means necessarily the parish in which one was born. The parish was obligated to provide relief, and poor people carefully preserved knowledge of their settlement so as to ensure their right to relief. A person could obtain a fresh settlement in a variety of ways, but mere change of residence in and of itself was not sufficient, which could lead to difficulties and conflict between parishes. To take a simplified example, sometimes individuals maintained residences in their settled parishes out of an abundance of caution or simply because of long ties with the community, even as they worked in an adjacent one.[102] Yet when an individual lost his or her job, the parish in which he or she had a settlement, rather than the parish of employment, was responsible for the costs of relief. To many ratepayers in the settled parish that seemed unfair: they were subsidizing the parish of employment, providing it with workers but freeing it of the responsibility to maintain them in hard times.[103] This was a frequent cause of complaint in urban areas with multiple, closely packed parishes.

The law of settlement and its associated problems did not change with the passage of the 1834 New Poor Law, which continued the ancient principle of parochial financial responsibility for relief of the settled poor even as it grouped over fifteen thousand parishes into six hundred or so unions for administrative efficiency. The grouping of parishes into unions in some ways heightened awareness of the differential costs of relief.[104] The Whitechapel Union in London's East End, for example, comprised nine parishes and places, ranging from the relatively densely populated and relatively poor St. Mary, Whitechapel to the much smaller and wealthier St. Botolph without Aldgate to the St. Katharine's Dock Precinct. The Dock Precinct had very few settled poor and consequently a very low poor rate, in contrast to St. Mary, Whitechapel. This would have been apparent every time the Guardians gathered to raise a rate. The fact that a number of St. Mary's settled and irremovable poor worked in the Dock Precinct made the situation more inequitable, at least from St. Mary's perspective.[105]

One solution to the inequity in parochial costs for relief was the equalization of poor rates throughout the metropolis, effectively doing away with the law of settlement and having all parishes pay according to the value of their property for the support of all metropolitan poor. Efforts to alter the mode of financing the New Poor Law's operations began soon after the passage of the law and continued unsuccessfully in the 1850s.[106] In London, an organization devoted to the reform of metropolitan Poor Law taxation formed in 1855.[107] In 1857, Parliament got a major advocate of poor rate equalization when Acton Smee Ayrton was elected MP for Tower Hamlets.[108] Ayrton immediately moved for a select committee on metropolitan poor rate inequalities, but the measure was defeated. Undeterred, Ayrton introduced a metropolitan poor rate bill in 1858; although fully debated, it was also defeated.[109]

Poor-rate equalization was thus widely discussed and debated at Westminster and throughout the metropolis in the mid-1850s.[110] The MCS raised equalization in the context of sewer funding in the early 1850s, and as we have seen the 1858 and 1862 acts equalized intercepting and main drainage rates across

London.[111] Equalization of local drainage charges also was part of the debate over the working of the 1855 MMA. This came about largely as a result of the structure of the submetropolitan district boards of works. Whereas large parishes were often constituted as single vestries, smaller parishes were grouped with larger ones to form multiparish DBWs.[112] Given that these district boards comprised several parishes or places, some arrangement as to how to pay for expenses had to be organized. The DBWs did not raise rates from individuals but from parishes. However, Parliament did not require the DBWs to raise the money they needed from all parishes in an equalized manner, with each parish raising a sum in proportion to its assessed value. The 1855 MMA (s. 159) gave district boards (and vestries, for that matter) the power to rate parts of their districts if the expenses were for the exclusive benefit of part of a district. Yet once again that power was discretionary, and the statute did not require parishes to bear, as near as possible, the cost of their own improvements.[113]

It was probably obvious at the time that section 159 would lead to conflict. Any decision to rate an entire district equally for works invited the objection that the constituent parishes that had spent money in the past maintaining their roads and drains would now be taxed to spend on behalf of their neighbors who had not done so. The other objection that some parishes had was that parishes with higher rateable value would contribute proportionately more to the expense than poorer parishes, thereby equalizing the cost of urban improvement within the district. This section, as seen above, also was an early object of judicial attention. The Queen's Bench initially stressed that apportioning on the basis of benefit was a duty of the vestry, although it retreated to the position that apportioning was at the discretion of the vestries and district boards.[114]

In the absence of research into the minutes of every vestry and district board, it is very difficult to know how they responded to section 159 or to these decisions, though we can have little doubt that their clerks would have drawn their attention to them. In the Whitechapel DBW, the decision about how to allocate the costs of metropolitan improvement was contested from the start.[115] The Whitechapel District Board Finance Committee initially decided that all expenses should be paid for on the basis of a uniform rate on all parishes in the district.[116] When this was proposed to the whole Whitechapel DBW, one member immediately gave notice of motion that all necessary sums should instead be collected and spent "in the manner as is the practice of the Guardians of the Whitechapel Poor Law Union," that is, on a parish-by-parish basis.[117] When this motion finally came before the DBW, it was roundly defeated. Perhaps as a gesture of conciliation, the DBW resolved to shift the costs of bringing parts of the district up to a common standard of paving onto the parishes concerned, although the DBW reaffirmed its support for raising all other expenses—of which drainage would have been by far the largest—on the basis of the rateable value of the district.[118] This was union chargeability by another name.

The Whitechapel DBW's decision meant that parishes like St. Botolph without Aldgate would be saddled with much higher rates. Its rateable value per head ranked well above the metropolitan average and was among the highest in the metropolitan area.[119] And smaller parishes in the Whitechapel District Board immediately noticed that their rates increased dramatically. Holy Trinity, Minories saw its contribution increase nearly fivefold.[120] The Precinct of Saint Katharine saw its sewer rates more than triple.[121] When Holy Trinity, Minories appealed to the DBW against the rates, it was informed that the DBW had fully considered the principle on which the rate was based and had decided that such a distribution of costs was "undoubtedly the intention of the Act."[122] Perhaps it is not surprising that when the Whitechapel District Board levied a uniform rate based on the principle that all parishes and places should contribute according to their rateable value, smaller parishes refused to pay, with St. Botolph without Aldgate appearing as the test case. The magistrate in charge sent the case up to the Queen's Bench, where it was argued in June 1860.[123]

The St. Botolph case is analyzed in the next section, but I raise it here, because the relevant section of the statute became part of the 1860 select committee hearings and the Commons debate over the amendment of the MMA. The issues that section 159 raised dominated in particular the early testimony of William Durrant Cooper, a solicitor from St. Pancras involved in drafting the 1855 act. On the basis of section 159, Durrant Cooper testified, St. Pancras Vestry chose very early in its life to exempt parts of the parish from the cost of works done to benefit other parts.[124] Yet St. Pancras's system proved difficult to implement in practice. Durrant Cooper, who was a member of the vestry before becoming its solicitor, testified that it was nearly impossible to allocate benefit under section 159 and that it was nearly impossible precisely to specify the area benefited.[125] Durrant Cooper's opposition to the clause rested, however, on more than concerns of practicability. He also held a much broader, and politically controversial, notion of benefit—one that required equalized rating as a result of the political economy of metropolitan labor. St. Pancras, he noted, was "very much" benefited by sewers works carried out by the MBW; Paddington was not. Yet, he claimed, poor people who lived in St. Pancras worked in Paddington. St. Pancras raised poor rates to pay for those people when they were thrown out of work for whatever reason; Paddington did not. It seemed as though Cooper suggested that equal sewers rates like those levied by the MBW were Paddington's subsidy for St. Pancras's poor rates.[126]

Coming as it did from someone involved in drafting the original act, this was a striking admission. Durrant Cooper's reference to London's laborers and their support agreed very strongly with arguments made by promoters of an equalized metropolitan poor rate. Counsel for the City immediately asked him, Was it "desirable to have a general rate for the poor?" If such a rate was subject to certain safeguards, Durrant Cooper had "no objection."[127] Taking a different tack, another questioner pressed him on the justice of having districts that had done their duty in the past to subsidize now those that had not. Durrant Cooper again reformulated the issue in terms of London's labor market. The City of London, he noted, had paid for all its own sewers, but it sent all the people who worked in the City back to St. Pancras at night.[128] Durrant Cooper agreed with the principle enunciated by the MBW that everybody benefited from the MBW's works.

St. Pancras Vestry might not like it, but "having been concerned for the whole metropolis" he "most certainly" did.[129]

Though it made no specific appearance at the 1860 Select Committee, the Whitechapel District Board of Works, one of the sources of trouble around section 159, similarly framed the financing of metropolitan improvement in terms of the political economy of metropolitan labor markets. The Whitechapel DBW carefully followed the progress of the 1860 amending bill through Parliament and recruited its MPs into the battle on the floor of the Commons when the St. Katharine Docks Company sought to amend the bill to exempt its property from the rates.[130] In a lengthy letter to the MPs, the Whitechapel DBW's clerk, Alfred Turner, argued that the Docks Company required a reserve pool of laborers who remained semipauperized due to the fluctuating demand for their work.[131] Yet the laborers could not live in the Docks Company precincts, where the company would at least be forced to pay for the poor rates raised to relieve them if they could not work. If the company's attempt to secure an exemption from local improvement rates succeeded, it would ensure that it would not have to pay any rates that might benefit its workers.[132] In Whitechapel, public health and the Poor Law were as tightly linked as ever.

Durrant Cooper's testimony before the select committee brought to the fore the equalizing issues arising from section 159 and their manifest connection with London's labor market. The 1860 amending bill did not propose any change in section 159, because the vestries and the district boards evidently did not want the section changed and the MBW had no specific interest in it. After the select committee passed the bill, it moved to the floor of the House, where opponents used its appearance as their last chance to secure favorable amendments. One amendment proposed to force district boards to assess parishes only for work done within those parishes, thereby effectively turning the discretion given to DBW under section 159 into a requirement. Debate on this amendment turned into a wide-ranging discussion of the nature of benefit and the legitimacy of the old parochial principle. Some MPs were all too aware of the link between sewers rates and poor rates and the possible consequence of abandoning the parochial principle in one for the other. Sir Fitzroy Kelly argued, "If the principle of the Bill were affirmed, he saw no reason why hon. members who were favourable to an equalization of poor-rate should not demand, with precisely the same justice, that, although Aldgate might have very few poor and [St. Mary] Whitechapel a great many, yet that Aldgate should pay 17,000*l* a year for poor-rates, and Whitechapel only 6000*l* or 7000*l.*"[133]

The proposed amendment was roundly defeated on the floor of the House. A subsequent amendment seeking to exempt dock properties from the rates was spared the same fate only by being withdrawn. The scale of the defeat of the amendment suggested something of the degree to which parliamentary thinking on equalization in general had changed by 1860. In 1861, in what Anne Digby calls the most radical change in Poor Law finances in the nineteenth century, Parliament made the charge for certain categories of pauper an equal one among parishes within a union, thereby significantly reformulating a major part of Poor Law union expense.[134] In 1865, Parliament completed this project, equalizing all expenses for poor relief among the parishes in a given union. Although the history of poor relief in London followed a different trajectory, in 1864 Parliament likewise equalized some poor expenses among metropolitan poor authorities.[135] In 1867, Parliament returned to London's poor relief with an even more dramatic equalizing measure, the Metropolitan Poor Act.[136] This act's most striking innovation from this perspective was the creation of the Metropolitan Common Poor Fund, raised on all places according to rateable value.[137] This fund significantly redistributed the costs of medical care in the metropolis.[138]

The 1860s thus were a watershed in metropolitan (and national) Poor Law financial history. This metaphor is equally apt for the financial history of London's drainage. Health provided a powerful rationale for change in both cases. Metropolitan sewerage authorities, in particular, had been using health to argue for equalized improvement costs for decades, and the MBW and V/DBW had been particularly active in so doing since 1855. Given the long history of agitation in favor of poor rate equalization, Fitzroy Kelly's claim that sewers equalization was a slippery slope to poor rate equalization was overstated; each movement, as it were, had its own history. Yet the nearly simultaneous achievement of these two long-sought goals probably was not entirely coincidental. The debate over the equalization of sewer rates clearly reflected and possibly reinforced metropolitan and parliamentary willingness to consider other limited approaches to equalization.[139] The conversion of metropolitan and parliamentary opinion, furthermore, was only part of the story. As was the case for Epsom in the previous chapter, the advocates for equalized sewer rating also succeeded in convincing judges. Indeed, Fitzroy Kelly's intervention in the 1860 debate involved more than an appeal to the old principles; he was also concerned with rectifying what he saw as an ill-conceived judicial interpretation of the 1855 MMA.[140]

The Courts, 1860–65: Equalization, Benefit, Liability

Although the 1858 and 1862 Metropolis Local Management Amendment Acts settled rate issues for the future, the amended acts did not resolve ongoing legal conflicts that arose out of the 1855 MMA. From 1860 to 1865, the Queen's Bench revisited the traditional law of sewers on three different occasions in 1855 MMA sewer-rate cases.[141] These cases dealt with the same issues that initially stimulated the MBW to amend the 1855 act, the courts having delivered unsatisfactory rulings on them in 1857 and 1858. In these three cases, however, the justices ruled in favor of the MBW and the vestries and district boards. And in so doing, the court gradually accepted the MBW's determination to redefine of the costs of urban improvement.

The first case—*The Overseers of Saint Botolph without Aldgate v. the Board of Works for the Whitechapel District*—revolved, as already noted, around the Whitechapel

DBW's decision not to divide its district for the purposes of some rates under section 159. The significance of the case to both parties was indicated by the Whitechapel District Board's retention of Attorney General Sir Richard Bethell and St. Botolph without Aldgate's retention of the former attorney general and soon to be Chief Baron of the Exchequer Sir Fitzroy Kelly. Both parties agreed that Parliament permitted district boards to rate as the Whitechapel District Board did; the only argument that St. Botolph without Aldgate could make was that such a decision flew in the face of the historic principle of parochial financial responsibility. Kelly thus argued that the 1855 MMA did not replace parochial financial responsibility, even as it grouped parishes together for administrative convenience. The Whitechapel District Board argued that it did.[142]

The judges found themselves forced to decide parliamentary intention. Two of the judges noted that the act was silent as to the principle that should guide the allocation of charges among parishes. Given that silence, one might have expected the justices to fall back on historic precedent, as Sir Fitzroy Kelly argued, and have each parish pay its own way. Otherwise, he claimed, large parishes would be able to plunder small ones, or, to decode his language, poor parishes rich ones.[143] Kelly argued that if the statute was intended to equalize expenses among parishes within a district board, the statute would have said so explicitly. He compared the rating policy of the Whitechapel District Board with poor-rate equalization, calling the proposal "revolutionary." The justices, however, were unconvinced. If the MMA permitted the possibility of equalization within district boards, it must reflect parliamentary intent. The Poor Law, they noted in 1860, did not even give unions the possibility of rating over the entire union. The justices unanimously ruled in favor of the Whitechapel DBW.[144]

Whitechapel's victory was significant for several reasons, but I want to draw particular attention to it as the first rating case in which the Court revised its original interpretation of the 1855 MMA. In the 1857 *Vauxhall Bridge* case, the Court claimed that "it might be considered fair to distribute equally over the district all expenses incurred with a view to the general health of the district," but they could see no statutory justification for it.[145] But the 1860 Whitechapel verdict implicitly permitted that very scenario to occur. In so permitting, the Court accepted the argument that sewers in 1860 were different things from sewers in, say, 1800. Justice Charles Crompton noted in the Whitechapel case that a "rate levied for defraying what are called sewerage expenses, under an Act of Parliament of the kind before us, is a very different thing from a sewers' rate strictly so called." The difference, in Crompton's mind, lay in the fact that the "indirect benefit arising to a parish in the district from that expenditure may be very much greater than that which is direct."[146] In the Whitechapel case, the requirement for direct benefit, the foundation of the old principle, was explicitly breached.[147]

In 1863, the Queen's Bench revisited its extrajudicial remarks in the (1857) *Vauxhall Bridge* case, providing a fresh interpretation of benefit.[148] The Imperial Gas-Light Company had property rated for the poor, including buildings and underground gas pipes and mains. The company believed that the underground mains did not derive a full benefit from drainage works carried out by the MBW and accordingly appealed to the quarter sessions against a rate made under the 1855 Metropolis Local Management Act. The sessions ruled that the pipes did not derive the same benefit as other property and reduced the assessment by 50 percent. In oral argument in Queen's Bench in support of the sessions' decision, counsel for the gas company laid stress on the Court's *Vauxhall* opinion that the old principle of rating had not been repealed and that the MBW had to take benefit into account when rating. Mr. Clerk, counsel for the gas company, argued that the statute itself suggested that the amount of benefit needed to be considered.[149] In rating lands used for agricultural (and other) purposes for the sewers rate at one quarter the annual value, Parliament quantified the extent to which benefit varied among different sorts of property. It seemed strange, Clerk argued, that land through which gas mains passed might be rated at one quarter annual value, whereas the mains themselves were rated at full value.

The Court must have realized it was in a bind. The gas company, relying on the statute and quoting almost exactly the Court's own opinion in *Vauxhall*, produced a very strong argument in favor of the reduction. Charles Crompton was the only member of the Court who had been present at *Vauxhall* and, in order to preserve the principle so recently articulated by the Court, claimed that the Court did not intend that the amount of benefit would be taken into consideration, only the fact of it. In delivering the judgment of the Court in the *Queen against Head*, Chief Justice Cockburn stressed that he too did not disagree with the opinion in *Vauxhall* or even, reaching back to the seventeenth century, with Callis; benefit was still the condition of rateability. This position agreed with the Court's opinion in *Vauxhall*, but everything depended on how one defined benefit. The Court claimed that in *R v. Head*, the test of benefit was the drainage of the district. If the property was drained, mediately or immediately, it was benefited and was fit to be rated.[150] It did not matter what kind of property it was or the use to which the property was put or even whether it needed drainage or not. On the basis of this new test, the Court ruled for the MBW: the gas company's mains were fully liable.[151]

The decision in *R v. Head* thus significantly redefined benefit yet again. Even if a property did not need to be drained, and even if that property, like impervious pipes, could not be benefited in any common sense understanding of the term, the Court decided that it legally benefited.[152] The climax of the Court's rejection of the traditional view of the benefit of drainage came in 1865, in *Pew v. MBW*, the last of the cases dealing with rating I will consider here.[153] Pew's complaint arose out of the Rock Loan.[154] As we have already seen, the repayment provisions for this loan were extremely controversial, and the MBW and Parliament spent years trying to fix the problem. At the same time, local ratepayers fought their own battles against these charges. St. Giles, Camberwell was one of the disadvantaged parishes in the loan repayment scheme, having derived, according to the case agreed on by the parties, about £1,000 benefit for £9,000 expenditure. The parties to the case thus agreed that Camberwell was being rated well beyond any benefit it derived. Camberwell sought to force the MBW either to spread the loan over the entire metropolis or to assess parishes within the old, separate Surrey and Kent sewerage district according to benefit, not rateable value, as the MBW in fact had proposed to do in 1859 and 1860. The MBW, in contrast, argued against an apportionment based on benefit, claiming that the 1855 MMA changed the old law of sewers. *Pew* marked the third time since 1860 that Queen's Bench was asked to consider whether the MMA had fundamentally changed it.[155]

The Court ruled against the appellants and in favor of the MBW.[156] The Court found that the MBW was not obliged to inquire as to the amount of benefit that parishes obtained. Furthermore, the Court claimed that if the appellants' argument, and the opinion in *Vauxhall*, were carried to their logical conclusion, the MBW would have to assess the amount of benefit on every single property in the district, and the Court found no power in old or new statutes to conduct that kind of inquiry.[157] In a striking exchange during oral argument, the Chief Justice wondered whether it was not contrary to the old law that lowland Bermondsey required new sewers, whereas upland Camberwell, which did not, had to pay for them. Justice Colin Blackburn interjected that it "certainly is contrary to the principle of the old law as it was understood and expounded in various cases in this court."[158] In deciding for the MBW, the court signaled that its acceptance of the MBW's understanding of the law of sewers was complete.[159] Parliament was not, it seems, the only body willing to tolerate greater degrees of equalization during the 1860s.

❧ ❧ ❧

All of the bodies mentioned in this chapter—the old separate commissions of sewers, the Metropolitan Commission of Sewers, the MBW, and the vestries and the district boards that worked in conjunction with it—have suffered, at one time or another, from very bad press, and some of them have never had a good reputation.[160] The charges levied against these bodies range from incompetence to corruption, sloth, parsimony, and self-interestedness, singly and in combination. Historians have recently, in different ways and to different degrees, revisited the shortcomings of these bodies, and this chapter contributes to that trend.[161] Its narrative describes the final years of what was a decades-long struggle, started by the old separate commissions of sewers in the early nineteenth century. This chapter has focused on the words and legal deeds of the various bodies responsible for urban improvement in mid-century London, highlighting the political, legal, and ideological work they undertook in order to finance London's drainage. Historians have sometimes lost sight of this topic, given the parliamentary and ministerial challenges the project faced and the enormous technical and logistical efforts needed to complete it. This chapter also argues that particular actors played crucial parts in this drama, especially the elected and indirectly elected members of the various boards, and to a lesser extent the officers who worked for them.[162]

The question remains, though: Why did they do it? The forces of parochialism were very strong in London, and it must have taken considerable commitment to pursue this redistributive agenda, particularly as some of their MBW colleagues were uninterested. The board members were going to benefit from the completion of London's drainage as much as everyone else was, but that motivation, it seems to me, is limited. It is more likely that the experience gained through years of being unable to respond to repeated demands from their constituents and communities for improved drainage contributed significantly to a sense that change was required. By the mid-1860s, key members of the MBW had been working on drainage for over a decade. John Thwaites, for example, was active in Southwark Vestry during the 1840s and served on the Metropolitan Commission of Sewers before being elected first chairman of the MBW, a post he held until 1870.[163]

But equalized drainage rating was not the inevitable outcome of contemporary dissatisfaction with drainage. In both 1848 and 1855, Parliament believed that the administrative integration of sewers management did not imply equal rating, and Queen's Bench supported that view prior to 1860. Even interception as a method did not demand integration as a financial strategy. As we saw in the previous chapter, Bristol divided its drainage into six different self-financed projects; at the very least London could have managed with one financially distinct drainage scheme on each side of the river, as the MCS advocated in 1853.[164] The MBW did not advocate two separate districts, and we must regard that as an explicit decision, presumably informed even if not determined by the poverty of the southern districts. London's main drainage rates were not equalized because of systemic exigency. They were equalized because the MBW made it happen, given the board's conviction that the benefits of drainage, especially health, accrued to people, not property, including and perhaps especially people who were not direct ratepayers. If they were going to get this benefit, well-to-do property was going to have to pay for it, and that meant metropolitan-wide, equalized rating.[165]

The effect of the MBW's success in this endeavor varies, depending on whether we look at the first or second tier. As John Davis notes, one of the reasons that the unequalized vestry system survived as long as it did was because so many important metropolitan activities were first-tier (MBW) charges, supported by a common rate.[166] The significance of establishing main drainage as a common first-tier charge in the 1858 and 1862 amending acts, implicit in this claim, was thus immense. For vestries and district boards, the amending acts introduced no new rating principle, but by fighting off parliamentary attempts to convert the "may" contained in section 159 to a "must," the MBW and its second-tier partners at least kept the possibility of equalizing expenditure within V/DBWs alive, and the 1860 Whitechapel decision gave V/DBWs a legal rationale for seizing that possibility. The practical significance of the Whitechapel decision in terms of second-tier metropolitan sanitary work is more difficult to assess.[167] Some vestries and district boards probably hesitated to embark on major local drainage projects until the Metropolitan Board of Works completed plans for London's main drainage. That decision was not made until August 1858; the work itself was not completed until 1865.[168] Eventually the vestries and district boards constructed over eleven hundred miles of sewers. The principles that financed them remain in many cases still to be determined.[169]

Chapter Five

Healthy Domesticity, 1848–72

Previous chapters in this book have argued that local authorities actively and effectively used new or newly conceived concepts of the public's health to redefine healthy things, places, and properties. In this chapter, I explore the boundaries of healthy domesticity. I focus on quotidian practices of private rights, using the drainage of private property and the control of lodging houses as my examples. I choose these two examples because although in each case the state crossed a domestic threshold, it did so in different ways.[1] Healthy drainage allowed the state into the home, as it were, shifting the boundary between the state and the individual, while healthy lodging houses drew a new if ill-defined boundary between individuals, demarcating those entitled to certain private rights from those not.[2] Healthy boundaries were exclusive as well as inclusive.[3]

I also choose these examples because they illustrate the different sorts of difficulties that the central and local state confronted in regulating aspects of domestic life. Active opposition in both cases was rooted in long-standing concerns over the sanctity of domestic arrangements and the rights of private property.[4] But those anxieties were inflected by supplementary concerns. In the case of private drainage, opposition was exacerbated by the identification of house drainage as a private benefit.[5] This fundamentally ideological identification was formalized for the first time in 1848.[6] It structured and seriously limited the provision of house drainage for the entire nineteenth century, and it triggered, yet again, local debate about how the costs of delivering health to the poor were going to be distributed.[7] Traditionally conceived private property rights also did not fully determine the boundaries of healthy lodging. The emergence of "common lodging houses" as the only houses with lodgers regulated at mid-century, and the form that regulation took, cannot be understood apart from an ideology of domesticity that simultaneously prohibited and permitted regulation, policing some domestic arrangements even as it protected others.[8]

In the first three sections of this chapter, I focus on the history of private drainage. When looked at from a national perspective, this history is complex. Towns employed a wide variety of waste-management systems, from cesspits to dry conservancy to water carriage with water laid on or not, with each of these arrangements potentially inside or outside the house. Different towns moved through different phases and stages of waste removal at different times and to different degrees, following no one path to sanitary modernity.[9] Historians have been appropriately sensitive to this uneven development, recognizing that uniformity was impossible and hesitating to identify different local authorities as leaders or laggards. This is entirely understandable: the earliest generation of public health historians condemned the delinquency of many localities, ignoring the range of difficulties they faced. It was to be expected that later generations focused less on the fact that some local authorities did not act than on the difficulties they encountered when they did.

The desire to avoid Whiggish history has led, however, to a relative neglect of the work carried out by those we might call early adopters. They faced the same difficulties that many local authorities faced and, indeed, actually triggered some of them. The features that slowed down change in any given town were varied, but historians recognize that local authorities simply did not have the power to do all that they may have wanted to do. That legal inability was, in certain cases, constructed after the fact. The public health statutes passed at mid-century gave local authorities various powers, but the limits of those powers had to be worked out. As the early adopters tested the limits of the legislation, the courts occasionally pushed back and established the legal parameters within which change would take place.[10] Besides triggering these difficulties, early adopters sometimes found ways to circumvent them. Local authorities did not always convince Parliament or the courts of the wisdom of their approaches, and they were in general less successful in this area than in taxation, but the record of their successes and, just as important, their failures nonetheless suggests a revision in the model of inevitably piecemeal progress that dominates current historiography of domestic sanitary reform.

In the last section I turn to lodging. Under the 1851 and 1853 Common Lodging House Acts, police could enter common lodging houses without a warrant and without notice, at all times of the day or night.[11] This extraordinary police power itself had to be policed, because it was inconceivable that all houses in which people lodged could be dealt with in this way.[12] The control of lodging houses presupposed the construction of a new legal boundary, encircling those persons and properties subject to relatively unrestricted inspection.[13] That was not an easy matter. Parliament wrestled with several different definitions of "common lodging houses" in seven different bills in the space of a decade. It passed three of the most important acts controlling common lodging houses with no definition at all. The inability statutorily to define lodging houses did not, however, prevent certain houses with lodgers from being regulated.[14] These houses were, as many historians have noted, filled with the poorest people, but class alone cannot explain this development. Control of lodging illustrates the complex ways in which ideologies of domesticity, health, and property informed public health, intersected in the control of domestic spaces, and helped define an outcast group.[15]

This section also revisits the boundary between central and local initiative. In chapter 1, I argued that through their bylaw-making authority, municipal corporations creatively reshaped nuisance law in the second quarter of the century. Their freedom of legal movement was always under threat of a central veto, but this veto was initially deployed inconsistently and irregularly. By the late 1840s, the central government began to exert its authority more firmly. The regulation of common lodging houses reiterates this shift in power, with the impetus coming largely from the center. Although the acts gave local authorities the power to make regulatory bylaws, the bylaw-making process in 1851 could hardly have been more different from that of 1835. The Home Office exerted much tighter control over the process from the start. Health was a pivotal arena for resetting boundaries between central and local governments.[16]

Compulsory Private Drainage: The Ideological, Structural, and Statutory Contexts

One of the principal objectives of the Public Health Act (PHA) in the provinces and the Metropolis Sewers Act/Metropolis Local Management Act (MMA) in London was the improvement of urban drainage. In the second half of the nineteenth century, London's intercepting and main drainage was completed, and provincial towns had constructed miles of main sewer lines.[17] In addition to authorizing the creation of main sewer systems, the legislation permitted local authorities to compel the drainage of private property.[18] It also permitted them to ensure the sufficiency of sanitary accommodation for any new and existing houses.[19] In this section, I review briefly the ideological, structural and financial, and statutory problems that local authorities encountered as they extended their work onto private property. I do so not because these difficulties have not been recognized before, as they have,[20] but because a focus on them furnishes evidence of the political and sometimes extralegal ways that local authorities found to work within or around the obstacles they encountered.

Some of the ideological difficulties associated with private house and property drainage were well known in the early 1840s. The Health of Towns Commission in 1844 and 1845 provided the opportunity to air them again.[21] The inspection of insanitary dwellings, for instance, was condemned as un-English in the 1840s.[22] Even if property was insanitary, testimony reveals that individuals ostensibly officially concerned with public health had not fully reconciled themselves to compulsory state intervention. The pre-1848 metropolitan sewer commissions, for instance, did not have the power to compel householders to drain into their sewers.[23] Yet when the Health of Towns Commission inquired whether sewer authorities should be able to compel attachment, the answer was by no means unanimously yes. Joseph Daw, the Clerk to the Commissioners for the City of London, agreed that compulsory power would be useful in many instances and would undoubtedly benefit the public health and even the health of the occupants, but he worried that the power was too "arbitrary and despotic." He questioned "whether we have a right to go into the house of a man, and compel him to drain his premises."[24] Richard Kelsey, the surveyor to the City Commission, also believed that "it would be very obnoxious for public officers to break into a private house and make drains for them."[25]

This was not a concern merely of some of the metropolitan commissioners of sewers. According to Thomas Sworder, the solicitor who led Hertford's opposition to adopting the Public Health Act, the notion that the local board of health could tell a resident to have a drain if he did not was, "very objectionable."[26] In Aylesbury, opposition to the Public Health Act was grounded in fear of expense, but a local editor also worried about inroads the PHA made into the rights of property. He wanted a cheap copy of the PHA printed so that every man would know that "every bit of property he possessed . . . belonged to the local board as well as himself and the public." This was a serious blow to the rights of property: "It is putting all we have . . . under the care of other parties, armed with the full prerogatives and penalties of the law."[27]

These claims highlighted one ideological obstacle to the compulsory improvement of private property that concerned contemporaries: the sanctity of private homes. A second aspect was the expense to which such a power exposed homeowners.[28] This included not just the cost of doing *de novo* work but also the cost of undoing old work. It is easy to forget that local authorities such as local boards of health or the metropolitan commissioners of sewers (and its successor bodies) did not descend on towns that had never so much as heard of drains before and that would be amazed and delighted at the authorities' ministrations. Local residents had decided whether and how to drain their premises long before any authorities appeared on the scene. The status quo thus did not reflect absolute neglect of sanitary arrangements but rather the deliberate judgment of property owners as to the needs and requirements of their property, either the property they lived in or the property they rented to others. When local boards of health arrived and told local residents that this or that aspect of their property had to be changed, they occasionally rendered all prior arrangements, however costly, null and void.

At the root of the cost objection was the structural division between drains and sewers. The 1848 metropolitan and provincial legislation marked the first time that Parliament defined drains as serving individual properties and sewers as serving many.[29] Both terms had existed and to some extent had been used interchangeably for centuries; in the mid-nineteenth century, the terminology was still in flux.[30] The distinction was hardly crucial before the late 1840s, and there was little need to formalize it.[31] In the late 1840s, however, circumstances called for a clarification, probably because so many more sewers were being built, so many more houses were being connected to them, and so much more water was being piped into houses. But the mere fact that circumstances changed did not compel any particular kind of distinction between the two. Parliament made the distinction it did because Parliament believed that drains were a private improvement for which private individuals should pay. The imperative for Parliament was less to standardize terminology than to map the terminology cleanly onto the structural distinction between public and private property.

Parliament presumably believed that the distinction was helpful, but it created several fresh problems. In the first place, there was no clear difference between drains and sewers from an engineering standpoint. Edward Cresy, one of the surveyors of the Metropolitan Commission of Sewers, noted that the distinction between them was meaningless.[32] Although it might seem obvious that the line demarcating a stretch of pipe belonging to the homeowner from that belonging to the local authority would be the property line, in the circumstances of nineteenth-century urban Britain, drawing that line was not as easy as it might sound. Furthermore, this distinction and its associated statutory provisions forced local authorities to individualize the costs of house drainage. This put them in a bind, because they wanted the potentially expensive work of private drainage done, but not at the cost of bankrupting property owners, some of whom were themselves of limited means.[33]

These linked ideological and structural/financial problems were compounded, in some local authorities' eyes, by statutory limitations. One important example was the inability to order the compulsory mass conversion of privies to water closets. Water closets are the gold standard today, but in Victorian Britain there was no consensus around their desirability. Water closets were controversial for a range of reasons. In many places they were a nonstarter in the middle of the century, because many had no sewers or water with which to flush them. In keeping with this reality, the 1848 PHA, the 1848 Metropolis Sewers Act, and the 1855 MMA granted local authorities control of sanitary accommodation in new and existing houses. However, these statutes only permitted local authorities to ensure "sufficient" accommodation, which could be a water closet or a well-maintained privy and ashpit.[34] For many authorities, this was unobjectionable, and the powers the PHA gave them were more than adequate to regulate the local environment. Yet for some local boards of health that had sufficient water supplies and branch drains to enable house owners to connect, water closets were "an object of the first importance in a sanitary point of view."[35] The inability to compel their adoption en masse as a matter of policy was a serious problem.

What the statutes did not authorize was, in some ways, made worse by what they did. Although the main pieces of legislation passed in 1848 permitted a wide range of compulsory interventions, Parliament incorporated multiple safeguards into public health legislation. Under the Public Health Act, magisterial permission was often required to allow local boards of health to act; appeals to the quarter sessions and ultimately Queen's Bench protected ratepayers against illegal charges. Property owners could claim a credit if they could demonstrate that their property was already adequately drained before the PHA came into effect.[36] The PHA also gave residents the right of appeal directly to the General Board of Health (GBH) if they were ordered to undertake private improvements.[37] This last safeguard was extraordinary; the fact that Parliament believed that the GBH should have the final say on, for example, the drain of a single property was an indication of parliamentary distrust of the local bodies it had created and anxiety over the powers it had granted them.[38]

Local authorities encountered each of these three related kinds of difficulty, usually in combination, as they drained their districts. For determined local authorities, these obstacles were not insurmountable. Nor were they meant to be. In permitting compulsory drainage, Parliament obviously expected it to happen, but it also insisted that property be protected from arbitrary and unreasonable interference. That is, Parliament expected a balance between the promotion of health and the protection of property. There were boundaries of health, but these had to be forged. There was nothing inevitable about the way these boundaries would be drawn, and the outcomes were unpredictable.

Public Health and the Rights of Property

Underlying many of the legal difficulties, each of which was grounded in a statute, was the shape-shifting right of property. In this section, I bring forward some necessarily anecdotal evidence from Eton, Ware, Windsor, and the metropolis in order to illustrate the differential impact the rights of property had.[39] In the absence of a much greater body of cases to analyze at all levels, it is difficult to generalize, but the ritual invocation of the "rights of property" did not invariably shut a project down, although it certainly slowed it down, whether the resistance expressed itself to the GBH or the courts.[40]

Dr. Edward Eton was one of Eton's sanitary enthusiasts. When he acquired some cottage property along the riverfront in Eton in Spring 1855, he immediately set about rectifying the defective sanitary arrangements of the court. At what must have been no inconsiderable expense, Dr. Eton abolished the open cesspools that still existed and constructed three water closets for the inhabitants. Yet rather than draining the property into the Eton Local Board of Health's sewer, which emptied into the Thames, he drained it directly into the river. Although Dr. Eton seems to be, in retrospect, something of a model sanitary citizen, the Eton Local Board of Health was not happy with his decision to drain directly into the Thames. In June 1855, shortly after he took control of the property, the board ordered him to connect with its main sewer.[41]

Dr. Eton's sense of outrage is palpable in the ensuing correspondence, as perhaps it should have been. He had completed a good-faith effort to improve his tenants' property and was penalized for it. He immediately appealed to the GBH for protection against the arbitrary interference of the Eton Local Board of Health, rhetorically linking his appeal to what he called "private rights so dear to every Englishman."[42] The GBH, as was its habit, referred the matter back to the LBH for comment. Although the LBH believed it was justified, it agreed to submit to the GBH's recommendation. The GBH was loth to intervene in local sanitary battles but sent Inspector Alfred Dickens to Eton; Dickens agreed that the property was fully drained.[43] However, he also claimed that Dr. Eton's drain could become a nuisance and that the situation would improve if Dr. Eton simply complied. Thus the GBH notified Dr. Eton that it would not interfere, and the Local Board of Health accordingly proceeded.[44] Dr. Eton was reduced to pleading with the GBH that he at least be allowed to choose the contractor who would do the work.[45]

Even though Dr. Eton did not win his case, central officials certainly took his complaint seriously. His initial letter of complaint was referred to the president of the General Board of Health for his opinion.[46] The president required an on-site inquiry, the recommendations of which he also vetted.[47] Unfortunately, we cannot determine with any degree of accuracy the frequency with which property owners complained or challenged local action: so many of the discussions would have been off line, as it were. Others, although recorded in GBH and LBH records, were not collected or otherwise reported for any particular purpose and so can be recovered only by tedious archival and newspaper research. Indirect evidence tells us that property owners certainly objected to being told that their existing arrangements were unsatisfactory. The section of the PHA (86) that allowed local boards of health to credit property already drained before they began their work was, according to one informed commentator, "the foundation of much erroneous reasoning and unfounded claims for exemption."[48]

Of course not all local residents pleaded to the GBH. Some ended up in the courts, although they, too, did not always secure the outcome they sought. The brothers William and Charles Vaughn had spent £140 draining their property only to have the Eton Local Board's sewer cut through it and render it useless. The undrained land was then summoned as a nuisance. When the brothers challenged the summons, the magistrates were unsympathetic.[49] In 1859, the Windsor Local Board of Health ran a sewer through Joseph Berlin's property, thereby preventing him from building any structure on top of it without the board's permission.[50] Berlin sought compensation, as he was entitled to do under the law. His solicitor argued that all of the restrictions the local board of health placed on him would "interfere, and that seriously, with the rights of ownership."[51] Yet although Berlin won his compensation claim, he was forced to pay the professional costs he incurred in bringing the case. The local magistrates noted that his inconvenience was no greater than that which many other residents incurred, and none of them sought compensation. In the context of mid-Victorian England, the infringements on Berlin's freedom were not trivial, and his case suggests that even the local propertied class accepted substantial restrictions on the rights of property in the name of health.[52]

The local authorities' mandate to ensure adequate drainage extended beyond existing homes and properties and also permitted them to control new building. According to the Public Health Act, any new house constructed in a local board of health's district had to be approved by the board. The LBH could fine individuals whom it found in violation and in extreme cases could demolish the property.[53] This power terrified local property owners. In Hertford, Thomas Sworder, the solicitor who had led the opposition to the adoption of the PHA, claimed that the local board of health's power to tear down a house built without its permission was "different from any thing I ever read of."[54] Sworder must have felt that his opposition to the PHA was vindicated when the Ware Local Board of Health, just two miles downriver from Hertford, asserted its regulatory control over builders in May 1850. The board notified local builders that they were required to deposit plans of buildings with it and that the board could sanction them or not.[55]

Not all builders in Ware initially cooperated with the local board of health. Although one local builder, George Hitch, deposited plans, two others, Arthur Reason and John Francis, refused, A third, Thomas Webb, appeared before the board but declined to produce acceptable plans.[56] The correspondence of these builders with the Ware Local Board of Health and the GBH makes clear that they were stunned at the power that the local board presumed to take. When Francis replied to the board's initial request for plans, he disputed the board's right even to ask for them let alone to approve them and told the board that he considered the matter closed. Webb appealed to the GBH for protection, noting that "it is a matter of considerable importance to myself & other builders here to know what the local board can require."[57] The GBH, flush with its first power, cautioned Webb that he defied the local board of health at his peril. Webb remained uncooperative, and the local board finally took him to court. Wanting only to demonstrate its legitimacy, the board did not seek the full penalty, because Webb was suitably deferential and apologetic, and the magistrates convicted.[58]

Builders were not likely to find themselves accidentally in violation of the Ware Local Board of Health's building code. The rules were simple: submit plans before breaking the ground. That builders continued to have trouble with the Ware LBH suggests that resistance to the new regime persisted.[59] In 1854 the Ware Local Board of Health stayed proceedings against a builder who had constructed cottages without a permit, he having agreed to tear them down.[60] Yet the power to demolish houses seemed to be a limit beyond which many contemporaries were unwilling to go. When local boards invoked these powers, they sometimes found themselves opposed by magistrates and media.

The 1855 MMA gave London's local authorities similar control over new building.[61] In an early case in the Poplar district, Nicholas Knight and Henry Weitzell constructed some houses on top of a seawall that they partially destroyed in the process. They had obtained a permit to build from the DBW in September 1856 but claimed that through an error they had not indicated the full scope of the plan. After lengthy negotiations with Knight and Weitzell, the board demolished the houses, charging more than £40 to do it. Because the houses themselves cost over £100, the total cost to the defendants in this case was substantial.[62] The magistrate refused to allow the charges. The Poplar DBW was vilified by the *East London Observer.*[63]

Although the Poplar DBW won its case on appeal, in other cases and courts the demolition power caused more consequential judicial alarm. In early 1859, Paddington Vestry, acting under a misapprehension of their powers with respect to sewer building, threatened a builder with the destruction of his houses. Vice-Chancellor John Stuart not only issued a perpetual injunction restraining the vestry but also delivered a scathing indictment of the vestry's behavior, noting the "enormous" and "very large and arbitrary" power the vestry possessed and advising the members to be sure what they were about.[64] In an 1863 metropolitan case, the Queen's Bench argued that the power of demolition was so "enormous" and could inflict such "grievous injury" that it had to be qualified.[65] The 1855 MMA gave any person a right of appeal to the MBW, but the court inserted an additional layer of review.[66] The bench felt so strongly about this that each member spoke. Three of them delivered relatively lengthy rationales, one reaching back more than a century. Private property rights were so self-evident that the court unanimously decided that although the statute was deficient, "the justice of the common law will supply the omission of the legislature."[67] The court could not eliminate the section, but it could force delay.

With such a limited sample, the force of any conclusions must also be limited, but these examples show that the rights of property were an uncertain resource for opponents of local board of health drainage activity. Property rights were routinely invoked, yet either a clear statutory warrant for the action or a different local magisterial interpretation of them meant that opponents who grounded their appeal on them did not necessarily prevail in the lower courts.[68] Magistrates were not the only local elites who disagreed with the law's opponents. It is important to remember that local board of health members invariably believed as strongly in the rights of property as anyone, but in the abstract these rights provided little guidance. Whatever meanings they had were forged not in the abstract but in local adversarial fora.[69]

Structural and Statutory Barriers and Burdens

Just as challenging to local authorities were the structural obstacles they encountered. In the first place, the structural division between drains and sewers seriously interfered with the ability to construct what some thought was the most efficient way of draining certain houses in urban settings. The distinction did not envision the practical reality of urban drainage in many neighborhoods, where occasionally each house in entire rows and blocks required amendment. The statute, rather than combining the drainage of all of them, required each property to be separately improved and connected to the sewer.[70] This meant, in many cases, that owners required to drain their properties were faced with significant expenditures, in contrast to a combined drainage plan taking in the whole block.[71] The surveyors of the Metropolitan Commission of Sewers reported on the difficulties that this structural distinction caused in London as early as 1851.[72] Only the fear associated with an anticipated 1855 reappearance of cholera induced Parliament explicitly to authorize combined works in the metropolis.[73] The four-year delay in granting this power was a function of a multilayered debate over the merits of combined versus separate drainage, but the structural division was intimately bound up with the issue.[74]

The power to build drainage works was only one of the problems the structural division created; the other was paying for them. Whether individual or combined, house drainage was not meant to be paid for by local authorities but rather by property owners. This posed further problems, and local boards of health found themselves in some difficulty over the matter.[75] This issue emerged most prominently in the debate over converting privies to water closets. We have already noted that the law around water-closet mass conversions was weak; the GBH cautioned local boards of health that their powers were limited.[76] At the same time, the GBH noted that local boards were empowered to judge the sanitary sufficiency of any given situation and that it was within their power to decide that a supply of water was necessary for flushing.[77] The GBH appeared to suggest that local boards could finesse their way around the problem of converting individual properties to water closets.[78] But some local boards of health wanted unambiguous power to convert entire neighborhoods, and they peppered the GBH with queries about the need for more power if they did not have it.[79] Under prompting from local boards of health, the GBH suggested that the power to convert might be revisited in an amended PHA, though no such revision happened in the short term.[80]

The GBH's resolve would not have been strengthened by judicial rulings on related cases in London. The courts were called on to decide a water-closet-conversion case shortly after the 1855 MMA became law. The Wandsworth District Board of Works had resolved to do away with privies in its district and ordered a Mr. Tinkler to convert thirty-nine privies to water closets. When he refused, arguing that the privies he provided were not a nuisance, the DBW threatened to do the work itself, and Tinkler obtained an injunction restraining the DBW.[81] The Lords Justices upheld the injunction on appeal; the DBW had no statutory sanction for its decision to adopt the abolition of privies as a policy, independent of any review of the sufficiency of particular privies.[82] In coming to his initial decision, Vice-Chancellor Sir John Stuart was apparently deeply struck by the powers conferred on the district boards by the Metropolis Local Management Act. He referred to them as "enormous," "extraordinary," or "arbitrary" seven times in the space of a page and a half.[83] In the Court of Appeal in Chancery, the Lord Justice Sir James Knight-Bruce, too, found some of the provisions of the MMA "remarkable," and Lord Justice George Turner observed that the DBW would be well advised to exercise its "very extensive powers" with caution. Knight-Bruce thought that the provisions of the MMA did not "deal with the rights of property" in the manner that the DBW contended.[84]

This case was widely noticed in London, and the GBH could hardly have been unaware of the implications for the similarly drafted PHA, so its cautious advice made sense.[85] In the face of the General Board of Health's trepidation, some local boards apparently took matters into their own hands. In reply to repeated queries from the Swansea Local Board of Health about the ability to order conversions, the Local Government Act Office (LGAO)—which succeeded the GBH in 1858—drew up a list of twenty-two towns that had largely completed the task, suggesting that Swansea contact them, and drawing particular attention to Croydon.[86] Cuthbert Johnson, the author of an influential edition of the PHA and still the chair of the Croydon Local Board of Health, presumably told them—if they asked—what he subsequently told a clearly surprised Royal Sanitary Commission (RSC): that Croydon had abolished cesspools within its district, and virtually all parties had water closets, notwithstanding the lack of statutory sanction for such a policy.[87] The Swansea local board evidently moved ahead with conversions in its district: one of the county members, Evan Richards, MP, testified to the RSC that the large majority of privies had been converted into water closets even as he acknowledged that the law was deficient.[88] The strategies that local authorities apparently employed included a mix of threats and bluffs. The Croydon Local Board told anyone with insufficient accommodation that whenever the town got a water supply, they would be forced to convert, so they might as well do it now.[89]

Liverpool, operating under local acts, also skirted the margins of legality. The desirability of water closets was a particularly disputed matter in Liverpool and in Lancashire in general. Some large towns such as Manchester were opposed to them, committing significant resources to other waste-control measures.[90] Liverpool, in contrast, embraced water closets, partly because it had an adequate water supply and partly because it had an outlet for sewers in the tidal Mersey River.[91] Liverpool did not begin to convert until 1857; its large-scale conversion did not begin until 1863, the year a new medical officer of health (MOH), William Stewart Trench, took up his position.[92] Although Liverpool's local acts did not make explicit the power to order a conversion, when the Health Committee, acting on the recommendation of the MOH, certified that a particular privy was a nuisance or likely to be a danger to health, the committee routinely told owners that the only way to make it better was to convert it into a water closet.[93] Yet the Health Committee's ability to order these conversions apparently did not receive judicial sanction until 1868, more than a decade after the committee had started its work on the project.[94] In Liverpool, "compulsory" conversion was an ambiguously legal endeavor.[95]

Converting to water closets was thus a legally fraught goal for local authorities, but paying for these private works required even further legal gymnastics; statutory inadequacy was exacerbated by structural assumptions that drainage was a private benefit. That meant that the expense of conversion had to be borne by the individual, and that meant it would be difficult to enforce in low-value housing. At Sandgate, the LBH decided to provide rate assistance to proprietors of small houses to aid them in effecting household drainage, "for the general welfare of the Town."[96] This decision created serious legal difficulty for the LBH but raised in an acute form the ongoing problem of paying for residents too poor to pay for themselves.[97]

In London, Parliament tacitly acknowledged this problem during the passage of the 1855 Sewers (House Drainage) Bill. The initial version of the bill allowed the MCS to recover the costs from owners, as was typical. A revised version of the bill, however, allowed the commission to collect "the whole or Part of the Expenses."[98] The change, which did not survive passage, was not trivial. Had only part of the costs been recovered, the public would have partly subsidized the costs of private improvement. Given the paucity of debate on the measure, it is impossible to know the reason for the change.[99] But based on Lord Ebrington's remarks to the House when it was introduced, the measure was clearly intended to apply to low-value housing, which may well explain the attempt partially to offset the costs.[100] This change suggests a behind-the-scenes debate over the boundary between public and private benefit and burden, and an acknowledgment that low-value housing, with its poorer tenants and possibly poorer owners, required some collective assistance.[101]

The strategy only contemplated in London was followed almost exactly by Liverpool.[102] A Liverpool Health Committee officer mooted the idea of using public money to pay for conversion to water closets in low-value housing in the early 1860s; the Town Council itself seriously discussed the matter in 1864.[103] Initially, the suggestion arose as a means of compensating owners who had drained their properties according to previous local specifications. As early as 1846, Liverpool's Health Committee obtained authority to regulate house construction, including sanitary arrangements. However, the arrangements that the committee sanctioned at that time were not water closets with water laid on but impervious cesspools or properly drained middens.[104] For some Liverpool property owners the order to convert their privies to water closets in the early 1860s was as intolerable, and unreasonable, as was the order for Dr. Eton to connect his drains to Eton's sewers. They had done what was asked of them in the past, but now that the standards had changed, they were now required to undo and remake that work.[105]

The suggestion that owners be compensated for this work was hotly contested. When the Health Committee debated a motion to pay partially for private conversion, one member exclaimed that it was the "most ridiculous" thing he had ever heard.[106] Opponents of public funding argued that the retroactive conversion of privies was no different from the retroactive conversion of factory chimneys that were newly required to consume their smoke, and nobody expected the public to pay for that.[107] Furthermore, they argued, individuals who had purchased low-end property knew what they were buying and had to accept the consequences of that decision; property had its costs as well as its rewards.[108]

Proponents of public funding never abandoned the argument that the Town Council was responsible for these newly unacceptable middens in the first place, but they also developed additional arguments in favor of their position. If conversion was for public as opposed to private benefit, the public, they argued, should pay.[109] That kind of expenditure, proponents claimed, was not substantially different from paying for public water standpipes in courtyards, something the Town Council already did.[110] One member pointed out that the council already paid for part of the work of private drainage. The Health Committee was in the habit of paying for the cost of running a drain up to the house, leaving the owner to pay for further renovations. There was no clear statutory authority for doing this, and it was not even clear if it was legal, but the fact that the committee did this gave proponents of public money an in; the principle of public payment for private improvement had already been established.[111]

The debate over these private improvement costs occupied the Health Committee and the Town Council for several years leading up to the inquiries conducted by the Royal Sanitary Commission.[112] The debate crossed the usual party lines. Joseph Robinson, a leader of a new generation of reformers on the council who had made improvement of Liverpool's dreadful housing courts a plank in his platform, was bitterly opposed to paying for conversions, as was Robertson Gladstone, another Liberal.[113] It is perhaps unsurprising that the opponents of compulsory water-closet conversions—the normally reactionary spokesmen of small property owners—were the strongest supporters of public payment. Yet interested parties were by no means the only supporters of public funding. One of the most ardent supporters was the medical officer of health, Dr. Trench. He strongly argued for public support of the costs in the Health Committee, before the full Town Council, and in front of the RSC.[114] The council ended up subsidizing property owners significantly.[115] By the end of 1866, 750 privies were converted at the owners' expense, and nearly 2,500 were converted or in process at the public expense.[116] By mid-1869, the Health Committee had converted more than 13,000 privies, spending more than £40,000.[117]

The Liverpool Health Committee's policies on paying for conversions were consistent with pre- and post-Reform council action. Liverpool's local laws provided, or provided cover, for public expenditure on public sewers, on drains into those sewers, and on water-closet conversions, all in the name of health.[118] We should not underestimate the importance of Liverpool's decision to fund some or all of these activities out of rates or other public sources as Health of Towns Commission investigators in the 1840s were not even unanimously in favor of rate-funded sewers, let alone drains or water closets; Lyon Playfair claimed that Liverpool's comparative failure to build sewers was precisely due to the fact that they were paid for out of rates rather than individually assessed frontage fees, and parties were disinclined to pay for that from which they did not derive direct benefit.[119] Liverpool's Town Council and Health Committee clearly had a different conception of benefit and burden. That William Trench did not succeed in getting statutory sanction for their strategy of paying for conversions with public funds is immaterial.[120] What the Health Committee did was impressive; what Trench and others wanted to do was remarkable.[121] The boundaries of private property in Liverpool were, in the eyes of some, fluid.

❧   ❧   ❧

The successes and failures of some local authorities under the Public Health Act, the Metropolis Local Management Act, and local acts encourage us to revisit some of the conventional judgments in the historiography of domestic sanitary reform. Historians recognize that even well-intentioned local authorities were not in a position to provide water closets, even if a consensus had existed that they were the gold standard—and it did not. Piecemeal progress was unavoidable. That is absolutely true, but the story of private drainage outlined above suggests an overlapping narrative, not of inevitably halting progress but of politically determined action and reaction. The legislation under which local authorities operated was not congenial. Public health laws exposed local authorities to individual complaint, central oversight, judicial scrutiny, and media attack; opponents occasionally scored major victories in the courts. The surprising thing is that when faced with this formidable array of potential and actual opponents, local authorities, who broadly supported private rights and who were themselves occasionally divided, did anything. Yet they did. And what Swansea, Liverpool, Croydon, and numerous other towns did in converting to water closets could have been done by any other similarly situated town.[122] Local political commitments were an important part of local sanitary reform.

Common Lodging Houses

Houses let in lodgings were a common and important part of the housing landscape in nineteenth-century Britain. On any given night at mid-century, tens of thousands of people in London stayed in lodgings.[123] The range of lodgings varied tremendously, from a house including a single room let to a single lodger to dormitories occupied by the most impoverished people in extremely overcrowded conditions, and with every gradation in between. Lodgers were themselves quite varied, ranging from the adolescent Charles Dickens, who lodged in Lambeth while his parents were housed in the Marshalsea debtors' prison, to Charles Darwin, who lodged under considerably more pleasant circumstances after he returned from the *Beagle* voyage.[124]

Lodging acquired a fresh political salience during the second quarter of the nineteenth century because of links forged between certain houses with lodgers and crime, immorality, and disease.[125] These concerns gave an impetus to regulation, and in the late 1840s and early 1850s, Parliament passed several different measures to regulate what came to be called "common lodging houses."[126]

The control of common lodging houses has not attracted much historical attention, as Tom Crook has noted.[127] I want to approach this regulation through its legislative history. The control of lodging houses presupposed the construction of a new boundary, encircling those properties and people subject to regulation. But the process of defining an acceptable object of regulation (the common lodging house), and of demarcating a group suitable for control, was surprisingly contested and complex, because overlapping anxieties about lodging houses suggested different kinds of problems and solutions.

Lodging houses were initially problematized as the "haunts" of vagrants, criminals, and prostitutes; the 1824 Vagrancy Act provided police with a means to enter them.[128] The 1831–32 cholera outbreak furnished an occasion to link lodging houses to health, although they were apparently not made a particular object of medicolegal concern until the 1840s.[129] A Glasgow local act recognized the public health significance of lodging houses, permitted their regulation, and authorized the removal of sick residents to other establishments.[130] Edwin Chadwick devoted a chapter to lodging houses in his 1842 *Report on the Sanitary Condition*, popularizing Glasgow's work and drawing attention to lodging houses' insalubrity and their role in spreading infection to nonresident individuals and around the country. Chadwick recognized that lodging houses had multiple functions and served multiple constituencies.[131] He was hesitant about giving them a rigid definition, and although he thought it beneficial to extend rather than narrow any definition, he believed that discretion should be left to local magistrates.[132]

Chadwick's recommendation for flexibility and magisterial discretion in the control of lodging houses was not, however, taken up by the Health of Towns Commission, which was designed to flesh out the ideas contained in the *Report on the Sanitary Condition*. The commissioners recommended that only lodging houses for the reception of "vagrants, trampers, and other such wayfarers" be controlled.[133] Prepared in the aftermath of the HOTC, Lord Lincoln's 1845 Health of Towns' Bill, which did not become law, seemingly shared the HOTC's focus and permitted the control of low-value houses let to "mendicants, strangers, and other persons."[134] These two documents marked a move away from Chadwick's recommendation, more precisely stipulating the establishments to be regulated and the individuals imagined to be part of the problem. The emphasis, furthermore, was on transients or migratory individuals, primarily as importers and spreaders of disease. Neither the HOTC nor Lord Lincoln explained this narrowing of the problem, although it may well be that the legislative precedent provided by vagrancy acts was critical.

The period from 1847 to 1851 was a turning point in the control and conceptualization of lodging houses. As table 5.1 shows, Parliament repeatedly revisited different definitions of lodging houses as it struggled to reconcile the rights of property and privacy with the desire to control and compel. In 1847, Parliament passed the Towns Improvement Clauses Act, the first general, albeit permissive, control measure for "public lodging-houses." Parliament dropped any explicit reference to vagrants or other presumably identifiable social actors, opting instead to regulate houses valued at less than £10 that were let in whole or in part for less than a week.[135] Although this definition did not reappear in any other general statute, it was an interesting, even astonishing, broadening of the "lodging house,"[136] which was no longer defined exclusively by the category of people who lodged but by objective characteristics of the place itself.[137] This act also added new responsibilities for the authorities in charge of the houses, requiring them to promote cleanliness and ventilation as well as fixing the number of lodgers, an imperative reiterated in the 1848 Public Health Act.[138] In 1847–48, lodging houses were objects of health regulation, not simply of crime control.[139]

It is hardly surprising that lodging houses, or common lodging houses as they were called after 1848, were objects of health regulation in an act intended to promote the public health, but health was always about more than simply cleanliness and drainage.[140] Attempted definitions after 1847 drew attention to other features of common lodgers and their houses, particularly the relationship to people with whom they shared accommodation (unmentioned by the 1845 HOTC, the 1845 Health of Towns Bill, or 1847 Towns Improvement Clauses Act). An important characteristic of several attempted legislative definitions

Table 5.1. The definition of lodging houses and lodgers, 1845–57

	House value	Occupants	Length of stay	Co-occupants
1845 Health of Towns Commission[1]		"vagrants, trampers, and other such wayfarers"		
1846 Health of Towns Bill[2]	Less than £15	"mendicants, strangers, and other persons"	One night or short periods	
1847 Towns Improvement Clauses Act[3]	Less than £10	"persons"	Less than a week	
1848 Public Health Bill[4]		Persons	Less than a week	More than one family
1848 Public Health Act[5]				
1848 City Sewers Act[6]		Persons	Less than a week	More than one family
1851 Common Lodging House Bill[7]		Persons	Less than a week	More than one family
1851 Common Lodging House Act[8]				
1851–52 Home Office advice[9]		Lowest classes	Very short periods	Strangers to each other
1853 Common Lodging House Bill (1)[10]		"Wayfarers, Vagrants, or Mendicants"		
1853 Common Lodging Houses Act[11]				
1857 Crowded Dwellings Bill[12]				Outside close consanguinity

Notes:
1. Second Report of the HOTC, PP 1845 (602), 66–67.
2. A Bill for the Improvement of the Sewerage and Drainage of Towns and Populous Districts, PP 1845 (574), s. 179.
3. 10 & 11 Vict., c. 34, s. 116.
4. Lawes, *Act for Promoting the Public Health*, 104–5, note *d.*
5. 11 & 12 Vict. c. 63, s. 66.
6. Lawes, *Act for Promoting the Public Health*, 104–5, note *d.*
7. PP 1851 (272), s. 2.
8. 14 & 15 Vict., c. 28.
9. Hundred House Division magistrates to HO, November 28, 1851, minute, HO/45/os4427/103, NA. 1852, minute, HO/45/os4427/103, NA. PP 1852–53 (573), s. 20. Udsey Petty Sessional Division to HO, January 21,
10. PP 1852–53 (573), s. 20.
11. 16 & 17 Vict., c. 41.
12. PP 1857 sess. 2 (160), s. 3; (187), s. 2.

of the common lodger and hence the common lodging house after 1847 was shared accommodation with non-family members.

The importance of the family in the definition highlights the public health movement's concern with domesticity, to which Mary Poovey has drawn our attention.[141] As the move to regulate compulsorily common lodging houses gathered momentum, the parliamentarians involved inflected domesticity with the moralizing concerns that Frank Mort has highlighted.[142] The 1851 Common Lodging Houses Act, for instance, allowed local authorities to make regulations "for the separation of the sexes" in common lodging houses.[143] This stress on the separation of the sexes was another statutory novelty in terms of lodging house control; it had not appeared before, and not even the 1848 PHA had made any explicit reference to separating the sexes.[144] The model common-lodging-house regulations that the Home Office prepared for local guidance accordingly stipulated that unmarried adults of the opposite sex could not share a sleeping apartment even if they were related, nor could parents share a sleeping room with their children unless under fourteen years of age in the provinces or under ten years of age in London. Even children of the opposite sex could not share sleeping apartments unless they were under ten years of age.[145]

It is important to note that these regulatory features were not implicit in earlier definitions; even if many of the same houses would have been captured by pre- and post-1851 definitions and regulations, the conceptualizations were not synonymous. Lodging houses and lodgers were different things and persons in 1851 than they were in 1824 or even in 1845. Lodgers, in 1851, were not simply the comers and goers so evocatively described by Ralph Samuel.[146] They were not defined solely by their residential instability, their structural location, or their putative criminality but by their domestic arrangements as well, a difference that reflected the concerns of the parliamentarians involved. The 1851 Common Lodging House Act and its regulations promiscuously mingled sex and sanitation, perfectly modeling the anxieties of those such as the evangelical Lord Ashley, who inspired and probably helped draft them.

We can see this process at work in the formation of the GBH Lodging House Regulations. Ashley's interest in lodging houses clearly predated his 1848 appointment to the GBH. In 1847 he penned an article in the *Quarterly Review* and in 1848 gave a long speech on them in the Commons on the "juvenile population." His interest in 1847 was in lodging houses as sites of moral degradation of young people. He was not interested in them as sites of disease control, and even in his 1848 speech it was a very minor concern.[147] Chadwick was interested in disease control and paid less attention to sex. When the two men came together on the GBH, these concerns fused. By late 1850, when the GBH prepared its draft of common lodging house regulations for Home Office approval, the separation of sexes was part of them.[148]

Although heteronormative middle-class domesticity crucially informed common lodging house regulation, it did not determine the scope of the legislation. The fact that there was some measure of consensus around the issues at stake in the regulation of common lodgers and their houses did not mean that

Parliament agreed on a definition of them. With the exception of the 1847 Towns Improvement Clauses Act, no general legislation defined a common lodger or common lodging house.[149] This deficiency certainly was not for lack of trying. As the Public Health Bill passed through Parliament in 1848, the Commons repeatedly tinkered with the definition before effectively abandoning the attempt as the bill was sent to the Lords.[150] A Lords Select Committee arrived at a definition "after much discussion," according to the legislative draftsman, but the Commons believed that houses not meant to be regulated would have fallen under the definition and hence expunged it.[151] The Lords' definition appeared again in the 1851 common lodging house bill but again was rejected, this law too appearing without any meaningful definition.[152] Parliament evidently wanted discretion left to magistrates.[153]

The inability to reach parliamentary consensus on the boundaries of domestic regulation also stymied attempts to extend the acts. In 1853, Lord Shaftesbury (as Lord Ashley had become), the sponsor of the 1851 act and an enthusiastic advocate of lodging-house regulation, promoted an amended bill that granted a number of new powers, several of which Parliament accepted.[154] The bill also attempted to extend the scope of the act, allowing a greater number of houses to be inspected as common lodging houses.[155] This feature of the bill ran into trouble immediately. Lord Beaumont stressed that all inspection was undesirable, and the bill needed a definition to restrain it to "lodging houses of a certain class."[156] Beaumont's call for a clear definition was not, however, easily met, as he probably had anticipated. In a vain attempt to preserve the bill, Shaftesbury, echoing the recommendations of the HOTC, defined a lodging house as any house let out to "Wayfarers, Vagrants, or Mendicants."[157] This gambit, tacked onto the end of the bill, did not succeed, and the definition was expunged along with the clause that had made it necessary. The bill passed without any definition or interpretation clause.[158]

Shaftesbury's final and most dramatic attempt to redefine the boundaries of healthy lodging was also a failure. The 1857 Crowded Dwellings Bill would have permitted the control of rooms in private houses let to individuals who claimed to be members of the same family. These rooms were often badly overcrowded and were exempt from regulation, a fact long lamented by reformers, the police, and medical officers of health.[159] The Crowded Dwellings Bill proposed to regulate these rooms and to define a "family," stipulating the kinds of relationships that would exempt one from control, and laying the burden of proof on people claiming to be members of the same family.[160] The Crowded Dwellings Bill was extremely controversial in the Commons[161] and the press.[162] The government accepted an amendment to the bill that would have restricted its application to common lodging houses only, thereby hoping to placate MPs who saw it as extending to all the homes of the poor.[163] Even with this concession, objections continued, and the bill was withdrawn. Its defeat marked the last attempt to redefine the boundaries of healthy lodging for nearly a decade.[164] Shaftesbury's repeated failures highlighted the complex and unpredictable ways in which class, sex, and property intersected during this period and around this problem.

Parliament's refusal to extend the scope of regulation during the 1850s did not, of course, mean that regulation did not take place; the statutes passed between 1847 and 1851 authorized regulation.[165] It meant that regulation was negotiated outside of Parliament, between the Home Office and magistrates. These negotiations gave the Home Office, the controlling party, tremendous leeway and effectively allowed them to define common lodging houses outside of the legislative process, as their correspondence with local magistrates made clear.[166] Local magistrates were not so enthused about the absence of a definition of common lodging houses as the acts' framers were. They wanted clarity as well as discretion. The GBH issued an unhelpful notification that common lodging houses should be understood as the "houses now in use, and practically known under that name."[167] The Home Office too received queries about what constituted a common lodging house. Were beer shops and pubs, for example, common lodging houses? They were, the Home Office replied, if they were common lodging houses. This non-answer probably also was unhelpful. The Home Office quickly began to advise correspondents that what really mattered was short-term, shared accommodation among strangers of the lowest classes.[168] The Law Officers of the Crown agreed that common lodging houses did not include "hotels, inns, public-houses, or lodgings let to the upper classes or middle classes."[169]

The guidance provided by the Home Office and the GBH clearly seems structured around class in theory, but class and domesticity were linked; even class was an ambiguous marker in practice. The effective exemption for accommodations rented by the week (or longer) ensured that many if not most working people did not fall into the regulatory net; many were paid and rented lodgings by the week.[170] Other working-class lodgers were also effectively exempted from control. One group of magistrates, for example, was interested in the Common Lodging Houses Act's implications for housing their region's short-term labor force. Laborers engaged in specific tasks such as church building routinely lodged with cottagers in the neighborhood. According to the Home Office, these workers and the cottages they lodged in did not seem to fall under the act. The Home Office thus implied that short-term lodging with strangers was, in itself, not always a problem. Nor apparently, according to the same letter, was migration in search of labor, previously regarded with some degree of skepticism in official circles.[171]

In addition to defining the common lodging house, the central government controlled the nature of the regulation that local authorities exercised. As common lodging-house regulations or bylaws began to flow into the Home Office, the Office frequently found itself forced to reject them or require amendments, including additions to and deletions from the recommended code. In most cases, the Home Office did not save the original bylaws and regulations a local authority submitted, so the objectionable regulations must be sought among local records. The letters transmitting the draft codes, however, were usually saved, and the minutes on them occasionally described their "inquisitorial" or other objectionable additional features.[172] Sometimes local authorities attempted to use their codes for purposes other than those intended by the leg-islation. The Leek Improvement Commission's attempt to use the regulations to make it an offense to lodge prostitutes or thieves was rejected.[173] Salisbury wished to prohibit particular individuals from being lodging-house keepers, and that too was rejected, because the 1851 Common Lodging Houses Act was not meant to exclude individuals from being in the trade.[174] It is interesting to note that the evidence rarely suggests that local authorities wished to strike some reg-ulation, although in one case the Devizes Town Council struck three regulations for reasons which the Home Office insisted were "insufficient." The regulations in question included a requirement to provide dustbins and water closets, so the Home Office had a standard below which it refused, in theory, to allow lodging houses to fall.[175]

❧   ❧   ❧

I have made no attempt to explore the enforcement of the various acts that permitted the regulation of lodging; Tom Crook's work suggests something of the problems of that task. But we can imagine some effects on keepers, lodgers, and regulators. Lodging-house keepers certainly felt the acts' effects. A num-ber of establishments were driven out of business or further underground by the requirement to upgrade. This must have resulted in less accommodation for lodgers, even if it was substandard accommodation.[176] Lodgers felt the laws' effects in other ways, too. Imagine a London family, headed by one of Captain Hay's industrious laborers, passing through a rough time but wanting nonethe-less to avoid the workhouse. If they did not have the money to sublet a room or part of a room from some relative, friend, or stranger, a lodging house was their best option. Henry Mayhew claimed in the 1840s that about 10 percent of the lowest lodging houses had separate sleeping quarters for families, but the 1851 regulations precluded that option unless the children were under ten years of age.[177] If they were not, the family was segregated into different sleeping quar-ters, with all of the heartache and hazard that implied.[178] And it was not only lodgers who were affected. Like the workhouse, the common lodging house was a disciplined space. And again like the workhouse, which, as Lynn Hollen Lees has noted, was meant to frighten, the common lodging house disciplined people outside as well as inside.[179] The common lodging house was the penalty for being unable to afford even to sublet rooms, just as the workhouse was the price of failing to work at all. The common lodging house had its own standard of less eligibility, albeit one that the state worked through the private rather than the public sector. In several ways, then, common lodgers were casualties of the attempted middle-class construction of respectable working-class domesticity.[180]

A different legacy of this exercise was the way in which the Home Office's reg-ulations and advice divided the poor, demarcating those subject to unrestrained domestic inspection, those not entitled to privacy rights. Common lodging-house regulation was part of a cluster of state practices that analyzed, catego-rized, and marginalized.[181] These regulatory practices and their taxonomic implications reflected and reinforced the idea of an underclass or residuum, a quasi-biologically imagined subpopulation. The Home Office's attempt at social taxonomy linked its work with the rich literature of metropolitan social inquiry from Edwin Chadwick to Henry Mayhew to Charles Booth and beyond.[182] The Home Office's contribution to this taxonomic project was not insubstantial, even if it was incomplete and fraught with controversy.

Regulating lodgers and keepers was not the only project at work here. Any local bylaws for regulating lodging houses had to be submitted to the Home Office or the GBH for approval.[183] The Home Office and the GBH appeared unwilling to allow provincial local authorities to take the initiative in this matter and prepared a draft code that was sent not only to those jurisdictions that asked for it but to any jurisdiction that submitted bylaws.[184] This mechanism of requiring central approval of bylaws and regulations powerfully strengthened bureaucratic and ministerial hands. Home Office records reveal that the Office effectively enforced conformity with its own model code.[185]

This technique of governance had been pioneered to a certain extent in the model clauses acts of the late 1840s, but those were permissive, and no local authority was required to adopt them. In the case of common lodging houses, they had no choice. Central (and local) authority was thus considerably strengthened by this approach. The value of the model bylaw approach was obvious; when the 1858 Local Government Act passed, the Local Government Act Office quickly prepared model bylaws.[186] The LGAO stressed that they were permissive only, but given the increasing attention paid to bylaws after mid-century, this discretion usually implied the discretion voluntarily to obey.[187] The central state regulated the local governors as well as the local governed.

Conclusion

One of the defining features of nineteenth-century urban development in Britain was the growth of public health. The centrality of public health to modern urban life derives from the effects it had on mortality rates, but these effects do not exhaust its significance. As I have argued in this book, among the most important legacies of the early English and Welsh public health movement were the redefinitions of property it promoted. I have framed these redefinitions as a series of boundary shifts between healthy and unhealthy things, between public and private services, between taxable and nontaxable property, between cities and suburbs, and last, between healthy and unhealthy domesticity. Parliament and the courts permitted or sanctioned all of these boundary shifts, but they were largely driven, I stress, by provincial and metropolitan local authorities of one sort or another.

This interpretation suggests a revision in our ongoing revaluation of local authorities in this period. Their current somewhat unfavorable reputation rests on the slow rate of change in urban death rates and the incremental progress made in building sanitary works. Although both observations are correct, they may not tell the full story. Public health measures may well have contributed to the decline of some infectious diseases, even if overall mortality did not decline.[1] And the record of sanitary works, if taken as a metric for evaluation, needs cautious interpretation. We need to take stock not only of how many nuisances local authorities abated, how many privies they converted into water closets, or how many miles of sewer they laid but also of the fact that there was even a category of nuisance to abate, that they controlled private domestic arrangements in any way, and that they were able to build healthy infrastructure on a financially sustainable and more equitable basis than in the past. Each of these activities required some readjustment of the salubrity, sanctity, and liability of property. In some cases, decades of legal labor were necessary to achieve it. All of these legal accomplishments mattered. They set the stage for the more rapid growth of healthy cities during the last quarter of the century. This interpretation takes the edge off the discontinuities implied in recent analyses of Victorian local government, connecting mid- and late century while recognizing that much more remained to be done.[2]

It is important to consider these achievements in evaluating mid-century local authorities, because in some cases had they not occurred, circumstances on the ground would have changed at a much slower pace. In the judgment of many contemporaries, the common law of nuisances was manifestly ineffective in remedying environmental nuisances they increasingly regarded as problems. Parliament's 1846 creation of a statutory health hazard, largely driven by reaction to local developments and pressure, significantly enhanced the ability to control local environments. Influential contemporaries believed that the law governing drainage was also deficient. In London, parochial financing of sewers in the 1850s would almost certainly have accelerated the differential development of infrastructure among parishes and across the metropolis. The Metropolitan Board of Works did not have to change this financing arrangement in 1858. Parliament had endorsed it in 1855, and the board could have muddled through. The board decided, however, that the status quo was unworkable. But as the Metropolitan Board of Works struggled to escape the straitjacket of parochial benefit, there was more than one way forward. They could have created a small number of subdivisions based, for example, on the boundaries drawn up by the old Commissioners of Sewers, or they could have created an even smaller number of subdivisions. Had the Metropolitan Board of Works, as some suggested, divided the metropolis into two financially autonomous drainage districts on either side of the river, it is virtually certain that southern residents would have spent more and thus waited longer than they otherwise did for their main drainage. One financially unified district was a much more progressive option.[3]

The story of London that this book tells connects the history of financing healthy infrastructure to the long, contested history of local rate equalization and the redistribution that flowed from it. Equalization was increasingly important in debates over Poor Law financing in the metropolis during the late 1850s. The victories of the Metropolitan Board of Works and the Whitechapel District Board of Works at that time reflected and reinforced a new political and judicial sensibility around the issue. In one sense, London's history was distinctive. Although interparochial transfers occurred in the provinces, they did not occur on such a scale. But in another sense parochial equalization in London had effects analogous to the redistribution that Epsom's and Cheltenham's rates effectively accomplished on a smaller, intraparochial scale.[4] What mattered in both London and the provinces was redistribution on any scale. This book has argued that this redistribution was legitimated by a change in the legal doctrine of rating, distinguishing indirect health benefits from the direct benefits on which the rate was historically based. The shift to indirect benefit was itself grounded, I suggest, on an implicit right to health for those unable to procure the necessary infrastructure themselves. The most important legacy of public health, examined through this lens, was not health but redistributive taxation.

These inter- and intraparochial transfers had another legacy. Rates were collected from individuals, but they were based on areas, and they also helped redefine the nature of the area. Establishing new administrative boundaries was (and is) always controversial for more than one reason. But struggles over rates forged a new kind of community, even if on the basis of historic boundaries originally created for other purposes. The community they created was united not by a service, because the infrastructure for which property was rated often did not extend to all of the places within the area. Nor were they stitched together by underground drainage pipes. They were imagined communities, united by a new kind of benefit and burden, a new shared liability.[5] The significance of this idea for the increase in municipal initiative, associated with the civic gospel, in the last quarter of the century remains fully to be explored.

Because I argue that particular local authorities played a crucial role in creating "public health," some comment on why they did it is called for. To state the obvious, they did it in part because it was their responsibility in the statute or commission from which their authority derived. In this study, epidemic diseases such as typhus and cholera and changing demographics provided the initial context for action. To this it might be objected that I have merely revived an older explanation: that public health happened when well-meaning local authorities responded rationally to bad conditions. Although that charge is to some extent true, so, I believe, is the claim against which the charge is raised. And in any event, the mere fact that local authorities responded tells us nothing about the character of the response or the work that went into it. Epidemics did not transform society, like some *deus ex machina*, but public bodies in whose environments they occurred responded creatively to them in very specific short- and long-term ways.

Although I have focused on accomplishments, I do not claim that local authorities did not have shortcomings. Even when they had power they often did not use it; not all authorities equalized rates. And the power that they did not have they did not always seek; public health had boundaries that were not crossed. Houses, for example, might be bad but virtually no one believed before mid-century that anyone but the private and the voluntary sector should remedy the situation. Edwin Chadwick drew an important boundary, as Christopher Hamlin has convincingly argued, around private wage relations and the labor market; if the poor were sick, it was not because they did not make enough to buy sufficient food or medicine or to procure sufficient accommodation. There is little evidence that local authorities contested these boundaries, even if some individuals, such as local medical men, did.

Mention of Chadwick highlights the way in which my emphasis on the local roots of reform meant that the story made little space for the usual leaders of the early public health movement. To be sure, Chadwick's ideas formed a backdrop for work that was going on in local areas, especially after 1842. The 1848 Public Health Act likewise crucially shaped local action, although Chadwick's role in framing the key provisions is not completely clear. But in this story Chadwick accompanied developments as often as he led them. Physicians, such as Dr. William Farr, played key roles in aspects of the early public health movement, but in the developments traced here their role was developing, perhaps peripheral. The early public health movement is a story of parallel, partially overlapping narratives. The miasmatic medical theory so strongly championed by Chadwick and his associates, and on which local authorities relied, illustrates the point. Given the legal constraints under which they acted, metropolitan sewer commissions seeking to reframe liability for drainage, and provincial municipal corporations creating bylaws governing the summary control of nuisances, needed a theory of disease transmission like miasmatism. Indeed, had the concept of miasma not already existed, they probably would have invented it—which, in a legal sense, they did. Of course, physicians' miasmatic theories predated both Chadwick and the relevant local authorities, but both probably initially acted independently of each other in forming their versions.

A reconsideration of Chadwick's role highlights another theme in this book: shifting central–local relations. I have argued that local initiative played a major role in the evolution of early English and Welsh public health, although that initiative was always constrained by Parliament and the central state. Neither provincial nor metropolitan authorities could have effected local rate equalization had not Parliament passed a statute that permitted the possibility. And in both cases, when subsequently presented with the possibility of amending the statutes to prevent equalization, Parliament did not take the bait. Nor was Whitehall by any means hostile to equalization, and it referred several other local authorities to Epsom's case for guidance. On balance, Parliament and Whitehall left the issue to localities. The emphasis on local initiative in this study is consistent with the claim that the centralizing ambitions of some political actors were thwarted during the mid-Victorian period. But although central control was thus in some ways limited, in others it was steadily augmented. Whitehall increasingly exerted control over local authorities, especially when local regulatory regimes enacted local bylaws. Whitehall's oversight of them illustrates the complexity of nineteenth-century government growth and the difficulty of characterizing this period in terms of central or local dominance. In sanctioning bylaws, Whitehall implicitly controlled the local population, but in rejecting them Whitehall explicitly controlled the local councils.

Public health was thus a fulcrum on which central and local government were balanced; this study's end point marks another rebalancing in that relationship. In 1872, after four years of annually debating and rejecting motions and resolutions concerning central financial support for locally funded and locally provided "national" services, Parliament voted in favor of such support, decisively defeating William Gladstone's government on a nonbinding resolution.[6] In a direct response, the Exchequer began supporting local public health work for the first time, acknowledging at least implicitly its national significance.[7] The debates in Parliament over national and local responsibilities are often analyzed in terms of the politics of taxation of real and personal property, as they should be.[8] Yet I am not convinced that support for central funding in 1872 was solely political. The local creation of communities of health may have played a role in the evolution of local and hence national opinion. The significance of the boundaries of health formed by local boards of health and the Metropolitan Board of Works remains fully to be determined.

Notes

Introduction

1. For various versions of this account see Finer, *Life and Times*; Frazer, *History of English Public Health*; Hammond and Hammond, *Bleak Age*; Lewis, *Edwin Chadwick*; and Glyn Roberts, *Municipal Development*.

2. Mumford, *City in History*; Polanyi, *Great Transformation*, especially 141–57; Ringen, "Edwin Chadwick, the Market Ideology, and Sanitary Reform," 107–20.

3. Mandler, "Introduction: State and Society in Victorian Britain"; D. Porter, *History of Public Health and the Modern State*, 1–5; Wiener, "The Unloved State." Public health always found a place in welfare-state narratives: D. Fraser, *Evolution of the British Welfare State*.

4. Ayers, *England's First State Hospitals*; Brand, *Doctors and the State*; Hodgkinson, *Origins of the National Health Service*.

5. Lubenow, *Politics of Government Growth*.

6. The debate can be reviewed in Cromwell, "Interpretations of Nineteenth-Century Administration," 245–55; MacLeod, *Government and Expertise*.

7. Lambert, *Sir John Simon*.

8. In early studies, this typically was connected to the development of industrial society. See Mumford, *City in History*; Polanyi, *Great Transformation*; Rosen, *History of Public Health*. Wrigley argues that population growth in England around the turn of the nineteenth century was without precedent in English history and was markedly asymmetric; Wrigley, "Coping with Rapid Population Growth," locs. 800–820, 1014.

9. Cook, *Routledge Companion to Britain*, 105.

10. Emsley, Hitchcock, and Shoemaker, "London History—A Population History of London." Part of the increase obviously reflects boundary changes. Dennis, "Modern London," 95–99.

11. Rodger, "Slums and Suburbs"; F. M. L. Thompson, "Rise of Suburbia."

12. Dyos and Reeder, "Slums and Suburbs," 359–86, especially 381.

13. E. P. Thompson, *Making of the English Working Class*, 352–56.

14. Briggs, *Victorian Cities*; Dyos, *Victorian Suburb*; Sheppard, *London, 1808–1870*.

15. D. Fraser, *Power and Authority*; D. Fraser, *Urban Politics*; Hennock, *Fit and Proper Persons*.

16. Garrard, *Leadership and Power*; Hamlin, "Muddling in Bumbledom."

17. Owen, *Government of Victorian London*. See, more recently, Halliday, *Great Stink*; Platt, *Shock Cities*; D. H. Porter, *Thames Embankment*.

18. On the exclusions, see Hamlin, "State Medicine in Great Britain"; Poovey, "Domesticity and Class Formation." Gareth Stedman Jones's indictment of the Metropolitan Board of Works and its second-tier partners' housing policies drew

attention to one of the blind spots of the early public health movement; Stedman Jones, *Outcast London*.

19. I exclude here any discussion of treatment delivered in the workhouse per se or via the poor law medical service. See Flinn, "Medical Service Under the New Poor Law"; Hodgkinson, *Origins of the National Health Service*; Reinarz and Schwarz, *Medicine and the Workhouse*. On the Poor Law, see Green, *Pauper Capital*; Lees, *Solidarities of Strangers*.

20. The best overview is Wohl, *Endangered Lives*. See also Frazer, *History of English Public Health*.

21. Eyler, *Victorian Social Medicine*; Lilienfeld, "Greening of Epidemiology"; Wolfenstein, "Recounting the Nation."

22. Brunton, *Politics of Vaccination*; Durbach, *Bodily Matters*; Mooney, *Intrusive Interventions*; Mooney, "Public Health Versus Private Practice."

23. Perren, "Meat and Livestock Trade"; Perren, *Meat Trade in Britain*.

24. Bartrip, *Home Office and the Dangerous Trades*; Gray, "Medical Men, Industrial Labour and the State in Britain"; Kirby, *Child Workers*; Malone, "The Gendering of Dangerous Trades."

25. Arnot, "Infant Death, Child Care and the State"; Marks, *Model Mothers*.

26. Arnot, "Infant Death"; Davies, "The Health Visitor as Mother's Friend," 39–59; Marks, *Model Mothers*.

27. S. D. Chapman, *History of Working-Class Housing*; Stedman Jones, *Outcast London*, chapters 8–9; Wohl, *Eternal Slum*; Wohl, "Unfit for Human Habitation."

28. Hamlin, *Public Health and Social Justice*. See also Pelling, *Cholera, Fever and English Medicine*; Pickstone, "Dearth, Dirt and Fever Epidemics"; Pickstone, "Ferriar's Fever to Kay's Cholera."

29. Ogborn, "Law and Discipline." Histories of smallpox and sexually transmitted infections have been particularly useful in analyzing the gendering of patients, therapies, and institutions: Cox, "Compulsion, Voluntarism, and Venereal Disease"; Dunsford, "Principle Versus Expediency"; Durbach, *Bodily Matters*; Howell, "A Private Contagious Diseases Act"; Mort, *Dangerous Sexualities*; F. B. Smith, "The Contagious Diseases Acts Reconsidered"; Spongberg, *Feminizing Venereal Disease*. The classic study of Victorian prostitution is Walkowitz, *Prostitution and Victorian Society*. See also Gilbert, *Cholera and Nation*.

30. Baldwin, *Contagion and the State*.

31. Osborne, "Security and Vitality"; Otter, "Cleansing and Clarifying"; Otter, "Making Liberalism Durable."

32. Joyce, *Rule of Freedom*.

33. For recent overviews of English and Welsh public health during the period covered by this study, see Hamlin, "State Medicine in Great Britain"; D. Porter, *Health, Civilization and the State*, 46–96; D. Porter, "Public Health."

34. Wiener, "The Unloved State." See also Mandler, "After the Welfare State," 382–88; Mandler, "Introduction: State and Society in Victorian Britain."

35. Gunn, "From Hegemony to Governmentality," 716–17; Mandler, "Introduction: State and Society in Victorian Britain," 13–21; Taylor and Trentmann, "Liquid Politics."

36. Joyce, *Rule of Freedom*, 7–8, 112.

37. See the collections of essays in Clark and Crawford, *Legal Medicine*; Goold and Kelly, *Lawyers' Medicine*.

38. There is a large historical literature on medicine and the legal system oriented around psychiatry, forensic medicine, and, more recently, malpractice: Crawford, "Patients' Rights"; Crowther and White, *On Soul and Conscience*; Fullmer, "Technology, Chemistry and the Law"; Golan, "History of Scientific Expert Testimony"; Hamlin, "Scientific Method and Expert Witnessing"; C. Jones, *Expert Witnesses*; Ward, "Law, Common Sense and the Authority of Science." .

39. Taggart, *Private Property*. See also Brenner, "Nuisance Law and the Industrial Revolution"; Daunton, "Taxation and Representation in the Victorian City"; Dingle, "The Monster Nuisance of All"; McLaren, "Nuisance Law and the Industrial Revolution"; Mosley, *Chimney of the World*. Hamlin demonstrated that fora of conflict provided the context for reconciling diverse interests in water and occasionally in forcing local policy change. Hamlin, *Science of Impurity*. For a magisterial legal analysis of water rights, see Getzler, *History of Water Rights*.

40. Atkins, *Liquid Materialities*; Benidickson, *Culture of Flushing*.

41. Practitioners and contemporary professionals often include historical sections; Cocks, "Statutes, Social Reform, and Control," 535–57; Kessel, *Air, the Environment and Public Health*; Malcolm and Pointing, *Statutory Nuisance*.

42. Chambers, *Digest of the Law*. Obviously this timing is to be expected. There were no national public health laws before 1848, so there would hardly be much jurisprudence. This is not to overlook the existence of the Vaccination Act, 1832 Cholera Act, the 1846 Nuisances Removal Act, or the 1847 Clauses Acts, several of which addressed matters in classic public health.

43. Baker, *An Introduction to English Legal History*, 178–86.

44. Dicey, *Lectures on the Relation Between Law & Public Opinion*, 362.

45. Atkins, *Liquid Materialities*; Benidickson, *Culture of Flushing*.

46. See chapters 1, 3, and 5 for examples. Cases also appeared, at least for a time, in the Annual Reports of the Association of Municipal Corporations or in periodicals such as the *Public Health: A Record and Review of Sanitary, Social, Medico-Legal and Municipal Affairs*, which started publication in 1868. The records of the Association of Municipal Corporations are held at the National Archives. See, for example, the Sixth Annual Report appendix, ii–xii, PRO/30/72/9, NA.

47. Clifford, *History of Private Bill Legislation*, vol. 2. For one such example, see Sheard, "Water and Health."

48. Hamlin, *Science of Impurity*.

49. Hanley, "Bye Laws, the Environment, and Health before Chadwick." Later nineteenth-century bylaws have attracted much more attention, particularly with respect to housing: Gaskell, *Building Control*; Harper, *Victorian Building Regulations*.

50. This attempt is reminiscent of Peter King's argument that the central government increasingly sought to rein in local criminal-law initiatives in the second quarter of the nineteenth century: King, *Crime and Law in England*.

51. For other revaluations of the local state, see Harling, "The Centrality of Locality"; Harling, "The Powers of the Victorian State"; Thane, "Government and Society."

52. Szreter, "Economic Growth, Disruption, Deprivation, Disease, and Death," 705; Hennock, "Finance and Politics," 212–25; T. Hunt, *Building Jerusalem*, 259–312; Jenson, "Getting to Sewers and Sanitation," 532–56.

53. T. Hunt, *Building Jerusalem*, 313–80; Wohl, *Endangered Lives*, 173–79. For London, see Clinton and Murray, "Reassessing the Vestries"; Luckin, "The Metropolitan and the Municipal."

54. Bell and Millward, "Public Health Expenditures"; Daunton, Introduction, 21–29; Daunton, *Trusting Leviathan*, 269–85; Millward and Sheard, "The Urban Fiscal Problem." For a slightly different argument, see Platt, *Shock Cities*, 394–406.

55. Szreter, "Economic Growth, Disruption, Deprivation, Disease, and Death," 711; Szreter, "The Importance of Social Intervention."

56. Frazer, *Duncan of Liverpool*; Hamlin, *Public Health and Social Justice*; D. Porter, *Health, Civilization and the State*, 119–20; Sheard and Power, *Body and City*.

57. This rested on the doctrine of *ultra vires*. *Ultra vires* became especially important in the second quarter of the nineteenth century: De Smith and Brazier, *Constitutional and Administrative Law*, 518–25; G. Roberts, *Municipal Development*, 31–32. For further discussion, see chapter 1.

58. The GBH had to sanction any mortgage of local rates under the 1848 PHA. The board also had a number of other control functions assigned to it. See chapter 5.

59. Lambert, "Central and Local," 130–31. This routinized central oversight was a much more important point of connection between the center and the periphery than the very rarely used ability of the center to compel local action, a power in any event not obtained in public health law until 1866. The process at work here was the growth of a bureaucratic element in the English state, and both Mark Harrison and Dorothy Porter draw attention to bureaucracy as one of the constitutive elements of the modern state: Harrison, *Disease and the Modern World*, 2; D. Porter, *Health, Civilization and the State*, 7. See also MacLeod, *Government and Expertise*. Not only was the balance shifting between central and local but it was shifting, as Joyce notes, within the central apparatus: Joyce, *Rule of Freedom*, 112–13.

60. Joanna Innes's work on Parliament has highlighted the multiple kinds of relationships between central and local governments and the inadequacy of the dichotomy implied by the central/local label, a theme developed by numerous other historians. See Innes, "Local Acts." See also Bellamy, *Administering Central-Local Relations*; Davis, "Central Government and the Towns"; Eastwood, *Government and Community*; Morris and Trainor, *Urban Governance*. This book builds on that reconsideration of the relationship. Parliament and Whitehall controlled the governors as well as the governed.

61. Fee and Porter, "Public Health, Preventive Medicine and Professionalization"; Lawrence, "Sanitary Reformers and the Medical Profession"; Marland, *Medicine and Society in Wakefield and Huddersfield*. But see Hardy, "Public Health and the Expert."

62. Brown, *Performing Medicine*; Fee and Porter, "Public Health, Preventive Medicine and Professionalization"; Hardy, "Public Health and the Expert"; Lawrence, *Medicine in the Making of Modern Britain*; Lawrence, "Sanitary Reformers and the Medical Profession"; Novak, "Professionalism and Bureaucracy"; Rose, "The Doctor in the Industrial Revolution"; Wohl, *Endangered Lives*, 142–49. This increase in medical participation coincided with the professionalization of both medicine and public health: Fee and Acheson, *History of Education*.

63. Hamlin, *Public Health and Social Justice*, 112–20; R. K. Webb, "Southwood Smith." On Simon, see Lambert, *Sir John Simon*. I use "medic" following Gilbert, *Cholera and Nation*, 2.

64. Eyler, *Victorian Social Medicine*; Szreter, "The GRO and the Public Health Movement in Britain."

65. Frazer, *Duncan of Liverpool*; Kearns, "Town Hall and Whitehall"; Laxton, "Fighting for Public Health."

66. Hardy, *Epidemic Streets*. For a Scottish example, see Laxton and Rodger, *Insanitary City*.

67. Of course, medical men testified at hearings on bills directly affecting the profession of medicine, such as the 1833 Anatomy Act, various bills regulating medical practice, and asylum bills.

68. Hamlin, "State Medicine in Great Britain"; MacLeod, "Anatomy of State Medicine"; D. Porter, *Health, Civilization and the State*, 121–27; D. Porter and R. Porter, Introduction, 3–4.

69. See chapter 2.

70. Dr. John Snow famously testified at a parliamentary select committee in 1855, yet when one recognizes the way in which other medical witnesses at the same hearing were excluded and ignored, Snow begins to look less like an acknowledged medical expert and more like a hand-picked witness.

71. In a related development, physicians failed to ensure that coroners had medical qualifications: Burney, *Bodies of Evidence*.

72. D. Porter, Introduction, 24. Although Thomas Wakley's 1836 attempt to secure payment for professional services rendered during inquests was successful, attempts to make investigations and certification of death reliant on medical expertise were not: Burney, *Bodies of Evidence*, 108–9.

73. Bynum, *Science and the Practice of Medicine*; Pelling, *Cholera, Fever and English Medicine*. For two different biographies, see Hamlin, *Cholera*; Longmate, *King Cholera*.

74. Durey, *Return of the Plague*, 185–200; Evans, "Epidemics and Revolutions," 123–46. But this disease certainly had social effects most often linked to dissection: Burrell and Gill, "The Liverpool Cholera Epidemic of 1832," 478–98; Durey, *Return of the Plague*, 155–84. On dissection, see Richardson, *Death, Dissection, and the Destitute*.

75. Gilbert, *Cholera and Nation*, 7–8; D. Porter, *Health, Civilization and the State*, 87–96. Sigsworth, "Cholera in the Large Towns of the West and East Ridings, 1848–1893" charts the response after 1832. Hardy, "Cholera, Quarantine and the English Preventive System," 250–69, expertly covers the post-1866 period. See also Hanley, "Parliament, Physicians, and Nuisances."

76. For an analysis of the role of fever, especially typhus, in creating a sympathetic basis for collective action, see Hamlin, *More than Hot*, especially locs. 1500–1555, 1720.

77. William Laurence Burn was an early advocate of the view that localities could not reasonably have been expected to make much more rapid progress than they did. I agree, though for different reasons; Burn, *Age of Equipoise*, 137.

78. Hamlin, "Predisposing Causes."

79. The congruence between anticontagionism and sanitary reform has long been recognized, but this connection tells us little about the means by which the medical theory was translated into a legal doctrine. See Ackerknecht, "Anticontagionism between 1821 and 1867," 562–93; Cooter, "Anticontagionism and History's Medical Record."

80. Nuisance laws could also be seen as a tax: Daunton, "Taxation and Representation."

81. This work might be compared with Kearns's analysis of the work in which Chadwick was engaged in 1842. Chadwick had to construct arguments that he could use to get around the obstacle to sanitary reform posed by private property rights. This involved more than a journalistic exposé of bad conditions. Chadwick, Kearns argued, constructed excess mortality as a consequence of market failure. Commissioners and councillors, too, struggled to justify their actions, though I see less evidence of concern with market failure. See Kearns, "Private Property and Public Health Reform."

82. Indeed, William Gladstone refused to consider giving tax credits for charitable donations: Daunton, "Payment and Participation," 270–71. On eighteenth-century hospitals and their voluntary funding, see Fissell, *Patients, Power, and the Poor*; Hamlin, *More than Hot*, loc. 2720; R. Porter, "The Gift Relation." On later nineteenth- and twentieth-century funding, which included state support, see Cherry, "Before the National Health Service"; Waddington, "Paying for the Sick Poor."

83. Kearns, "Private Property and Public Health Reform," quotation on 197. See also Bellamy, *Administering Central-Local Relations*, 8–13; Morris, "Externalities"; Rodger and Colls, "Civil Society," 17.

84. Hennock, "Finance and Politics"; Kearns, "Private Property and Public Health Reform"; Szreter, "Economic Growth"; Wohl, *Endangered Lives*, 166–79.

85. Hamlin, *Public Health and Social Justice*; Rodger, "Political Economy." These examples scarcely exhaust the subject, and we could add nuisance and workplace health to this list. See also the interesting Crowther and White, "Medicine, Property and the Law."

86. My use of boundary shifts as the framing device for the developments I trace is, of course, part literal description and part metaphor. The shift of taxation boundaries was real enough, but that between public and private services is obviously not illuminated by an image of lines shifting on a map. An alternative framing device could be the changing meaning of the public sphere or civil society or the social. As Pamela K. Gilbert, Jose Harris, and others have noted, these ideas, deployed in a variety of not entirely compatible ways, have attracted much historical attention among British urban and medical historians: P. K. Gilbert, "Producing the Public," locs. 43–44; Harris, "Introduction: Civil Society in British History." For some useful studies, see also Brunton, "Policy, Powers and Practice"; Luckin, "Shaping of a Public Environmental Sphere"; Otter, "Cleansing and Clarifying," 63; Rodger, "Common Good"; Rodger and Colls, "Civil Society."

87. Daunton, *Trusting Leviathan*. For a briefer account, see Daunton, "Trusting Leviathan."

88. Daunton, *Trusting Leviathan*, 274, 282. There are echoes here of Hamlin's "social capital": Hamlin, *Cholera*, 104.

89. Daunton, *Trusting Leviathan*, 275–76. To be sure, healthy drainage was hardly provided the first occasion when rates were raised for all ratepayers for general benefit. County rates paid for jails and bridges; parish rates paid for highways and relief. These were historic burdens, although even they were being challenged during the 1830s. Adding a new category of expenditure that was redistributive was not a simple matter. For example, provision of highways was rarely discussed in terms of access for the poor.

90. Though I agree with Bellamy that private property rights militated against community interest, I do not entirely share her view that local possessive pluralism

contradicted "the notion of a unitary or transcendental 'community'": Bellamy, *Administering Central-Local Relations*, 12.

91. This was not the first time that national or local taxes had been used to support health beyond the Poor Law. According to Dorothy Porter, though, central state involvement in the late eighteenth century was rare, and local state involvement was episodic: D. Porter, *Health, Civilization and the State*, 54–57. For examples of central involvement, see chapter 2n111.

92. One of the features of the management of paupers around mid-century was the development of new institutional provision for education, mental health, and sickness. For the metropolitan perspective, see Green, *Pauper Capital*, 115–56. See also Brundage, *English Poor Laws*, 92–100; Lees, *The Solidarities of Strangers*, 275–81. For a recent evaluation of workhouse schools, see Humphries, *Childhood and Child Labour*, 323–28. On Poor Law institutions, see Hodgkinson, *Origins of the National Health Service*.

93. This right was qualified in various ways. The poor had no right to housing or to decent accommodation or to a living wage or sufficient food. Even the right to be free of preventable epidemic disease did not lay an obligatory duty on local authorities before 1866 and for some time thereafter. Probably the best analogy is smallpox. In 1840, Parliament, in compelling the provision of vaccination free of charge, effectively gave individuals the right to freedom from this disease: Brunton, *Politics of Vaccination*, 21. As is well known, during the 1850s this was an ambiguous good.

94. My argument is influenced by Lees's account of social citizenship and the Poor Law. Even as it reinforced division, in practice the Poor Law created communities: Lees, *Solidarities of Strangers*, 7–12. On the right to relief, see Charlesworth, *Welfare's Forgotten Past*. On the right to health, see D. Porter, *Health, Civilization and the State*, 57–64.

95. Rodger, "Taking Stock," 56. This was obvious in the case of political citizenship: Hall, McClelland, and Rendall, *Defining the Victorian Nation*. But it is equally obvious in the case of what historians variously identify as cholera citizenship or sanitary citizenship: Hamlin, *Cholera*, 57, 95, 103–5; Hamlin, *More than Hot*, locs. 2108, 2673; Jenson, "Getting to Sewers and Sanitation."

96. Durbach, *Bodily Matters*; Hamlin, *Cholera*; Poovey, "Curing the Social Body"; Walkowitz, *Prostitution and Victorian Society*. In several international and colonial contexts, historians have increasingly drawn attention to public health's role in drawing literal and metaphorical boundaries and borders between and among places and peoples. Recent work exploring these themes, primarily in the twentieth century, includes Bashford, *Imperial Hygiene*; Molina, *Fit to Be Citizens?*; Shah, *Contagious Divides*.

97. P. K. Gilbert, *Citizen's Body*; Hamlin, *Cholera*, 87–96; Hamlin, *More than Hot*, loc. 2673; D. Porter, *Health, Civilization and the State*, 57–64. For a discussion of changing notions of citizenship among historians, see Mooney, *Intrusive Interventions*, 1–4.

98. Hamlin, "Public Sphere."

99. My focus here is on the 1848 Public Health Act (11 & 12 Vict., c. 63), the 1848 Metropolis Sewers Act (11 & 12 Vict., c. 112) and the 1855 Metropolis Local Management Act (18 & 19 Vict., c. 120). I also consider a small number of local acts.

100. Hamlin, *Cholera*. An 1863 drainage case yielded a legal principle still cited in 2006: *Tinkler v. The Board of Works for the Wandsworth District*, 44 English Reports

989–94; *Cooper v. The Board of Works for the Wandsworth District*, 143 English Reports 414–21. *Cooper* was cited as a crucial case for the "fair hearing rule" in a 2006 speech by Justice Steven Rares of the Federal Court of Australia; see "Blind Justice," 1. Benidickson describes the legal difficulties associated with the water-closet revolution in *Culture of Flushing*, 78–97.

101. Scotland has a distinctive statutory, institutional, and legal history. In addition to sources cited above, see Hamlin, "Environmental Sensibility in Edinburgh," 311; Hamlin, "William Pulteney Alison"; Laxton and Rodger, *Insanitary City*; White, "Medical Police, Politics and Police." For aspects of Irish medical history, see G. Jones and Malcolm, *Medicine, Disease and the State in Ireland*.

102. Davis, "Central Government and the Towns"; Green, *Pauper Capital*; Schwarz, *London in the Age of Industrialisation*.

103. Bell and Millward, "Public Health Expenditures and Mortality"; Hamlin, "Sanitary Policing"; Luckin, "Pollution in the City"; Millward and Sheard, "Urban Fiscal Problem."

104. Lewis, *Edwin Chadwick*; Frazer, *History of English Public Health*.

105. Keith-Lucas, "Some Influences"; Hennock, "Urban Sanitary Reform," 113.

106. D. Porter, *Health, Civilization and the State*; Rosen, *History of Public Health*.

107. Christopher Hamlin and John Pickstone both chart the shift from a moral economy of medicine to a political economy of public health. Hamlin, "State Medicine," 19, 25; Pickstone, "Dearth, Dirt and Fever Epidemics"; Pickstone, "Ferriar's Fever to Kay's Cholera"; D. Porter, *History of Public Health and the Modern State*, 54–57.

108. Piketty, *Capital*; Szreter and Hardy, "Urban Fertility and Mortality Patterns." This period also witnessed a peak in the incidence of child labor: Humphries, *Childhood and Child Labour*. Classic treatments of what came to be called the Condition of England include Hobsbawm, *Industry and Empire*, 79–96; Harrison, *Early Victorian Britain*, 63–90; Thompson, *Making of the English Working Class*, 347–66.

109. I have used, among other sources, Chase, *Chartism*; Drescher, *Abolition*; Gray, "Medical Men"; Green, *Pauper Capital*; Hobsbawm and Rude, *Captain Swing*; Poynter, *Society and Pauperism*; M. Roberts, *Political Movements*; Thompson, *Making of the English Working Class*.

110. For the longer history of the increasing concern with social issues, see Eastwood, *Government and Community*; Innes, *Inferior Politics*; Jupp, *Governing of Britain*, 147–76.

111. For various approaches to the high politics of social reform, see Eastwood, *Government and Community*; Eastwood, "Men, Morals and the Machinery of Social Legislation," 190–205; Hilton, "Whiggery, Religion and Social Reform," 829; Mandler, *Aristocratic Government*; Mandler, "Cain and Abel," 83–109. For a comprehensive survey of the ideology of social reform see F. D. Roberts, *Social Conscience*. One common response was to focus on educating the working classes, initially through voluntary means but quickly through state subsidy: Humphries, *Childhood and Child Labour*, 306–65.

112. The definitive study is Hamlin, *Public Health and Social Justice*. See also Brundage, *England's "Prussian Minister."* Still useful are Finer, *Life and Times*; Lewis, *Edwin Chadwick*. On the Poor Law in London, see Green, *Pauper Capital*. For

contemporaneous developments in France, see Coleman, *Death is a Social Disease*; La Berge, *Mission and Method*.

113. For a contemporary politico-medical analysis of the 1832 cholera epidemic, see Kay, *The Moral and Physical Conditions*. On Kay, see Mort, *Dangerous Sexualities*; Poovey, "Curing the Social Body." The Irish were a particular focus of Kay's; see MacRaild, *Irish Diaspora*. For some radical reaction linking cholera in 1832 to lack of political representation, see A. Fraser, *Perilous Question*, 208–9.

114. This was, as John Davis and David Green argued, crucial for metropolitan government and poor relief; Davis, *Reforming London*; Green, *Pauper Capital*.

115. Worboys, *Spreading Germs*. For a detailed analysis of post-1880 public health and the laboratory, see Hardy, *Salmonella Infections*.

116. A variety of authors identify a different kind of public health emerging in the last quarter of the nineteenth century. See Hamlin, "State Medicine"; D. Porter, *Health, Civilization and the State*, 128–46; Szreter, "Economic Growth." See also Mooney, *Intrusive Interventions*.

Chapter One

1. Nuisances Act 9 & 10 Vict., c. 96. On this law, see Lumley, *Act for the More Speedy Removal*. This law defined the sorts of things that might be health hazards and stipulated procedures for identifying and managing them. The enumerated items were, in the simplest terms, dwellings (filthy and unwholesome), drains (foul or offensive), and deposits (offensive or noxious). These nuisances had to be likely to be prejudicial to health and had to be certified as such by two medical practitioners. Historical treatment of statutory nuisance legislation is provided in Malcolm and Pointing, *Statutory Nuisance*, 19–29. This temporary law was made permanent in 11 & 12 Vict., c. 123 (1848).

2. On November 21, 1831, during the first cholera outbreak, the Privy Council ordered local boards of health to begin a summary program of nuisance abatement. The orders for cholera boards stipulated that they could abate a public nuisance if they received a certificate from a medical practitioner along with an oath from a credible witness testifying that a nuisance existed that was injurious to health: "From the LONDON GAZETTE," *Times*, November 23, 1831, 2, col. a. Durey notes that this order was deemed illegal: *Return of the Plague*, 79, 81. On July 19, 1832, the Privy Council again authorized local boards of health to abate certain listed nuisances duly certified as "dangerous to the public health" by two medical practitioners; Brockington, *Public Health in the Nineteenth Century*, app. 11, 129–35 reprints this order.

3. Chadwick, *Report on the Sanitary Condition*. For interpretations of Chadwick, see Brundage, *England's "Prussian Minister"*; Finer, *Life and Times*; Lewis, *Edwin Chadwick*.

4. In his introduction (35–37, 43–45) to Chadwick's *Report on the Sanitary Condition*, Flinn emphasizes Chadwick's significance. See also Finer, *Life and Times*, 147–63.

5. Hamlin, *Public Health and Social Justice*; Pelling, *Cholera, Fever and English Medicine*; Pickstone, "Dirt, Dearth and Fever Epidemics."

6. Hamlin, "Edwin Chadwick, 'Mutton Medicine,' and the Fever Question," 264. See also Hamlin, *Public Health and Social Justice*. For a different view of the ideological achievement Chadwick wrought, see Kearns, "Private Property."

7. Historians have long recognized that the provinces led the central government in health matters. Liverpool, for example, appointed the first medical officer of health: Frazer, *Duncan of Liverpool.*

8. Hamlin, "Public Sphere to Public Health"; Hanley, "Parliament, Physicians and Nuisances."

9. A small number of statutes dealt with nuisances; see Chadwick, *Report on the Sanitary Condition,* 348–54; J. T. Smith, *Laws of England,* 35–36.

10. For a general discussion of nuisance law, see Baker, *Introduction to English Legal History,* 422–35. Helpful contemporary discussion are in Blackstone, *Commentaries,* 3: 216–22; Paris and Fonblanque, *Medical Jurisprudence,* 1: 330–54; J. T. Smith, *Laws of England.*

11. Blackstone, *Commentaries,* 3: 216. The common law allowed different remedies for different types of nuisance. For a nuisance that affected an individual (a private nuisance), the law permitted the party to remove the nuisance him- or herself without further ado, or to sue for damages. A nuisance against the community, or at least a restricted geographic part of it (a public nuisance), was indictable, because it was a crime against public order. See Paris and Fonblanque, *Medical Jurisprudence,* 1: 334–54; Blackstone, *Commentaries,* 3: 220–22; J. T. Smith, *Laws of England,* 24–30.

12. Reflecting this broad sense of a nuisance, medical practitioners were not centrally involved in the determination of nuisances. In the common-law tradition, medical participation in nuisance proceedings was not necessary, though medical witnesses occasionally testified: Paris and Fonblanque, *Medical Jurisprudence,* 1: 330. On medicine in the courts in general see Jones, *Expert Witnesses;* Forbes, *Surgeons at the Old Bailey.*

13. See, for example, "Thompson *v.* Harris," *Times,* September 13, 1816, 3; *Rex v. Neil,* 172 English Reports 219–20.

14. On this point, see Daunton, "Taxation and Representation." For another context, see Atkinson, "The Impact of Cholera."

15. For a discussion of nuisance control by legal means, see Brenner, "Nuisance Law and the Industrial Revolution"; Dingle, "The Monster Nuisance of All." On air and water pollution, see Wohl, *Endangered Lives,* 205–56.

16. The implementation of nuisance law simply was a subsequent and additional layer of protection for property. An excellent local study from this period is Kearns, "Cholera, Nuisances and Environmental Management." On sanitary work of a later period, see Crook, "Sanitary Inspection"; Hamlin, "Nuisances and Community"; Hamlin, "Sanitary Policing." For an excellent account of sanitary work in a different context, see Davies, "Night Soil." On the related process of disinfection, see Whyte, "Changing Approaches to Disinfection."

17. Excellent surveys of pre-Victorian local government are Eastwood, *Government and Community;* Keith-Lucas, *Unreformed Local Government System;* Smellie, *History of Local Government.*

18. Webb and Webb, *Statutory Authorities.*

19. Keith-Lucas, *Unreformed Local Government System,* 15–16.

20. Some boroughs were unchartered: Innes, *Inferior Politics,* 86.

21. D. Fraser, *Power and Authority,* 2; D. Fraser, *Urban Politics,* 115–16; Keith-Lucas, *Unreformed Local Government System,* 15–16, 27.

22. Local functions of a quasi-judicial character, such as the management of public nuisances, could be discharged by counties or by municipal courts of long-standing jurisdiction, such as the Court Leet of Manchester Manor. Webb and Webb, *Manor and the Borough*, 26–27. The Webbs identify the Court Leet of Manchester Borough as a particularly active body and note the presence of comparable bodies in Lancashire.

23. For quantitative analyses of the number and kind of acts passed as well as the number of failures, see Hoppit, "Patterns"; Innes, "Local Acts." See also Innes and Rogers, "Politics and Government"; Jones and Falkus, "Urban Improvement."

24. For surveys see Clifford, *History of Private Bill Legislation*, vol. 2; Spencer, *Municipal Origins*. A list of local acts passed after 1800 is in the Commissioners for Inquiring into the State of Large Towns and Populous Districts, Second Report, Supplement, PP 1845 (602), 106. In 1847, Parliament responded to this avalanche of private regulation with a series of acts designed to simplify the local act process, including the Towns Police Clauses Act and the Towns Improvement Clauses Act. See Prest, *Liberty and Locality*.

25. Corporations often promoted local acts. For example, in 1835, Liverpool Corporation had thirty-eight local acts, Bristol fifty-eight: Keith-Lucas, *Unreformed Local Government System*, chap. 2. Where a local law was not promoted by an existing authority such as a municipal corporation, the resulting improvement commissioners coexisted with municipal corporations in the same location, the latter usually having a much narrower range of powers. The existence of two sources of authority in the same town could engender much controversy. See D. Fraser, *Urban Politics*, 91–102, 154–75.

26. Innes, "Local Acts," 30–37.

27. Foulkes, *Introduction to Administrative Law*, 78–87, quotation on 78. Foulkes outlines the ways in which this doctrine has been applied.

28. Paradoxically, for some advocates of local government, local acts set bad precedents. The champion of common law Joshua Toulmin Smith believed that these acts gave "powers the most arbitrary and grossly in violation of the liberty of the subject." The first thing a government preparing general legislation for sanitary matters ought to do, he believed, was to repeal and absolutely annul every one of them in respect of those matters; J. T. Smith, *Laws of England*, 9.

29. Hamlin, *Sanitary Reform in the Provinces*, 9–10; Webb and Webb, *Manor and the Borough*, 2:99–113.

30. According to long-established tradition, municipal corporations made bylaws for the good government of their cities on the basis of powers granted to them in their charters. These bylaws did not require central government sanction, though they were of course subject to legal challenge by local citizens: Merewether and Stephens, *History of the Boroughs*, 2:1443–52. For a listing of these bylaws, see Royal Commission of Inquiry into Municipal Corporations of England and Wales, Analytical Index to the Reports of the Commissioners Appointed to Inquire into the Municipal Corporations, PP (1839), 402, 83–85. Improvement commissioners also could make bylaws, but given the detailed character of their statutory nuisance provisions, for many of them bylaws for nuisances would have been somewhat superfluous. Courts leet also could make bylaws; Webb and Webb, *Manor and the Borough*, 2:105. I have not made any study of pre-1835 bylaws.

31. Spencer, *Municipal Origins*, 207–8; Keith-Lucas, "Some Influences"; Webb and Webb, *Statutory Authorities*, 235–349.

32. Dorchester Improvement (1834), 4 Will. 4, c. xvi, s. 55; Gravesend and Milton Improvement (1833), 3 & 4 Will. 4, c. li, s. 12; Tetbury Improvement (1817), 57 Geo. 3, c. ii, s. 23; Metropolitan Paving (1817), 57 Geo 3, c. xxix, s. 73. Short titles for statutes were not used consistently until the 1840s. I use short titles as given retroactively in Devine, *Index to the Local and Personal Acts*. As per convention, local act chapter numbers are given in Roman type.

33. Great Bolton Improvement (1817), 57 Geo. 3, c. lix, s. 6; Hastings Town and Port Improvement (1820), 1 Geo. 4, c. xii, s. 39; Bury St Edmunds Improvement (1820), 1 Geo. 4, c. lxi, s. 17; Stockton Improvement (1820), 1 Geo. 4, c. lxii, s. 21; Dorchester Improvement (1834), s. 53. Taunton Town and Market Regulation (1833), 3 & 4 Will. 4, c. xlvii, s. 12, and Gravesend and Milton Improvement (1833), s. 79 had more elaborate street codes. Sanitary nuisances in public streets occasionally were listed with other nuisances in clauses apart from the general street-nuisance clause: Hastings Town and Port Improvement (1820), s. 32.

34. Carroll, "Medical Police"; Hamlin, "Edwin Chadwick, 'Mutton Medicine,'" 257–64; Keith-Lucas, "Some Influences"; R. Porter, "Cleaning Up," 67; Webb and Webb, *Statutory Authorities*, 235–349.

35. Quotation from Stockton Improvement (1820), s. 24. See also Tetbury Improvement (1817), s. 26; Metropolitan Paving (1817), s. 67; Hastings Town and Port Improvement (1820), s. 37; Taunton Town and Market Regulation (1833), s. 13; York Improvement and Markets (1833), 3 & 4 Will. 4, c. lxii, s. 97; Gravesend and Milton Improvement (1833), s. 82; Bermondsey (St. Mary Magdalen) Improvement (1834), s. 70.

36. Quotation from Bury St Edmunds Improvement (1820), s. 17; see also Taunton Town and Market Regulation (1833), s. 12; Gravesend and Milton Improvement (1833), s. 79.

37. Hastings Town and Port Improvement (1820), s. 37; Stockton Improvement (1820), s, 24; Taunton Town and Market Regulation (1833), s. 13; York Improvement and Markets (1833), s. 97.

38. Paris and Fonblanque, *Medical Jurisprudence*, 1:330–54; J. T. Smith, *Laws of England*. Defined briefly, private nuisances affected an individual, and the remedy for them was to sue for damages (through an action on the case). Public, or common, nuisances affected the public, and the remedy for them was through indictment at the quarter sessions or other jurisdiction such as the courts leet.

39. Paris and Fonblanque and Smith did not discuss summary mechanisms found in local acts for dealing with common nuisances, but we would not expect discussion of the common law to refer to mechanisms contained in local acts, local acts not being common.

40. On this epidemic, see Brockington, *Public Health in the Nineteenth Century*; Durey, *Return of the Plague*; Morris, *Cholera, 1832*. Two more or less contemporary accounts of this epidemic are Kay, *Moral and Physical Condition*; and Shapter, *History of the Cholera*.

41. *Times*, November 23, 1831, 2, col. a.

42. Brockington, *Public Health in the Nineteenth Century*, 129–35.

43. On Cheltenham, see Hamlin, "Muddling in Bumbledom," 71–72; Hart, *History of Cheltenham*.

44. An Act for the Better Sewage, Cleansing, and Draining of the Town of Cheltenham, in the County of Gloucester (1833), 4 Will. 4, c. xxi. The local act constituting the street commissioners passed in 1821.

45. Liverpool Buildings Regulation Improvement &c. (1835), 5 & 6 Will. 4, c. liv, s. 37. Liverpool corporation's law harked back to the way in which seventeenth-century towns attempted to control the storage of potentially valuable human and animal waste. In seventeenth-century Liverpool, for example, dung could be stored on one's property as long as it was not permitted to obstruct passersby or run into the street and incommode movement along it. The easiest way to put this into practice was by fencing the dung or walling it in; King, "How High Is Too High," 446. Fencing or walling off was apparently a well-known and broadly accepted strategy in the 1830s for protecting private property from nuisance prosecution. The Metropolitan Police Act (1839), 2 & 3 Vict., c. 47, s. 60 (5) explicitly permitted pigsties that were shut out by a wall or fence.

46. The Liverpool Corporation was conscious of the health hazard posed by defective sewerage. The preamble of its 1830 local act explicitly drew attention to the defective quantity and quality of existing sewers and noted that "there is Reason to apprehend that the Health of the said Inhabitants may be seriously affected" by it: An Act for the Better Paving and Sewerage of the Town of Liverpool, 11 Geo. 4, c. xv. The "Reason to apprehend" formulation suggests something of the novelty or the contested character of this position.

47. For a recent and thorough exploration of the making of a new regulatory object, see Atkins, *Liquid Materialities*.

48. Though I have not made any study of it, it seems clear that not all common nuisances on private land were captured by these local acts. Apparently they could be dealt with only if they were next to a public street, so nuisances in private courts escaped. On this see Royal Commission for Inquiring into the State of Large Towns and Populous Districts, Second Report of the Commissioners for Inquiring into the State of Large Towns and Populous Districts, PP 1845 (602), 40–44.

49. Cooter, "Anticontagionism."

50. As a result of these problems, and in part to respond to increasing demands regarding representation, in 1830 the Tory government passed three acts that John Prest identifies as especially influential. They possessed three key features: they were permissive, they established some kind of ratepayer democracy, and they were meant to bypass the private bill procedure. Yet the democracy they established was hardly the radical reformers' dream; the 1830 Lighting & Watching Act, for example, laid down a plural voting scale (11 Geo., 4, c. 28, s. iii) based on property, like the sliding scale in William Sturges Bourne's Acts of 1818–19: Prest, *Liberty and Locality*, 9–13.

51. 5 & 6 Will. 4, c. 76, s. 90. Section 51 also permitted bylaws related to service on the corporation if elected; many codes included both kinds of bylaw.

52. Stedman Jones, "Rethinking Chartism," 102–7. For London, see Green, *Pauper Capital*, 82–94; Rees and German, *People's History*, 97–106.

53. E. P. Thompson, *Making*, 734–69; Hobsbawm and Rude, *Captain Swing*, 253–64.

54. This practice followed a parliamentary inquiry into the working (and potential abolition) of the Poor Law; Brundage, *English Poor Laws*, 44–52; Green, *Pauper Capital*, 88–89.

55. Dissenters had been subject to an annual indemnification before this time: Cannon, *Parliamentary Reform*, 191.

56. Jupp, *Governing of Britain*, 232–34; Macdonagh, *O'Connell*, 264–74.

57. On the parliamentary buildup to reform in the late 1820s, see Cannon, *Parliamentary Reform*, 187–241.

58. For vestries: 1 & 2 Will. IV, c. 60 (Parish Vestries Act). For poor relief: 4 & 5 Will. IV, c. 76 (New Poor Law).

59. Smellie, *History of Local Government*, 39–42.

60. There is no unanimity among historians about the significance of the 1832 Reform Act in terms of numbers, but at the very least the act offered a measure of standardization to the parliamentary franchise. For a debate on the numbers, see Beales, "The Electorate"; O'Gorman, "Reply: The Electorate." See also Jupp, *Governing of Britain*, 232–39; M. Roberts, *Political Movements*, 16–21.

61. 1 & 2 Will. IV, c. 60. See D. Fraser, *Urban Politics*, 26–28; Green, *Pauper Capital*, 93; Redlich and Hirst, *History of Local Government*, 166–69; Webb and Webb, *Statutory Authorities*, 449, 474–75. The 1833 Lighting and Watching Act also repealed the plural scale of voting in its 1830 predecessor: see 3 & 4 Will. 4, c. 90.

62. This practice was not changed until 1850, although the Small Tenements Rating Act of that year was permissive; D. Fraser, *Power and Authority*, 160. All compounders acquired the municipal franchise in 1869, assuming they were not disqualified for other reasons: Daunton, *Trusting Leviathan*, 270. See also Hunt, *Building Jerusalem*, 337.

63. M. Roberts, *Political Movements*, 21.

64. The plural scale was a major source of discontent in London; Green, *Pauper Capital*, 96–98.

65. D. Fraser, *Power and Authority*, 12.

66. Redlich and Hirst, *History of Local Government*, 137–38.

67. As was apparent in the Duke of Wellington's well-known claim that Hobhouse's Act left "the property of every man at the disposition of the rabble of the parish"; quoted in Green, *Pauper Capital*, 43. See also LoPatin-Lummis, "The 1832 Reform Act." Daunton discusses the tensions between power and franchise: *Trusting Leviathan*, 262–66.

68. Derek Fraser argues that Parliament's reluctance to give these corporations power was the single strongest argument that can be advanced against the claim that 1835 was a revolution in municipal government: D. Fraser, *Power and Authority*, 12, 164. But these bylaws granted real power, as contemporary commentators anxiously noted: H. Chapman, *Act for the Regulation*, 72.

69. My discussion in this section and the next relies on bylaws as they were submitted. As part III makes clear, the Home Office required many bylaws to be altered, and the bylaws as submitted often did not take effect, but I am interested in the original formulation.

70. See, for examples of different types of early nuisance bylaw, HO/70/1, NA Buckingham (November 9, 1836); HO/70/3, NA, Kingston-upon-Thames (August 10, 1836); HO/70/5, NA, Rye (October 20, 1836); HO/70/2, NA, Denbigh (July 4, 1836); HO/70/3, NA, Liverpool (October 29, 1836).

71. The argument here complements that developed in detail in Hanley, "Bye Laws, the Environment, and Health before Chadwick."

72. HO/70/4, NA, Pwllheli (November 26, 1836).

73. The Pwllheli council did not have to use health as a rationale and could have identified moving night soil as offensive, as was common. At local act hearings in the 1840s, these practices were also seen as morally objectionable: see, for one example, J. J. Rawlinson and William Hosking, Report from the Surveying Officers on the Sunderland Improvement, and Bridge Bills, in Copies of Reports for the Commissioners of Woods and Forests relative to Applications for Local Acts, PP, 1847, (124–86), xii, xvi. (The Sunderland Report is no. 48 of the 86 reports in paper no. 124.)

74. HO/70/4, NA, Pwllheli (November 26, 1836), bylaws nos. 5, 7, and 8.

75. Worcester Water and Improvement (1823), 4 Geo. 4, c. lxix.

76. "Meeting of the Town Council," *Berrow's Worcester Journal*, April 13, 1837, 3.

77. Compare Worcester local act 4 Geo. 4, c. lxix, s. 40 with bylaw no. 1. (The privately printed copy of Worcester's 1823 local act gives the same section as number 44.) The bylaws may be found at WCRO/b261.5/BA7123/parcel 10, City & Borough of Worcester, *Bye Laws made by the Council of the City and Borough of Worcester* (Worcester: T. Hayes, 1837), 3–4.

78. "Meeting of the Town Council," *Berrow's Worcester Journal*, April 13, 1837, 3. According to the *Journal's* report, this bylaw was meant to catch private and public nuisances. The corporation would not have involved itself in the prosecution of private nuisances, and the reporter or speaker must have meant public nuisances on private land; no other construction makes sense. The other health bylaw concerned the sale of unwholesome food.

79. The items were "any pig sty privy or necessary, improperly situated or not emptied sufficiently often—dunghills placed in unfit situations—stagnant drains or cess pools or other matters calculated to be prejudicial to the public health." Mayor to HO, October 23, 1838, HO/70/6, NA. A manuscript copy of the revised bylaw (WCRO/b261.5/BA7123/parcel 10) says, "Calculated to be prejudicial to the public health as a nuisance."

80. Worcestershire certainly had exposure to the epidemic; see British Library Add MS 39,167, fols. 158–71 for records of correspondence over the epidemic. On nuisance control during the epidemic, see Durey, *Return of the Plague*, 83; Hanley, "Bye Laws, the Environment, and Health before Chadwick."

81. For coroners' inquests at this time, see Burney, *Bodies of Evidence*, 4–6; Burney, "Medicine in the Age of Reform," 175. In a coroner's inquest, the coroner empaneled a jury whose members were required personally to view the matter at hand. Their decision, furthermore, determined the verdict. The coroner presented the facts to the jury and was empowered to call witnesses. The inspection inquest dispensed with these latter two components.

82. Worcester's bylaw committee may have developed the inspection inquest in part as a result of procedural considerations. Justices of the peace ruled on all cases before them in petty sessions, with witness testimony usually coming from the arresting officer. In the case of nuisances allegedly prejudicial to health, witnessing by police constables was perhaps more of a problem, although the constables were expected to be capable of identifying unwholesome food. Physicians would have

been more appropriate witnesses, but the committee undoubtedly realized that physicians could not be expected to do such work for free, and these procedural matters made the use of volunteers a sensible option. The Privy Council's 1831 anti-cholera proclamation required one or more credible witnesses in order to prove a nuisance to health; the committee may have seen the inspection inquest as a similar mechanism.

83. Another 1837 bylaw (no. xvi) permitted justices of the peace to destroy unwholesome food, and the committee believed no special protections for that form of private property were required: Worcester, *Bye Laws*, 18–19, at WCRO/b261.5/BA7123/parcel 10.

84. It is unlikely that Worcester's committee distrusted justices of the peace per se and wanted to circumvent them; bylaw committee members were eligible to be elected mayor and thus were eligible to become magistrates themselves. The borough bench was appointed by the Lord Chancellor, but the mayor was ex officio a justice of the peace and the chair of the borough bench: Moir, *Justice of the Peace*, 179. Councils recommended members for the bench: D. Fraser, *Power and Authority*, 10–11.

85. The process of ward making was one of the sticking points in the bill. The Whigs had wanted boundary commissioners to do it, but the Lords wanted to assign the task to revising barristers. The boundary commissioners John Aldridge and H. R. Brandreth disagreed with the revising barristers' recommendations on Worcester: Report of the Commissioners upon the Boundaries and Wards of Certain Boroughs and Corporate Towns, PP 1837 (238), part III, 368–72.

86. Liverpool Buildings Regulation, Improvement &c. (1835), 5 & 6 Will. 4, c. liv, s. 37.

87. Some of the local acts regulated the docks, some the old city limits. The corporate boundary under the 1835 Municipal Reform Act was the parliamentary borough: 5 & 6 Will. 4, c. 76, schedule A.

88. Report of Bye Law Committee, September 21, 1836, LRO/352 MIN/COU/II/1/1. Council meetings dealing with bylaws took place on September 30 and October 17, 18, 19 and 24–26.

89. "Council Proceedings," *Liverpool Mercury*, October 21, 1836, 374.

90. "Council Proceedings," *Liverpool Mercury*, October 28, 1836, 382. These bylaws, numbered 4 and 5, can be found at LRO/MIN/COU/II/1/1 (October 29, 1836), 299–334.

91. "Council Proceedings," *Liverpool Mercury*, October 21, 1836, 374. I will clarify that the 1835 act applied to the old, smaller corporate boundaries. The new 1836 bylaws applied to the new, larger corporate boundaries. The councillors could not amend an act of Parliament, but they could alter the language they drew from the act as they drafted new bylaws for a new jurisdiction.

92. By simultaneously widening and narrowing the field of regulation, the 1836 council constituted a new object, but one that still was largely defined by the imperative to protect private property against arbitrary or unreasonable attack. It is also important to recognize that the council, like the corporation before it, still declined to use health as a rationale. Yet that shared reluctance masked a more significant departure in 1836. In some ways the 1836 nuisance definition was a retreat from the implicitly health-based 1835 ten-foot nuisance, which clearly had been premised on

the notion of effluvia. The 1836 bylaw nuisance had no such premise built into it. It appears that in Liverpool in 1836, property trumped health for common sanitary nuisances.

93. But see Moore and Rodger, "Who Really Ran the Cities?" Gerry Kearns draws attention to the neglected aspect of interurban cooperation in "Town Hall and Whitehall," 108.

94. HO/70/4, NA (Newcastle, August 2, 1837); HO/70/5, NA, Stockton (sent March 10 1838), and Sunderland (October 5, 1837). It is not clear if Newcastle and Sunderland worked from Liverpool's bylaws or from some other local act or set of bylaws. The Hull council specifically worked from Liverpool's bylaws, and it would not be surprising if Newcastle and Sunderland did as well: "Town Council Meeting," *Hull, Rockingham . . . Gazette,* June 17, 1837, 3.

95. Tewkesbury was so enamored of Worcester's nuisance law process that it drafted a bylaw for destroying dangerous buildings that applied the same mechanism. Copies of Worcester's 1837 bylaws survive in the records of the Kidderminster, Droitwich, Bewdley, Evesham, and Tewkesbury corporations. I suspect that archives in other adjoining counties would yield more examples. Gloucester also corresponded with Worcester.

96. My interpretation is based on an analysis of the draft bylaws found at Shropshire Archives, 3365/2538, "Borough of Shrewsbury, Drt Bye Laws 1838." It appears that the council committee initially drafted a very short code containing only five bylaws, none of which made any reference to sanitary nuisances, in addition to twelve bylaws related to service on the council and other purely administrative matters. It is likely that Shrewsbury's committee members initially were confused about the provision in the Municipal Reform Act that gave councils the power to make bylaws for the suppression of nuisances not summarily provided for by any existing local act. Shrewsbury's local act had provisions prohibiting a number of nuisances; those provisions ultimately ended up in the bylaws. A list of nuisances provided for by the street act was annotated "omit these in by laws": Shropshire Archives, 3365/2538. "The following nuisances are provided against by the Street Act," n.d. The Shrewsbury committee members evidently then realized that the very short code they had initially contemplated was inadequate, because the street act pertained only to a restricted part of the borough, and they needed to make bylaws for the entire borough: Shropshire Archives, 3365/2538, draft letter to several other corporations, May 22, 1841; draft letter to HO, June 7, 1842. The first recorded correspondence with Liverpool came in late 1839. At this point, I believe, the committee carried out a detailed comparison with Liverpool's bylaw code. As a result, a further fifteen bylaws were added as a rider to the original draft. However, the committee saw this rider, too, as inadequate and made another comparison of existing municipal regulations with the Liverpool bylaw code. The committee added an additional forty-five bylaws, bringing the manuscript total up to eighty-five. Note that these bylaws were identified by the designation "L'pool," making the comparison explicit.

97. "Borough of Shrewsbury, Drt Bye Laws 1838," 3365/2538, Shropshire Archives. The initial five nonadministrative bylaws made no reference to sanitary nuisances. Given the bylaw committee's understanding of its task at that moment, this was somewhat understandable, although other places were by this time developing significant new bylaw powers over sanitary nuisances on private land. The twelve

"rider" bylaws subsequently added three separate bylaws about emptying night soil, moving it about, and cleaning it up after a spill. If my reading of this complex, extensively edited and assembled draft document is correct, the committee that drafted the rider did not believe that any further sanitary nuisance provision was necessary, because the rider proceeded immediately to deal with other matters. The bylaws taken to the full council, however, have inserted at this point another bylaw directed largely at sanitary nuisances.

98. The Carnarvon council, too, relied on a detailed engagement with Liverpool's code. The council began its bylaw-making process as did many other corporations by seeking models, choosing to consult Coventry, Denbigh, and Liverpool. Liverpool had produced the most complete code; the Carnarvon clerk evidently decided simply to go through it *seriatim*, ending up with forty-seven sections. The Carnarvon Corporation sent its first set of bylaws to the Home Office in June 1838: Carnarvon Corporation Minutes, XD11, September 11, 1837; September 29, 1837; November 21, 1837, May 21, 1838, Gwynedd Archives.

99. The list of banned substances is virtually identical to Liverpool's, right down to the order; Bye Laws as Revised by the Council, no. 22, Shropshire Archives, 3365/2538.

100. After revision of the 1838 draft, the Shrewsbury councillors seemed satisfied with the bylaws they produced in 1839. However, on submitting them to a barrister, they were advised to incorporate them into a local act, much as Liverpool had suggested. The expense deterred them, and the matter rested until 1841: Shropshire Archives, DA5/100/2, Shrewsbury Council Minute Book, February 3, 1840. Shrewsbury did not submit bylaws to the Home Office until 1842; see the printed copy in Shropshire Archives, 3365/2538 and the materials in HO/45/os 202, NA.

101. If my reconstruction of the chronology is correct, Bewdley's bylaw committee, like Shrewsbury's, initially prepared a very short, five-section bylaw code: Bye Law Committee Report, n.d., BA 8681/37 (ii) 5, WCRO. The Bewdley committee or the council apparently decided, however, that this short bylaw code was insufficient. A more extensive code was prepared and submitted to the Home Office (and rejected) in 1838. Bewdley Corporation's records contain extensive Liverpool material; see BA 8681/37 (ii) 10, (ii) 11, (ii) 12, WCRO, and I believe the bylaw committee then went through the Liverpool code, identifying possible articles for inclusion. The Kidderminster [?] Clerk reported to Bewdley's Clerk that he was much obliged for the loan of the Liverpool code: Kidderminster to Bewdley, May 7, 1838, BA 8681/37 (ii) 8, WCRO.

102. Borough of Bewdley, Drt Proposed Bye Laws, n.d. [1838?], BA 8681/37 (ii) 6, WCRO. Bewdley's approved 1843 bylaw code is at BA 8681/37 (ii) 21, WCRO.

103. Moore and Rodger, "Who Really Ran the Cities?" 50–51.

104. Hanley, "Bye Laws, the Environment, and Health before Chadwick." This process can be studied through examination of the annotations made on the draft bylaws and the letters sent by the Home Office to the relevant corporations. The documents do not, unfortunately, unambiguously identify the person responsible for the annotation. According to one historian of the Home Office, the Home Secretary in 1835 was expected to be involved in the response to every single letter that was sent to the office: Pellew, *Home Office*, 5–7. The Home Office history states that only the most senior officials would have been allowed to minute documents: HO/415/1, NA (accessed August 8, 2007).

105. On this point, see Hanley, "Bye Laws, the Environment, and Health before Chadwick."

106. Worcester's various bylaws may be found at HO/70/6, NA.

107. HO/70/2, NA for Droitwich's bylaws made on May 22, 1838. Letter from Home Office to Droitwich, May 26, 1838, 261.4/BA1006/parcel 29, WCRO.

108. Home Office to Worcester, July 23, 1838, at 496.5/BA9360/C8/Box8, WCRO, with annotations. This was an extraordinary departure from the statute, which permitted the HO to disallow bylaws only forty days after reception, not more than a year later. In contrast to other corporations confronted with demands to change their bylaws, Worcester was not inclined to be disagreeable, and after further negotiation the corporation secured new bylaws (see above). Other corporations challenged the Home Office's rejections: see Hull to Home Office, November 8, 1837, HO/70/3, NA; Congleton to Home Office, May 2, 1838, HO/70/1, NA. Congleton recruited its MP in the battle, though to little effect: G. Wilbraham to Home Office, July 29, 1838, HO/70/1, NA. Evesham also fruitlessly recruited its MP: Evesham to Lord Marcus Hill, February 25, 1839, 261.5/BA7123/parcel 10, WCRO.

109. Mayor to HO, October 23, 1838, HO/70/6, NA.

110. *Bye Laws, Passed by the Council of the Borough of Devonport, . . . 1838*, 17, bylaw VI.3, HO/70/2, NA.

111. *Supplementary Bye Laws, Passed by the Council of the Borough of Devonport . . . 1839*, 5, no. 2, HO/70/2, NA. See letter from Devonport to HO, April 16, 1839, HO/70/2, NA from Devonport's clerk explaining the council's response to the Home Office.

112. HO to Droitwich, May 26, 1838, 261.4/BA1006/ parcel 29, WCRO. The relevant draft bylaws may be found at HO/70/2, NA.

113. Tewkesbury Council Minutes, November 9, 1837, TBR/A1/9, Gloucestershire RO. After further deliberation, the council adopted bylaws including Worcester's inspection inquest: June 4, 1838. The Home Office disallowed them all: August 6, 1838.

114. Bylaws made March 23, 1840, no. 11, HO/70/6, NA.

115. HO to Great Yarmouth, April 3, 1840, HO/43/59, NA. Phillipps was the Permanent Under-Secretary; Michael Lobban, "Phillipps, Samuel March (1780–1862)."

116. Bylaw no. xi, Borough of Great Yarmouth, *Bye-Laws made and passed*, 6–7, at HO/70/6, NA.

117. "Copy of a bye law made . . . 9th October 1838 and 3rd January 1838," HO/70/3, NA. The framing of sanitary nuisance bylaws occupied Hull's attention again in 1847–48. See the correspondence of B. M. Jalland with the Town Clerk, Hull City Archives, Council Correspondence, TCC/669, 671. If Hull was given the HO advice, the town did not take it: see Borough of Kingston-upon-Hull, *Bye-Laws ordained by the Town Council*, 11, bylaw no. 15, TCR/4/2, Hull City Archives.

118. 2 & 3 Vict., c. 47, s. 60 contained one article controlling the emptying of privies and the movement of night soil (4), as was quite common in local acts of the period. The section also contained an article regulating the disposal of offensive matter in thoroughfares, also routine. The same article controlled noxious trades, prohibiting wastes from certain named trades from accumulating in any open or uncovered place, whether surrounded by a wall or not (3), echoing ancient regulations. Finally, one article prohibited pigsties not fenced off and any swine kept in

any house or near any street so as to be a common nuisance (5). The Home Office explicitly drew Great Yarmouth's attention to this act: HO to Great Yarmouth, April 3, 1840, HO/43/59. NA.

119. 9 & 10 Vict., c. 96.

120. Medical men were not defined in the 1846 Nuisances Removal Act and would not be until the passage of the 1858 Medical Act.

121. Hamlin, "Public Sphere"; Hanley, "Bye Laws, the Environment, and Health before Chadwick."

122. Joyce, *Rule of Freedom*, 76–89, quotation on 86; Ogborn, "Ordering the City," 517. See also Taylor, "Melbourne, Middlesbrough and Morality." The Webbs made a similar observation many years ago: Webb and Webb, *Statutory Authorities*, 273–75.

123. Michael Roberts makes this point with respect to vagrancy legislation: M. J. D. Roberts, "Public and Private." See also Ogborn, "Ordering the City," 509; Storch, "The Policeman as Domestic Missionary." V. A. C. Gatrell notes that controlling the streets was a major police function: "Crime, Authority and the Policeman-state," 244–45. For eighteenth-century Westminster, see Ogborn, *Spaces of Modernity*, 75–115.

124. Indeed, voluntary projects of moral reform were controversial, as was the enforcement of laws regulating morality. The existence of conflict between and within classes around issues of moral reform is well established: Cunningham, "The Metropolitan Fairs"; Innes, *Inferior Politics*, especially 215–26; Reid, "Praying and Playing," 758–67. Storch noted that there was no middle-class consensus on issues of working-class control. Different police forces had different approaches, councils different priorities, and magistrates different opinions: Storch, "The Policeman as Domestic Missionary." For a later period, see Petrow, *Policing Morals*. Within the middle class, conflict came from inside and outside moral-reform organizations and included both strategic and tactical considerations. Critics challenged the class bias of enforcement, the use of paid informers, the utility of test cases, and even the wisdom of legally controlling moral behavior. This can be approached in Hunt, *Governing Morals*; M. J. D. Roberts, *Making Victorian Morals*. For a study of enforcement, see Croll, "Street Disorder, Surveillance and Shame"; D. Taylor, "Crime and Policing in Early Victorian Middlesbrough."

125. In the case of noxious trades, enforcement was not solely about the rights of private property but also about the kinds of people entitled to the protection afforded by the common law. In an early articulation of the community standards argument, judges appeared to believe that filthy neighborhoods were fit places for noxious trades. Thus a judge in *Jones v. Powell* (1629) argued that butchers and hat makers could lawfully follow their trades in certain parts of London but not in other parts. In 1879, one justice observed that "a nuisance in Belgrave Square would not necessarily be so in Bermondsey." See *Jones v. Powell* in Baker and Milsom, *Sources of English Legal History*, 603. Belgravia quotation taken from Malcolm and Pointing, *Statutory Nuisance*, 50. On late-nineteenth-century sanitary enforcement, see Crook, "Sanitary Inspection"; Hamlin, "Sanitary Policing"; Otter, "Cleansing and Clarifying."

126. Christopher Hamlin contends that the 1840s and 1850s witnessed a transformation both in the nature of nuisances and in the character of the procedures available to deal with it. Newly medicalized nuisances, he persuasively argues, were increasingly identified through bureaucratic mechanisms characteristic of an urban and industrial society rather than through the procedures characteristic of

pre-nineteenth-century common-law nuisance practice. He maintains that the medicalization of nuisance, in the sense that health became the rationale for action, ostensibly was caused by cholera, though the context was set by the failure to develop mechanisms to deal with the problems of urbanization and industrialization: Hamlin, "Public Sphere to Public Health."

127. J. T. Smith, *Laws of England*, 53. Smith's enthusiasm suggests that even he was aware that at the very least more efficient machinery (v) was required even if most of the nuisances enumerated in the act were already provided for under common law (49).

128. Hanley, "Parliament, Physicians, and Nuisances," 728–31; Malcolm and Pointing, *Statutory Nuisance*, 19–29; Wohl, *Endangered Lives*, 310–22.

Chapter Two

1. Millward and Ward, "From Private to Public," 1; Hassan, "Growth and Impact," 533; Sheppard, *London, 1808–1870*, 109; Webb and Webb, *Statutory Authorities*, 182–83.

2. Hamish Fraser saw Glasgow as a pioneer: H. Fraser, "Municipal Socialism." See also the essays in Fraser and Maver, *Glasgow*. On Birmingham, see Briggs, *Victorian Cities*, 187–243; Hennock, *Fit and Proper*; T. Hunt, *Building Jerusalem*, 313–80. For more general perspectives, see Hassan, "Growth and Impact"; Millward and Ward, "From Private to Public"; Sutcliffe, "Growth of Public Intervention." The literature is surveyed in Millward, "Political Economy." For a fascinating look at the material politics of municipalization, see Daunton, "Material Politics"; Taylor and Trentmann, "Liquid Politics."

3. Webb and Webb, *Statutory Authorities*, 40n2, 152. Statutory sanction for public control came with the Tudor Law of Sewers (1531), 23 Hen. 8, c. 5.

4. Kellett, "Municipal Socialism," 40. For a fuller discussion, see Sutcliffe, "Growth of Public Intervention," 108–12. Neither Kellett nor Sutcliffe sufficiently scrutinize the limited character of public control around 1800 or acknowledge the presence of private models after that. Neither bases his argument on the analysis of any particular private failure. Kearns explores market failure, though I am not convinced that the commissioners of sewers are best seen as private: Kearns, "Private Property," 192.

5. In addition to the examples discussed below, during the 1840s Edwin Chadwick, one of the most prominent public health reformers, attempted (and failed) to create a private corporation to build private water and sewer supplies: Brundage, *England's "Prussian Minister,"* 101–12. In addition, several attempts were made at capitalist exploitation of raw sewage, especially in London. Some of these effectively were private sewer companies (although they proposed to fund their operations from the sale of a product to farmers rather than from fees collected from property owners or householders). The Metropolitan Sewage Manure Company, incorporated in 1846 (9 & 10 Vict., c. cccxcviii), proposed an intercepting scheme for some of the sewers of the Westminster Commission of Sewers: see Report by Sir H. T. de la Beche and F. L. Wollaston on the Metropolitan Sewage Manure Company's Amendment Bill, in Copies of Reports for the Commissioners of Woods and Forests Relative to Applications for Local Acts, PP 1847 (124). (This was report no. 59 of 86 reports

in PP 1847 [124], which will hereafter be cited as Copies of Reports, PP 1847 [124–59].) See also the Report by Sir H. T. de la Beche, F. L. Wollaston, Richard Phillips, and Dr. Lyon Playfair on the London Sewage Chemical Manure Company bill in Copies of Reports, PP 1847 (124–60), which intended to intercept some sewers of the Westminster and Surrey and Kent Commissions. A more complex case was the (unsuccessful) Great London Drainage Company Bill, which would have provided the company with a guaranteed sum (effectively a rate) from the Metropolitan Commission of Sewers in order to build its intercepting sewers: see Minutes of Evidence taken before the Select Committee on the Great London Drainage Bill, PP 1852–53 (629), qq. 2304–8. For a later venture, see Cottrell, "Resolving the Sewage Question." In the United States, private sewer companies existed at the end of the nineteenth century; New Orleans's was created in the late nineteenth century; see Melosi, *Sanitary City*, 149–52.

6. The fact that sewer rates were not municipalized may help explain why sewers were so uncontroversially assumed to be a public responsibility; only the people who directly benefited from them would pay for them.

7. Kellett, "Municipal Socialism," 140; Polanyi, *Great Transformation*, 154–56. For what Burn calls the interventionism of panic, see *Age of Equipoise*, 156–60.

8. Finer, *Life and Times*; Lewis, *Edwin Chadwick*.

9. See, for some examples, Hamlin, "Muddling in Bumbledom"; Hamlin, *Public Health and Social Justice*; Joyce, *Rule of Freedom*, especially 65–75; Osborne, "Security and Vitality"; Poovey, "Domesticity and Class Formation"; Szreter, "Economic Growth."

10. The funding of municipal projects often floundered precisely on the inability to rate all property. Ratepayers were considered consumers of services: Daunton, *Trusting Leviathan*, 275–76. These municipal services differed significantly from, say, poor relief or objects (such as jails and bridges) paid for out of the county rate and that were acknowledged in law as parochial or countywide services, notwithstanding ongoing controversy over financing, such as was seen with the Poor Law. Debates over how local and national revenue should be raised were, as Daunton shows, quite complex, reflecting profound structural economic and social changes, and alternately simmered and boiled over for most of the rest of the century. See also Beckett, *Local Taxation*. In this chapter, I am interested in how a service became municipal in the first place.

11. Daunton, "Taxation and Representation," 110.

12. The same could be said about water provision: Sheard, "Water and Health."

13. On the early legal history of commissions of sewers, see Webb and Webb, *Statutory Authorities*, 13–27. The statutes under which any given commission operated varied. For the Westminster Commission, the most complete list appears in the preamble of its 1847 local act (10 & 11 Vict., c. lxx).

14. Comyns, *Digest*, 6: 289. This statute did not imply that there were classes of exemption. Generally, juries had the discretion to determine liability, though even by the time of Callis in the seventeenth century, several classes of exemption appear to have established themselves in law. Land situated well above the level of the sewer, for example, was generally held to be exempt, as was land between the sea and the sea wall. The rationale whereby these lands were excluded was the statute itself; a party had to derive some benefit, or be likely to derive some benefit, or avoid

damage, in order to be liable. In Westminster, by the early nineteenth century juries simply endorsed the presentment: Webb and Webb, *Statutory Authorities*, 79–84.

15. A discussion of the processes of the Westminster Commission at this time, focusing on widespread corruption, is in Webb and Webb, *Statutory Authorities*, 79–84. The commissioners' view of their proceedings may be found at Opinion of Mr. Serjeant Taddy upon the Different Forms of Proceedings used in the Office of the Commissioners (case 6), p. 16, WCS/740, LMA.

16. Webb and Webb, *Statutory Authorities*, 79–84. Disputes about rates went to the Queen's Bench.

17. The fullest, if an unflattering, account of the metropolitan commissioners comes from Webb and Webb, *Statutory Authorities*, 57–106. Sheppard, *London, 1800–1870*, 255–56 reduces the space but keeps the tone. A more sympathetic account is Sunderland, "A Monument to Defective Administration?" See also Halliday, *Great Stink*; Hamlin, *Public Health and Social Justice*; Hanley, "The Metropolitan Commissioners."

18. J. T. Smith, *Laws of England*, 78, note *p*. Although the sewers tax struck some as perfect in theory, contemporaries noted that in practice it was often difficult to determine who benefited: Select Committee on Metropolis Sewers, PP 1834 (584), iv.

19. Innes, "Local Acts" argues that local legislation was not simply a barometer of parliamentary inactivity and local initiative. Indeed, Parliament took an active role in shaping local legislation before the reform era. As Innes suggests, during the 1830s this control shifted away from MPs and toward officials and other agents of government. The developments outlined in this chapter are broadly consistent with this view. See also Harling and Mandler, "From 'Fiscal-Military' State." On private bill legislation, see Prest, *Liberty and Locality*.

20. Innes and Rogers, "Politics and Government," 535–36; Jupp, *Governing of Britain*, 223–25. For surveys see Clifford, *History of Private Bill Legislation*; Spencer, *Municipal Origins*.

21. Spencer, *Municipal Origins*, 242–63 summarizes the drainage and sewerage provisions of a typical act.

22. The issue here is not whether these services were public or private, as the next section will show. As Millward noted, private ownership was perfectly compatible with public control as exercised through Parliament. Private control meant that rates could not be levied, and water companies were often taken into public ownership once they started to levy rates: Millward, "Political Economy," 329.

23. On pre-1835 local government, see Keith-Lucas, *Unreformed Local Government*; Redlich and Hirst, *History of Local Government*.

24. Taunton was not a corporate borough. Whatever charter it once had lapsed at the end of the eighteenth century. County magistrates administered justice. Parochial officers discharged Poor Law functions and carried out basic paving functions: Clark, *Report . . . on the Borough of Taunton*, 6–7.

25. Savage, *History of Taunton*, 578, 580; Report by John Maurice Herbert and Thomas Page, Esquires, on the Taunton Improvement and Market Bill, in Copies of Reports, PP 1847 (124–30), iii, vii, xiii.

26. Individuals could connect for a one-time payment of 2 shillings per £1 on the basis of the assessed value of the property for the poor rate: Minutes of Evidence . . .

upon a Preliminary Inquiry Respecting the Taunton Improvement and Market Bill, in Copies of Reports, PP 1847 (124–30), 99.

27. A duty on coal imported into London was suggested as the source for metropolitan improvements in 1836: Select Committee on Metropolitan Improvements, PP 1836 (517), iii–iv. See also D. H. Porter, *Thames Embankment*, 153–54 for coal duties used for funding metropolitan projects.

28. Daunton, *Trusting Leviathan*, 47–57; Matthew, "Gladstone, Disraeli, and the Politics."

29. The local police were also supported by a voluntary contribution: Clark, *Report . . . on the Borough of Taunton*, 14. For a more general view, see Innes and Rogers, "Politics and Government," 535.

30. Innes noted that these subscription or voluntary plans often floundered on the free rider problem: Innes, "Local Acts," 35.

31. The exact state of Rice's operations or finances was not clear, even at the time: Herbert and Page on the Taunton Improvement and Market Bill, in Copies of Reports, PP 1847 (124–30), viii. Rice expected to recoup his costs plus interest, but the interest rate was so high that the trustees objected to it. It seems that he did not expect merely to break even but expected a return on his outlay that presumably extended beyond what consols paid.

32. Minutes of Evidence, in Copies of Reports, PP 1847 (124–30), 99.

33. As will be discussed below, it was very common for public sewers commissions to allow private developers to build sewers in the first instance, with commissioners taking over maintenance thereafter. See note 100 below.

34. Report . . . on the Taunton Improvement and Market Bill, in Copies of Reports, PP 1847 (124–30), vii, xvi; Minutes of Evidence, in Copies of Reports, PP 1847 (124–30), qq. 5, 132–41.

35. These properties had to pay £100 (out of £400–500) total cost. This occurred with reference to a plan to drain the area around Church-square: Report . . . on the Taunton Improvement and Market Bill, in Copies of Reports, PP 1847 (124–30), vii; Minutes of Evidence, in Copies of Reports, PP 1847 (124–30), qq. 43–58.

36. I refer here to the "voluntary" contribution; the portion paid for with market duties was of course mandatory for all consumers who shopped at the market.

37. Minutes of Evidence, in Copies of Reports, PP 1847 (124–30), qq. 1723–24.

38. Clark, *Report . . . on the Borough of Taunton*, 10–12. The election of the local board of health did not initially improve matters: Austin, *Report on the Proceedings*.

39. Michael Williams makes the point that even in rural Somerset, "the administrative and financial problems were as important as the physical and technical problems of draining, and they were certainly no less difficult to overcome." See M. Williams, *Draining of the Somerset Levels*, 197–98. On the technical and legal complexity of some sanitary schemes, see Burn, *Age of Equipoise*, 137; Hamlin, "Muddling in Bumbledom."

40. In 1833, the trustees commissioned another plan to drain the town, but it was abandoned because their statute did not authorize a rate they believed was necessary to pay for it: Report. . . . on the Taunton Improvement and Market Bill, in Copies of Reports, PP 1847 (124–30), xiii. For the 1833 act, see An Act for Better Regulating the Market, and Cleansing the Streets, and Preventing Nuisances, in the Town of Taunton, 3 Will. 4, c. xlvii. The trustees floated a bill allowing them to

rate the town in 1839, but the measure was locally unpopular and did not proceed, apparently partly because of the trustees were not elected to their office: Minutes of Evidence, in Copies of Reports, PP 1847 (124–30), q. 1759 (pp. 104–5). The trustees were similarly unpopular in 1833, which may have contributed then, too, to the lack of any substantial attempt to tackle drainage: see letter to the editor from P. Q., a Parishioner, *Taunton Courier*, January 9, 1833, 7.

41. This question had several different aspects, including the appropriate distribution of charges between present and future beneficiaries and between owners and occupiers: Hamlin, *Public Health and Social Justice*, 255.

42. This was not an uncommon issue: Lyon Playfair, "Report on the Sanatory Condition of the Large Towns in Lancashire, in Second Report of the Commissioners for inquiring into the State of Large Towns and Populous Districts, Appendix, Part II, PP 1845 (610), paragraphs 8–10, 16–19.

43. Hart, *History of Cheltenham*, 282, 303. There is no indication that Cheltenham's elites were altruistically concerned about the health of the people. Cheltenham was already a fashionable location, and local promoters must have recognized that its salubrity was an important part of its appeal. Such concerns inspired public dissatisfaction with the private water supply: Hamlin, "Muddling in Bumbledom," 71–72.

44. An Act for better paving, lighting, cleansing, watching and improving the Town of Cheltenham &c. (1821), 1 & 2 Geo. 4, c. cxxi. Raising debt levels was a common and sometimes locally alarming occurrence: Jones and Falkus, "Urban Improvement," 139–40; Webb and Webb, *Statutory Authorities*, 273.

45. An Act for the better Sewerage, cleansing, and draining of the Town of Cheltenham in the County of Gloucester (1833), 3 Will. 4, c. xxi. Thus the law entitled the company to an annual rent charge only from customers voluntarily wishing to drain into some new sewer it constructed (s. 26). Any party already draining into any existing sewer that the company took over was allowed to continue to drain into it without charge, but the company did not have to maintain the drain (s. 29). The street commissioners could order any property not connected to the sewers to connect if they deemed that property to be a nuisance or a danger to health (s. 46). This provision presumably reassured the subscribers to the stock that their sewers would not go wanting. In addition, the cost of the service was modeled on a rent charge for water, with houses paying a rate based on their valuation (s. 43).

46. The *House of Lords Journal* does not record that the bill was opposed.

47. Cheltenham's act is an example of Millward's contention that anxiety over monopoly market position did not necessarily lead to public ownership but could instead mean public control. See Millward, "Political Economy," 325.

48. As it turned out, individuals were reluctant to pay for the privilege: see Report by John Maurice Herbert and Thomas Page on the Cheltenham Waterworks Bill, in Copies of Reports, PP 1847 (124–31), v; Minutes of Evidence, in Copies of Reports PP 1847 (124–31), q. 261. The Improvement Commission took over the company in 1857: W. Ranger to GBH, August 11, 1857, MH/13/49, NA for approval of purchase.

49. This was quite common: D. Fraser, *Urban Politics*, 28–29.

50. *Cheltenham Chronicle*, January 26, 1832, 3. See also *Cheltenham Journal*, January 23, 1832, 2. A correspondent to the *Cheltenham Chronicle* expressed approval, noting that the expense would fall only on those using the sewer: "Common Sewer," *Cheltenham Chronicle*, November 8, 1832, 3.

51. The unelected commissioners were a target of political reformers and later Chartists in Cheltenham. The commissioners' unwillingness to reform their constitution doomed their attempt to obtain a fresh act in 1839: Hart, *History of Cheltenham*, 309–13. The online index of the *Cheltenham Examiner* records Chartist meetings in 1839–40. For scattered references to Cheltenham and Chartism, see Chase, *Chartism*; D. Thompson, *Chartists*.

52. Select Committee hearings on Cheltenham local bills in 1851 and 1852 repeatedly state that the worst houses had no drainage and that the company had drained only the well-to-do neighborhoods: Select Committee on 1851 Cheltenham Improvement Bill (Commons), May 19, 1851, p. 52; May 27, 1851, p. 42 (C. Paul), HC/CL/PB/2/19/42 Parliamentary Archives (PA); Select Committee on Cheltenham Improvement Bill (Lords), May 12, 1852, p. 11 (Dr. W. Brooks); p. 17 (Charles Paul), HL/PO/PB/5/18/1, PA.

53. Both towns were early petitioners to adopt the Public Health Act: Clark, *Report . . . on the Borough of Taunton*; Cresy, *Report on . . . the Town of Cheltenham*. Cheltenham's situation is discussed at greater length in chapter 3.

54. These issues were raised in particular at Cheltenham when the Water Company obtained a new act in 1847; Herbert and Page on the Cheltenham Waterworks Bill, in Copies of reports, PP 1847 (124–31). See also Daunton, "Taxation and Representation," 107–10; Jenner, "Monopoly, Markets and Public Health."

55. Minutes of Evidence, in Copies of Reports, PP 1847 (124–30), 7–9.

56. The local promoters of this bill decided to insert a special clause stipulating that the "arterial" (or main) drains should be paid for with a districtwide rate. See Select Committee on Cheltenham Improvement Bill (Lords), May 11, 1852, pp. 21–25 (G. Williams), HL/PO/PB/5/18/1, PA; Select Committee on Cheltenham Improvement Bill (Commons), March 17, 1852, pp. 296–300 (John Bubb), March 18, 1852, pp. 135–36 (Charles Paul), HC/CL/PB/2/20/5, PA. See the Cheltenham Improvement Act, 15 Vict., c. l, s. cxiii.

57. Select Committee on Cheltenham Improvement Bill (Lords), May 12, 1852, pp. 138–40 (Admiral Lloyd); p. 162 (Charles Jones), HL/PO/PB/5/18/1, PA. Williams defended the decision in 1852; Select Committee on Cheltenham Improvement Bill (Lords), May 11, 1852, pp. 101–2 (G. Williams), HL/PO/PB/5/18/1, PA.

58. During an 1847 inquiry at Cheltenham, when government agents observed that few people had connected properties to the company's sewers, the agents claimed it was "not an unfrequent [*sic*] consequence of sewers being in the hands of a Company." Their comment suggests some wider familiarity with this situation: Report . . . on the Cheltenham Waterworks Bill, in Copies of Reports, PP 1847 (124–31), v. Tunbridge also had a main sewer paid for by public subscription: Royal Sanitary Commission, First Report, PP 1868–69 (4218), q. 3544.

59. Allen-Emerson, *Sanitary Engineering*, xii; Halliday, *Great Stink*, 29; Hamlin, "Edwin Chadwick and the Engineers."

60. On early postwar development in the West End, see F. H. W. Sheppard, *London, 1808–1870*, 112–16, 255. See also Benidickson, *Culture of Flushing*, 78–79; Halliday, *Great Stink*, 42–46.

61. The various metropolitan commissioners of sewers followed several strategies for increasing their revenue: Hanley, "Metropolitan Commissioners."

62. The casebook (WCS/740, LMA) contains fifty-four sequentially numbered cases and six unnumbered legal matters. The cases span the period 1760 to 1845, but only two date from before 1800 and only four from before 1810. The vast majority of the cases date to the postwar period, with spikes in 1817–22 and 1831–33. The early postwar period was evidently a time of great initiative by the commissioners. Although several of the cases were related to actions for liability for damage, they too were a by-product of the aggressive pattern of building that the commission engaged in at this time.

63. For some indication of the WCS's increased activity at this time, see Sunderland, "Monument to Defective Administration?"

64. The Westminster Commission had three districts, and within the Ranelagh district three further levels: Opinion of Mr. Serjeant Taddy upon the Different Forms of Proceedings used in the Office of the Commissioners (case 6), p. 16, WCS/740, LMA. The decision to divide the Ranelagh district into three parts, with land and houses separately rated in each, was taken before any legal controversy began: Orders of Court, May 16, 1817, WCS/65, LMA. Most but not all metropolitan commissions were divided up into several distinct divisions, or levels, as they were often called. In 1834, Tower Hamlets had eight levels and the Westminster Commission four. These levels, which did not necessarily concern elevation, usually maintained separate accounts with the commissions. Ratepayers in one level were not usually called on to pay expenses for works incurred in another level (although establishment charges were paid by rates levied on all levels). In theory, at least, levels were meant to be physically distinct lines of sewers. Often the system of the commission had grown up in such a fashion that levels or lines of sewers were physically distinct from each other: Select Committee on Metropolis Sewers, PP 1834 (584), qq. 59, 654.

65. Case as to the Liability of the Inhabitants of this Parish for Payment of Sewers Rates (case 18), WCS/740, LMA.

66. Case 18, WCS/740, LMA. Opinions dated late 1817.

67. Minutes, February 20, 1818, WCS/65, LMA.

68. Case and Opinion of Sir Robert Gifford as to the liability of the Inhabitants of Paddington to be Assessed to the Ranelagh Sewers (case 16), WCS/740, LMA. The commissioners did not stipulate what made sewers a common nuisance, but the law of nuisance was very clear that nuisances did not have to be unhealthy to be nuisances. See, for example, "Thompson v. Harris," Times, September 13, 1816, 3; Rex v. Neil, 172 English Reports 219–20.

69. Masters against Scroggs, 105 English Reports 678–79.

70. Case and opinion of Mr. Richardson as to the liability of the Inhabitants of Paddington to be Assessed to the Ranelagh Sewers (case 17), opinion dated April 25, 1818, LMA/WCS/740.

71. Case 16, opinion dated August 17, 1818, WCS/740, LMA.

72. September 18, 1818, Papers Presented 1818, WCS/224, LMA.

73. Ann Stafford was the occupier of a previously unrated house, and in 1817 and 1819 she was rated for the Ranelagh sewer by the WCS. She declined to pay, the commissioners accordingly distrained some goods, and she sued for trespass (as was standard).

74. "Stafford v Hamston, Further case," p. 6, WCS/745, LMA.

75. Letter to Dean and Chapter, December 21, 1816, Letter Books 1811–17, WCS/431, LMA.

76. Hamlin, *More than Hot*, locs. 1979, 2083; Hardy, "Medical Response"; R. Porter, "Cleaning up the Great Wen."

77. Pickstone notes that there were very few cases of typhus in mainland Britain from 1802 until 1816: Pickstone, "Dearth, Dirt and Fever Epidemics," 141. Certainly the commissioners would have been aware of the typhus outbreaks in London, which were well reported in the *Times*, especially in late 1817 and early 1818. A select committee reported on contagious fever in the Metropolis in spring 1818: Select Committee on Contagious Fever in London, PP 1818 (322). On typhus in an earlier period, see Pickstone, "Ferriar's Fever"; Risse, "'Typhus' Fever." Typhus and typhoid fever were not consistently distinguished until later in the century. See Hamlin, *More than Hot*, chap. 6; Hardy, *Epidemic Streets*, 151–53, 191–95; L. G. Wilson, "Fevers and Science."

78. The literature on medical ideas of contagionism lies outside my primary interest but is highly developed. See, for example, Ackerknecht, "Anticontagionism"; Baldwin, *Contagion and the State*; Cooter, "Anticontagionism"; Pelling, *Cholera, Fever and English Medicine*; D. Porter, *Health, Civilization and the State*, 81–87. For other approaches, see Hamlin, *Cholera*, 150–79; Hamlin, "Predisposing Causes"; Hamlin, *Public Health and Social Justice*, 63–66, 110–20; Pickstone, "Dearth, Dirt and Fever Epidemics"; Pickstone, "Ferriar's Fever." Recent works include Brown, "From Foetid Air"; Hamlin, *More than Hot*, locs. 1918–58, 3152–62; Kelly, "Not From the College."

79. Hamlin, *Public Health and Social Justice*, 63.

80. Select Committee on Contagious Fever in London, PP 1818 (322). The commissioners probably did not glean this belief from readily available sources such as the *Times*, which consistently published contagionist analyses at this time: "Typhus Fever," *Times*, October 1, 1817, 3; November 7, 1818, 3; "Contagious Fever," *Times*, July 24, 1818, 2.

81. An 1817 report to the WCS on the King's Scholars' Pond Sewer by four independent surveyors noted that the scouring of the sewers was essential for carrying off "all infectious Filth to which the Health of the Metropolis is so much attributed": Report of Daniel A. Alexander, Benjamin Bevan, John Farey, Senior, and Ralph Walker, June 24, 1817, p. 11, Papers Presented 1817, WCS 223, LMA.

82. "Stafford v Hamston, Instructions, Mr. Serj't Taddy to advise," n.d., WCS/745, LMA. I have not been able to locate this letter, but presumably it refers to William Wilberforce.

83. The Westminster Commissioners did not refer to miasma or effluvia in their briefs, only to unwholesome exhalations, suggesting a lack of medically informed advice. In addition, in a document containing questions that the commissioners proposed asking of witnesses, the two medical questions were answered, and were intended to be answered, by their surveyor: "Stafford v Hamston, Instructions, Mr. Serj't Taddy to advise," n.d., WCS/745, LMA.

84. Hamlin, *Public Health and Social Justice*, 119, draws attention to the locally universalizing character of this model of disease.

85. Jones and Falkus, "Urban Improvement." The WCS's silence with respect to the working classes or the poor is surprising. Presumably the obvious corollary of their miasmatic position that everyone potentially could be affected was not so

obvious, or perhaps the commissioners were still inclined to focus on their role in protecting property rather than people. Parliament investigated the provision of hospital care for the poor sick from typhus at some length. Typhus was part of a much wider crisis around the Poor Law during the postwar period, with expenditure peaking in London and across the country. In response, Parliament passed in 1818 an act to permit the removal of Irish unsettled poor, a major category of expense in some metropolitan parishes, and another act to provide funds for public works, again to relieve the rates. The Society for the Suppression of Mendicity was also founded in 1818. See Brundage, *English Poor Laws*, 44–52; Green, *Pauper Capital*, 9, 26–27, 30, 43–45; Hobsbawm and Rude, *Captain Swing*, 76.

86. "Stafford v Hamston, Instructions, Mr. Serj't Taddy to advise," n.d., WCS/745, LMA.

87. Taddy noted that the only thing that "medical gentlemen" would be allowed to testify to was the general unhealthiness of the stagnation of waters, and that was sufficiently well known. Presumably they would not be permitted to make claims about typhus or other diseases: "Stafford v Hamston, Instructions, Mr. Serj't Taddy to advise" Taddy's response appears to be dated October 3, 1821.

88. Court of Common Pleas, Stafford ver. Hamston, February 19, 1822, p. 28, WCS/745, LMA. The role of medical and scientific participation in court at this time is dealt with in Fullmer, "Technology, Chemistry and the Law"; Golan, "History of Scientific Expert Testimony." For a later period, see, among others, Burney, "Poisoning of No Substance"; Hamlin, "Scientific Method." Golan and Fullmer show that as early as 1820, disillusionment with science in the courtroom had already set in.

89. Perhaps, notwithstanding Hullock, the jury saw the facts as materially different and thought that Stafford benefited in more than a trivial way. But even the commissioners did not argue that, instead stressing that the quantum of benefit, even if insensible, did not matter, only the fact of it: Court of Common Pleas, Stafford ver. Hamston, February 19, 1822, p. 29, WCS/745, LMA.

90. Hullock claimed that Stafford derived no more benefit from the commissioners' works than any house in an elevated situation derived from the simple fact that water always found its level and, almost invariably, ultimately ran into a sewer somewhere. In his closing remarks, Hullock argued that if the jury found for the commissioners instead of for Stafford, then *Masters v. Scroggs* had been decided erroneously and thus every house in London would be liable to the sewers rate: Court of Common Pleas, Stafford ver. Hamston, February 19, 1822, pp. 60–65, especially p. 65, WCS/745, LMA.

91. Select Committee on Sewers in the Metropolis, PP 1823 (542), 49.

92. Select Committee on Sewers in the Metropolis, PP 1823 (542), 37–49, especially 39.

93. J. W. Unwin, the Tower Hamlets clerk, also noted that undrained land was a cause of pestilence: Select Committee on Sewers in the Metropolis, PP 1823 (542), 6. That the commissioners were increasingly seen as instruments of disease prevention was made clear in "Public Sewers," *Times*, August 30, 1823, 3: "This subject, so important to the cleanliness and health of the metropolis . . . Some legislative measure on a subject so important to the health of the metropolis."

94. There was some doubt about the commissioners' legal ability to build new works. In 1807, the commissioners instructed counsel to insert a clause in their new

local act unambiguously giving them this power: Case for the opinion of Mr. Wood as to the Power of the Commissioners to make New Sewers and to Alter and Divert the Course of Ancient Sewers (case 14), WCS/740, LMA. The 1807 local act appeared to give clear power to the commissioners to do so. However, for whatever reason, the commissioners did not attempt to take the power up until 1822, and the issue arose at that time only for new streets. As the commissioners noted, builders of houses in new streets usually built and paid for the sewers themselves, and the commissioners took them over once they were complete. In 1822, after what appears to have been significant debate, the commissioners resolved that for new streets and lanes, they would assume the responsibility of building sewers themselves. They asked counsel if they could do so and if they could charge for it. The commissioners were advised by two counsels not to assume the responsibility themselves: Case for the Opinion of Mr. Serjeant Lens as to the Legality of the Commissioners . . . Building . . . New Additional Sewers (case 11); Similar Case for Mr Marryatt (case 12), WCS/740, LMA. These cases were resent in 1841.

95. For a discussion of London's comparatively low mortality during the 1831–32 epidemic and the work of the metropolitan commissioners, see Durey, *Return of the Plague*, 53–59.

96. This clearly was a not uncommon idea at the time. We have already noted Liverpool's 1830 act.

97. See, for example, Board of Health, St Marylebone to WCS, Extract from a Report made by the Committee appointed by the Vestry of the Parish of St Mary le Bone, November 23, 1831, Papers Presented July–December 1831, WCS/248, LMA; Extract from the Reports of the Committees Respecting the Want of Proper Sewage in the Parishes of St Margaret and St John the Evangelist Westminster, read December 9, 1831, ibid.

98. Letter to Board of Health of Parishes of St Margaret and Saint John Westminster, January 24, 1832, Letters 1830–34, WCS/435, LMA.

99. Case for the Opinion of Mr. Serjeant Andrews upon . . . giving Authority to the Commissioners "to Order and Direct" the making of New Sewers (case 19), WCS/740, LMA. Opinion dated November 25, 1831.

100. In situations such as this, the commissioners typically split the cost of a new sewer with the owners of property, but the principal owners, the Mercers' Company, would not cooperate, and the commissioners needed to find some way to pay for the works: "Westminster Court of Sewers," *Builder*, July 10, 1847, 330. The rationale for the commissioners' contribution was that often parties had been contributing to the sewers rate for many years before they actually had a sewer into which they could drain, and it was only just that they should not be called on to pay the full cost when they had uncomplainingly paid rates for so long: Select Committee on Metropolis Sewers, PP 1834 (584), 33–34 (City of London), 93–94 (Surrey and Kent); P. J. Smith, "Before Bazalgette," 141.

101. Case for the Opinion of Mr. Serjeant Andrews as to who should be at the Expense of Building a Sewer in Long Acre (case 20), WCS/740, LMA. Opinion dated December 8, 1831.

102. Case for the Opinion of Mr. Campbell upon . . . giving Authority to the Commissioners "to Order and Direct" the making of New Sewers (case 21), WCS/740, LMA. Opinion dated December 28, 1831. Campbell became Chief

Justice of the Queen's Bench in 1850 and took part in crucial local board of health decisions. When he used the term *district*, presumably he meant the level, rather than the commission as a whole. On Campbell, see G. H. Jones and V. Jones, "Campbell, John."

103. Case for the Opinion of the Attorney General upon . . . giving Authority to the Commissioners "to Order and Direct" the making of New Sewers (case 22); A Similar Case for the Opinion of the Solicitor General (case 22), WCS/740, LMA. Joint opinion dated January 27, 1832. In 1833, Parliament passed a new General Sewers Act, which gave local boards explicit power to build new works. The commissioners hoped to make use of these powers, but they were again advised by the Solicitor General and the Attorney General that the act did not apply to them: Case for the Opinion of the Attorney General and the Solicitor General as to Whether the Saving Clause . . . Exempts the Commissioners . . . from the Operation of that Act (case 39), WCS/740, LMA. The Westminster Commission obtained a local act in 1834, though its sole purpose was to permit construction of a sewer in Bayswater. Even in this limited act, we can see the commission's deliberate strategy, intended to capture all property in the district. The act stipulated that all property in certain named parishes that "in any way benefited" (4 & 5 Will. 4, c. xcvi, s. 6) from the sewer would be liable. The Westminster commissioners' experience with *Stafford v. Hamston* undoubtedly made this clarification imperative.

104. The commission had a small number of ancient, decayed sewers that they could order repaired, simultaneously extending, deepening, and rerouting them. There were limits to the possible extent of this remaking.

105. Surveyor's Report, September 2, 1831, Papers Presented July–December 1831, WCS/248, LMA.

106. Select Committee on Metropolitan Improvements, PP 1836 (517), q. 290.

107. Sanitary matters were now clearly on the agenda; the Poor Law Commission sent a circular on the matter to the Greater London vestries in April 1838: Hamlin, *Public Health and Social Justice*, 108.

108. Report on the Portions of the District, Densely Inhabited by the Poorer Orders, January 15, 1839, WCS/881, LMA. Sixteen were noted as completed by January 1842.

109. Based on An Account of all Sums Rated by the Commissioners of Sewers for the City and Liberty of Westminster, PP 1822 (493).

110. Select Committee on Metropolitan Improvements, PP 1836 (517), 30; Hamlin, *Public Health and Social Justice*, 149, 241.

111. As in most European nation-states at this time, the British national and local governments were already involved to some degree in protecting the community against disease through, for example, quarantine. The national state also supported a variety of medical initiatives, many of which had the poor as their primary focus. The National Vaccine Establishment received support from the national state: Brunton, *Politics of Vaccination*, 14–16. The 1818 Select Committee on fever noted that Parliament gave £1,000 to the London Fever Hospital and proposed giving another £2,000: Select Committee on Contagious Fever in London, PP 1818 (322), 5, 7. Ireland was the subject of a number of provisions whereby Parliament granted local taxation powers for health (usually institutional provision) or in some cases provided direct support. For brief statements of some key measures see Nicholls,

History of the Irish Poor Law, 73–78; Hamlin, "Predisposing Causes," 59–62; Select Committee on Contagious Fever in Ireland, PP 1818 (285); Second Report from the Select Committee on Contagious Fever in Ireland, PP 1818 (359). Hamlin discusses the distinctiveness of Irish medicine's understanding of fever in *More than Hot*, locs. 1825–1913, 3133–3248. And of course the Poor Law raised funds at the local level for medical care of paupers. See, for example, Siena, "Hospitals for the Excluded or Convalescent Homes?" 17–18. On the state and health, see D. Porter, *Health, Civilization and the State.*

112. See, for example, Board of Health, St Marylebone to WCS, Extract from a Report made by the Committee appointed by the Vestry of the Parish of St Mary le Bone, November 23, 1831, Papers Presented July–December 1831, WCS/248, LMA; Extracts from the Reports of the Committees Respecting the Want of Proper Sewage in the Parishes of St Margaret and St John the Evangelist Westminster, read December 9, 1831, ibid. These voluntary committees were created because no official body existed that could be charged with responsibility for managing the epidemic at the local level. The voluntary committees were responsible for managing the local response to the epidemic, which mainly entailed the acquisition or very rarely the construction of adequate temporary hospital space, of which there was very little at the time, and the provision of medical and material support for sufferers unable to pay for it themselves. On local efforts during this outbreak, see Durey, *Return of the Plague*, 78–100.

113. Durey, *Return of the Plague*, 140–50, 154. For the early course of events in one northern town, see Morris, *Cholera, 1832*, 39–57.

114. The tension between individual and environmental approaches was apparent in the letters to the commissioners. The Committee for St Margaret and St John argued "that the want of a proper sewage appears to them to be one of the greatest & most lamentable obstacles to the ultimate improvement of the comforts of the poor." They agreed that "the inhabitants are of a class that cannot be expected to pay the same attention" to cleanliness as did other classes. Yet this committee noted as well that the "grievances in this District are such as it is not in the power of the Inhabitants to remedy," and they recommended that the government be approached: Extracts from the Reports of the Committees Respecting the Want of Proper Sewage in the Parishes of St Margaret and St John the Evangelist Westminster, read December 9, 1831, Papers Presented July–December 1831, WCS/248, LMA.

115. This period reminds us, as did chapter 1, that cholera had more effects than are sometimes suggested. Sigsworth, "Cholera in the Large Towns" charts the response after 1832. My argument complements Sigsworth's. The discourse, theory, and practice of filth underwent significant changes at this time: see Crook, "Putting Matter in Its Right Place"; Hamlin, "Public Sphere to Public Health"; Hanley, "Bye Laws, the Environment, and Health before Chadwick." Michael Brown argues that cholera "provided a focus around which new forms of medical identity and activity coalesced." See Brown, *Performing Medicine*, 152; Gilbert, *Cholera and Nation*. For more pessimistic assessments of cholera's effects in 1831–32, see Barnet, "The 1832 Cholera Epidemic," 37; Durey, *Return of the Plague*, 204; Kidd and Wyke, "The Cholera Epidemic," 56.

116. Extracts from the Charge delivered by the Chairman, Thomas Leverton Donaldson, Esq., to a jury Summoned to make Presentments on the Ranelagh and

Counters Creek Districts, on the 8th of April, 1842, p. 3, WCS/782, LMA. On property and cholera, see Kearns, "Cholera, Nuisances and Environmental Management"; Kearns, "Private Property and Public Health."

117. Case for the Opinion of the Attorney General upon . . . giving Authority to the Commissioners "to Order and Direct" the making of New Sewers (case 22); A Similar Case for the Opinion of the Solicitor General (case 22), WCS/740, LMA.

118. Indeed, at the beginning of the epidemic, a representative of the WCS had an audience with the Under-Secretary of State, George Lamb, about newspaper allegations that the commissioners were not doing their duty. After hearing the commissioners' side of the story, Lamb asked if Parliament could help. The offer was declined, although the suggestion was made that in a new metropolitan building act, builders should be forced to provide sewers for their houses: Memorandum, November 8, 1831, Papers Presented July–December 1831, WCS/248, LMA. It is not clear who was at the meeting, but anyone other than the Chair would be surprising. This interview took place early in the epidemic and before the commissioners confronted the drainage of Long Acre. One wonders what they would have wanted had they been interviewed after receiving the Law Officers' opinions in January.

119. The WCS did not give notice for this bill in late 1846, as the Standing Orders required, though the Commons voted to waive the Standing Orders and allow the bill in: *House of Commons Journal*, cii, March 26, 1847, 283. As a result, the bill did not pass through the Preliminary Inquiry procedure described later in this chapter. The government did not oppose the bill: "Westminster Court of Sewers," *Builder*, May 29, 1847, 258.

120. The 1847 Act (10 & 11 Vict., c. lxx) permitted the commissioners to order private property drained even if it was unconnected with any public street if they decided it was necessary for the health of the district (s. 20). It also gave the commissioners power to suppress nuisances such as stagnant ponds, even if unconnected with their works, if they were "likely to be prejudicial to Health" (s. 25). Both sections (ss. 20 and 25) required the presentment of the jury, making the process somewhat akin to a common-law conviction for public nuisance. The section dealing with nuisances was obviously predated by the 1846 Nuisances Removal Act, but the WCS 1847 act was the outcome of a long period of agitation by the commissioners. The WCS statutory health concern was anticipated by seventeen years in Liverpool, as we saw in chapter 1. We can see here the WCS moving toward a notion of what Hamlin has called cholera citizenship: Hamlin, *Cholera*, 95, 104, 145.

121. The relevant clause (s. 17) allowed the commissioners to rate parties "receiving Benefit or avoiding Damage" from the sewers. Given that the 1847 act explicitly kept all previous sewers statutes in force, including 23 Hen. 8, c. 5, the commissioners may also have decided not to vary the traditional wording.

122. Hanley, "Metropolitan Commissioners."

123. I make this claim on the basis of the clauses in the bill and the solicitors' report on them. Of course, the bill governed the drainage of new streets and houses, but the solicitors' report on these sections was mainly concerned with ensuring adequate publicity and avoiding conflict with builders and developers: Report of Solicitors with Forms, &c., July 15, 1847, WCS/756/108, LMA.

124. Draft of a Bill, s. 8, WCS/756/96, LMA. The act changed this provision to allow the commissioners to distribute the costs to the districts or levels in which the

sewer was located only; 10 & 11 Vict., c. lxx, s. 10. In the two clauses involving health hazards, the bill and the act also empowered the commissioners to distribute the costs of the work onto the district or level in which it was situated.

125. This concern was not uncommon among places contemplating sewerage. See, for two examples, "Special Meeting of the Leeds Town Council," *Leeds Mercury*, December 11, 1847, 7; St Pancras Vestry Minutes, July 13, 1857, Camden Local Studies Library.

126. Report of Solicitors, July 15, 1847, pp. 2, 13, WCS/756/108, LMA.

127. The commissioners had repeatedly presented proposals to the principal owner of houses fronting the street, the Mercers' Company, but the company had been unwilling to cooperate at all. See Report on the Portions of the District, Densely Inhabited by the Poorer Orders, January 15, 1839, WCS/881, LMA. The day the 1847 act received royal assent, the commissioners discussed the drainage in Long Acre: "Westminster Court of Sewers," *Builder*, July, 10 1847, 330. A coroner's inquest on a death in a court off the street later in the month triggered a recommendation that the surveyor report on the district: "Westminster Court of Sewers," *Builder*, August 28, 1847, 414. The surveyor's report triggered further debate, primarily because of disputes over the mode of payment for the sewer and house drains that the commissioners believed necessary. The surveyor was ordered to prepare plans, but the solicitors were asked to advise on various options for payment: "Proceedings of the Westminster Commissioners of Sewers," *Builder*, October 2, 1847, 473.

128. "Report of the Solicitors," October 15, 1847, p. 2, WCS/756/109, LMA.

129. This controversial conclusion at least had the merit of eventually suggesting a solution. By the early 1840s, Chadwick had arrived at the arterial system, linking high-pressure, constant water supplies to the flushing away of urban waste and the eventual irrigation of the countryside.

130. For the move to legislation, see Finer, *Life and Times*; Hamlin, *Public Health and Social Justice*; Lewis, *Edwin Chadwick*. For a political perspective, see Mandler, *Aristocratic Government*; Prest, *Liberty and Locality*.

131. Second Report of the HOTC, PP 1845 (602), 28–30.

132. Second Report of the HOTC, PP 1845 (602), 16–19.

133. Second Report of the HOTC, PP 1845 (602), 16, 24–25.

134. A Bill for the Improvement of the Sewerage and Drainage of Towns and Populous Districts, PP 1845 (574). This bill was not intended to pass but merely to generate discussion.

135. A Bill for the Improvement of the Sewerage, PP 1845 (574), ss. 126, 260. For paving and general purposes, the inspector was not empowered to divide the district. The local commissioners, however, were, but their decision to divide the district for other purposes required the sanction of the central inspector (s. 259).

136. A Bill for the Improvement of the Sewerage, PP 1845 (574), ss. 260, 253.

137. See, for example, the Sunderland bills submitted for the 1847 session; Report by J. J. Rawlinson and William Hosking, iii, in Copies of Reports, PP 1847 (124–48).

138. Finer, *Life and Times*, 295–96 describes Chadwick's involvement in the Parliamentary Select Committee but says nothing about the act. Brundage, *England's "Prussian Minister,"* 108–9, notes that Chadwick tried to use the Select Committee on Private Bills to the advantage of the Towns Improvement Company.

139. J. W. Philipps to D. Horne, December 12, 1846, December 18, 1846, Works 3/9, NA. The surveying officers took evidence locally and reported to the Office of Woods and Forests, which made the reports and the evidence on which they were based available to Parliament. Normally these reports were short, but the accompanying evidence, printed in whole for the first year of operation, could be quite substantial. The reports to Woods and Forests ran to more than five thousand pages. The town of Reading's improvement bill alone generated more than five hundred pages of evidence, though many improvement acts ran to fewer than one hundred pages (excluding water and gas bills). So voluminous was the evidence that after the first year Parliament printed only an abstract of the evidence in addition to the report.

140. Local Acts: Preliminary Inquiries, PP 1847 (33). There were separate sections for waterworks, drainage, gas works, paving, and sundry other matters. The drainage section imposed significant burdens on local promoters in terms of surveys and maps, among other things, and caused some alarm in some places.

141. De la Beche was one of the commissioners of the 1843–45 Royal Commission on the State of Large Towns. "Mr. Page" probably was Thomas Page, C. E., a successful engineer (see S. Smith, "Page, Thomas") and one of Woods and Forests' surveying officers. He later reported on the Croydon drainage: Hamlin, *Public Health and Social Justice*, 326–28. Hertslet was the Chief Clerk of the Westminster Commission of Sewers. He proposed to consult with John Roe, surveyor to the Holborn & Finsbury Commission of Sewers, although Roe's indisposition apparently prevented his participation: J. W. Philipps to Lewis Hertslet, November 18, 1846; Hertslet to Philipps, November 28, 1846, December 24, 1846, Works 3/9, NA. It is possible that other parties not represented in the surviving letter books were consulted, but it does not appear that Chadwick was consulted. He wrote to Woods and Forests asking for copies of the questionnaires: Works 3/9, January 4, 1847. It is interesting that apparently no medical men were consulted about the design, considering that questions were asked about health, nuisances, and unwholesome effluvia: Local Acts: Preliminary Inquiries, Special Instructions to the Surveying Officers, PP 1847 (33), section I-B, (i) qq. 5, 22, 27, 32.

142. Hertslet also queried the mode of rating: whether it would be based on frontage or net annual value. See extracts from Hertslet's letter of November 26, 1846; p. 48, Works/3/9, NA.

143. Suggestions by Mr. Page, p. 66, Works 3/9, NA.

144. Local Acts: Preliminary Inquiries, Special Instructions to the Surveying Officers, PP 1847 (33), section I-B, (i) q. 17; (ii) qq. 16, 22. There was no specific query relating to the rating of land, only premises and houses.

145. The preliminary inquiry procedure, as it turned out, did not answer the purposes for which it was intended. In 1851, Parliament removed the requirement for Woods and Forests to report on local bills but transferred some local bill oversight to the Admiralty, due to concerns with navigation at some locations: Brundage, *England's "Prussian Minister,"* 109; Clifford, *History of Private Bill Legislation*, 2:890–97.

146. The best treatment of this subject is Prest, *Liberty and Locality*.

147. 10 & 11 Vict., c. 34, ss. 23, 162.

148. 10 & 11 Vict., c. 34, s. 167.

149. Standing orders of the House required that local notice of bills be given in November and December. The 1847 bills thus had to be drafted by late 1846.

150. My use of the term *elites* derives from an assumption that Parliament expected local leaders to be the primary promoters of local legislative change and from the fact that only bills with such support were seriously examined. The Heywood local bill, for example, was promoted by a local Chartist but was abandoned, at surveying officer instigation, almost immediately: Copies of Reports, PP, 1847 (124–25). The term *local elite* is not meant to imply local elite unity or anything about the social and economic profile of such local leadership. On middle-class local divisions, see D. Fraser, *Power and Authority*; D. Fraser, *Urban Politics*. For a review of the literature on urban elites, see J. Smith, "Urban Elites."

151. The legislative framework for bills prepared for the truncated 1847–48 session was not significantly different. The government's Public Health Bill was not introduced until later in the session, and parties likely believed that the government would not pass a bill significantly different from the 1847 Towns Improvement Clauses Act.

152. A word about the choices I made here: of the eighty-six bills examined in 1847 under the Preliminary Inquiries Act, I have selected those that were identified as improvement bills. Because I am particularly interested in the drainage provisions, I omitted those concerned with gas, railroads, harbors, and even waterworks. I included sixteen bills in the sample, not all of which are discussed below.

153. Local Acts: Preliminary Inquiries, Special Instructions to the Surveying Officers, PP 1847 (33), section I-B, (ii) qq. 7, 8 assume possible corporate involvement.

154. But see Leeds, below.

155. Minutes of Evidence on the Bingley Improvement Bill, in Copies of Reports, PP 1847 (124–51), q. 497. Barr reiterated the point in a follow-up question.

156. Minutes of Evidence on the Rochdale Improvement Bill, in Copies of Reports, PP 1847 (124–26), q. 321. See also q. 369.

157. Minutes of Evidence on the Colchester Navigation and Improvement Bill, in Copies of Reports, PP, 1847 (124–50), q. 565.

158. Copies of Reports for the Commissioners of Woods and Forests relative to Applications for Local Acts, PP, 1847 (124). At Tunstall (Report no. 51), where the main issue was police, Charles Devenport, surgeon, appeared (qq. 712–40). At Bingley (Report no. 52), three surgeons testified: Henry Thomas (qq. 208–47, 265–86), George Dryden (qq. 287–306, 353–59), and John Dickson (qq. 307–28). At Lytham (Report no. 6), Mr. Houghton, surgeon, testified (qq. 78–81). At Blackburn (report no. 7), Thomas Dugdale, surgeon, testified (qq. 126–50). At Rochdale (Report no. 26), no medical man appeared as far as can be ascertained. At Saint Ives (Report no. 44) two appeared: John Leigh, "medical man" (qq. 338–93), and George Lonsdale Gurling, surgeon (qq. 465–512). At Sunderland (Report no. 48), William Mordey, surgeon, appeared (qq. 1862–1958). At Reading (Report no. 45), admittedly a very unusual case, seven practitioners appeared. At Colchester (Report no. 50), David Morris, surgeon, appeared (qq. 713–28). Question numbers refer in each case to the Minutes of Evidence.

159. Special Instructions to the Surveying Officers, PP 1847 (33), section I-B, (i) qq. 5, 27, 32, (ii) q. 44 drew attention to health or effluvia. Other questions refer to nuisances.

160. This raises the question of why local elites were themselves convinced. I have not explored this question, taking the evidence presented by the facts of the bills for granted. For discussion of the means by which Dr. William Farr and the General Register Office made local converts and empowered local coalitions, see Lewes, "The GRO and the Provinces"; Szreter, "The GRO and the Public Health Movement."

161. At Saint Ives, George Lonsdale Gurling, surgeon, was initially questioned about personal safety at night, the improvement in town lighting being one of the important objects of the bill: Minutes of Evidence, in Copies of Reports, PP 1847(124–44), qq. 470–80.

162. Minutes of Evidence, in Copies of Reports, PP, 1847 (124–44), q. 375.

163. Minutes of Evidence, in Copies of Reports, PP 1847 (124–7), qq. 150, 137, 134.

164. Even where medical men appeared, the testimony of laymen was often directed to medical matters, as Saint Ives showed: Minutes of Evidence, in Copies of Reports, PP 1847 (124–44), qq. 196, 262, 336, 573.

165. Minutes of Evidence, in Copies of Reports, PP 1847 (124–30), qq. 334–36, 463.

166. Minutes of Evidence, in Copies of Reports, PP 1847 (124–6), qq. 78–81.

167. Minutes of Evidence, in Copies of Reports, PP 1847 (124–30), qq. 1276–1306 (Henry Sterry), 2066–2108 (William Baimbridge).

168. Hamlin, *Public Health and Social Justice*, 278–82. The Reading bill hearing is a notable counterexample. It was an extremely controversial local bill proposal, and the contending parties mobilized all their resources.

169. The Improvement Commissioners and Town Council of Sunderland submitted rival bills in 1847–48. One of the important differences between the bills concerned the boundaries of the district: Copies of Reports, PP 1847 (124–48).

170. There were a variety of other exemptions as well, such as church and charitable property.

171. Thus Tunstall's act (10 & 11 Vict., c. cclii, s. 35) rated certain lands at one third net annual rateable value, Saint Ives (10 & 11 Vict., c. cclvi, s. 28) at one fifth. In Bingley's (10 & 11 Vict., c. cclviii, s. 32) and Blackburn's (10 & 11 Vict., c. cclv, s. 59) acts, certain lands were rated at two thirds net annual value, well above the Health of Towns Bill's one quarter and the Towns Improvement Clauses Act's one third.

172. The Leeds Town Council should have been able to construct all the drains it desired under its 1842 Act, but progress on the drainage was slow. Derek Fraser noted that technical difficulties were at the root of the problem. No fewer than four different reports on the drainage of the town were put forward at the time: Fraser, *Power and Authority*, 64–65. See also Wohl, *Endangered Lives*, 104–5. Technical complexity was a problem in a variety of locations: Burn, *Age of Equipoise*, 137; Hamlin, "Muddling in Bumbledom"; Luckin, "Pollution in the City," 213–17. Yet the Leeds council's final resolution of the technical debate by no means ended its problems, and once the technical debate was over, rating moved to the fore.

173. The Borough of Leeds was made up of eleven townships and four hamlets, each of which maintained its own poor and was financially distinct for various purposes: D. Fraser, "Areas of Urban Politics." (The 1842 Leeds act folded the hamlets

into the townships for rating purposes: see 5 & 6 Vict., c. civ, s. cccxxxvii.) The central townships to be drained were Holbeck, Hunslet, and Leeds.

174. Briggs, *Victorian Cities*, 142–43. In 1841, Hunslet and Holbeck were two of the poorest of twelve municipal wards in Leeds, ahead of only Leeds's eastern and northeastern wards: D. Fraser, "Areas of Urban Politics," 780; D. Fraser, *Urban Politics*, 217–19. On residential segregation in Leeds at mid-century, see D. Ward, "Environs and Neighbours."

175. "Leeds Town Council," *Leeds Mercury*, December 4, 1847, 11. There appears to have been some doubt as to the legality of the motion to seek a local act, and a special meeting of the council confirmed it: "Special Meeting of the Leeds Town Council," *Leeds Mercury*, December 11, 1847, 7. The special meeting added that owners of property in private streets should be spared the injustice of constructing sewers larger than necessary for their street.

176. Select Committee on Leeds Improvement Bill (Commons), April 7, 1848, HC/CL/PB/2/15/1, PA. Almost all the Select Committee's time was spent on the Calder and Aire Navigation.

177. H. Horn and A. Poynter, Report on the Huddersfield . . . Sewering Bill, in Report of the Commissioners, PP 1847–48 (135-19), 25–26. The 1848 Huddersfield act (11 & 12 Vict., c. cxl) itself was quite short, with most of the clauses coming from the various model clause acts it incorporated, but it explicitly allowed the Improvement Commission to subdivide the district for drainage purposes (s. 43). The newspaper report on the preliminary inquiry does not make explicit reference to this question: "Huddersfield Improvement Bill: Preliminary Inquiry," *Leeds Mercury*, February 12, 1848, 8.

178. The Taunton Market Trustees, as we have already seen, did not embrace sanitary reform with enthusiasm. Given what had transpired in Taunton, it is perhaps not surprising that some parties eventually stepped forward with a local bill to create a new body of commissioners. It is apparent from the hearing and the correspondence between the Office of Woods and Forests and the surveying officers that this bill was never going to have an easy passage. Taunton's bill was not returned from the Lords.

179. Minutes of Evidence, in Copies of Reports, PP 1847 (124–30), 77 (after q. 1539). Reeves drew attention to the fact that land was rated in other acts, although there was often a fixed distance beyond which it was not.

180. The inquiries at Huddersfield and Taunton (and at Leeds and in the Surrey and Kent Commission of Sewers examples discussed below) draw our attention to the way in which the surveying officers, emissaries of the central government, interpreted their brief. The preliminary inquiry procedure experiment was of such limited duration that it is difficult to generalize about surveying officers' importance, though they clearly were significant in particular instances. It is not clear to what extent this was a personal or political decision on their part. In terms of the subdivision issue under discussion here, their official instructions, the statutory environment (especially the 1847 Towns Improvement Clauses Act), and case law all pushed the barrister members, at least, in the same direction: toward subdivision.

181. Report on the Surrey and Kent Sewers Bill, in Copies of Reports, PP 1847 (124–61). The hearings lasted six days (from February 4 to February 13), in addition to tours of the district. The report was dated March 1, 1847. Henry Horn, a barrister, and James Walker, a civil engineer, presided: P. J. Smith, "Before Bazalgette,"

141. In addition, like all local acts, it was eligible for select committee hearings in Parliament, and both houses held hearings on it. The bill appeared before the House of Commons Select Committee on June 22, 1847, and before the Lords Select Committee on July 16, 1847. It received royal assent on July 22, 1847. The leading features of the Surrey and Kent Commission of Sewers bill are apparent from the Woods and Forests surveyors' report.

182. Dyos, *Victorian Suburb* covers an important, and as we shall see in chapter 4, litigious part of the commission, though his focus is on the later period. For his discussion of early nineteenth-century development, see pp. 36–50. In keeping with the view of his time, Dyos claimed that the Surrey and Kent Commissioners of Sewers discharged their duties with "quiet ineptitude" (140).

183. The half reduction pragmatically acknowledged that rating remote property at full value was a political nonstarter after 1846, especially given the rating provisions in the Towns Improvement Clauses Act and the Health of Towns Bill. The 1847 Westminster Commission of Sewers Act, in contrast, made no attempt to rate remote property, but the difference between the Surrey and Kent Commission's proposed bill and the 1847 Westminster Commission of Sewers Act partly related to the different topographical situation in Westminster. It too was a vast district, but its less-developed, outlying agricultural and rural areas did not drain into the central region, and the Westminster Commission of Sewers specifically reserved the right not to take up agricultural land until it saw fit. Its main concern was with the central part of the district. There was no novel general rate clause for Parliament to alter because the Westminster Commission of Sewers Bill adopted much of the 1833 general sewers law. That law, directed toward nonurban situations, gave owners of agricultural property a virtual veto over any new works, all such works requiring the consent of 75 percent of the property.

184. This was a long-standing concern for metropolitan commissions. The clerk of the Surrey and Kent Commission, Beriah Drew, and the surveyor, Joseph Gwilt, testified in 1834 that highlands in Camberwell benefited from the commissioners' works, and they stated that in justice they ought to be taxed: see Select Committee on Metropolis Sewers, PP 1834 (584), Drew, qq. 1294–97, 1364, 1489–93; Gwilt, ibid., qq. 1580–2. The Chair of the Holborn and Finsbury Commission testified (q. 225) that inhabitants in that commission's part of Hampstead benefited from the sewers, but "it is not such a benefit as the court . . . considered rendered them liable."

185. The integrated character of lowland and higher ground in the Surrey and Kent Commission of Sewers replayed the argument made in Liverpool in 1830, whereby all property owners were made to pay when new works needed to be constructed in the higher parts of the town: "Sewerage of the Town," *Liverpool Mercury*, September 25, 1829, 312.

186. Minutes of Evidence on the Surrey and Kent Sewers Bill, in Copies of Reports, PP 1847 (124–61). See, for example, qq. 25, 196, 259, 409, 668–74, 703–28, 755–61, 765, 779–87, 879–81, 1121–22, 1146–52, 1737, 1964–73, 2006, 2305.

187. Minutes of Evidence on the Surrey and Kent Sewers Bill, in Copies of Reports, PP 1847 (124–61). The medical witnesses were Henry Sterry, surgeon (qq. 1276–1306), and William Baimbridge, surgeon (qq. 2066–2108). Neither was particularly impressive. Baimbridge ended up arguing that bad drains may "produce any disease." The disease in question was ophthalmia (qq. 2100–2103).

188. Report by H. Horn and J. Walker on the Surrey and Kent Sewers Bill, in Copies of Reports, PP 1847 (124–61), vi, x–xi.

189. For the post-1846 context of taxation see, for example, the discussion in Offer, *Property and Politics*, 161–70.

190. Smith, "Urban Elites," 274–75. Colin Pooley stresses that even the residential segregation implicated in several of the boundary disputes was limited at mid-century; Pooley, "Patterns on the Ground," 438–39. Simon Szreter provides the best general explanation for the overall evolution of local services in the nineteenth century: Szreter, "Economic Growth," 702–7; see also Daunton, *Trusting Leviathan*, 265–73; Luckin, "The Metropolitan and the Municipal."

191. The bill had a number of controversial aspects; here I refer only to the territorial and financial expansion sought by the commission.

192. Report by H. Horn and J. Walker on the Surrey and Kent Sewers Bill, in Copies of Reports, PP 1847 (124–61), vi. For highland support, see Minutes of Evidence, qq. 676, 738, 770, 1264.

193. For an example of hostile questioning from riverside opponents, see Minutes of Evidence, in Copies of Reports, PP 1847 (124–61), qq. 1399–1403. Opposition often emerged in the context of parishioners' complaints that they had paid more than they had received in benefit: see, for example, qq. 631, p. 104. (Comments do not appear under any question but are between qq. 2318 and 2319.)

194. Horn and Walker explicitly rejected this claim: Report by H. Horn and J. Walker on the Surrey and Kent Sewers Bill, in Copies of Reports, PP 1847 (124–61), iv.

195. Minutes of Evidence, in Copies of Reports, PP 1847 (124–61), q. 1237.

196. Dyos and Reeder, "Slums and Suburbs," 381. Morris also argues that Victorian urban history was conditioned by the intensification of externalities and the collective measures to mitigate them: Morris, "Externalities"; Rodger, "Slums and Suburbs." Green makes a comparable argument with respect to metropolitan poor rates: Green, *Pauper Capital*.

197. F. M. L. Thompson, "Rise of Suburbia."

198. Select Committee on Metropolis Sewers, PP 1834 (584), 185. The committee returned to this issue in 1847. One commission's surveyor argued that many people who kept neither horse nor carriage paid the highway rates nonetheless: First Report of the Metropolitan Sanitary Commission, Minutes of Evidence, PP 1847–8 (895), 169. On highways, see Guldi, *Roads to Power*. In 1855, counsel for the Epsom Local Board of Health compared drainage rates with police rates, drawing attention to a service for which people were taxed but from which they benefited only indirectly, or perhaps directly but infrequently: "Surrey Quarter Sessions," *County Chronicle, Surrey Herald, and Weekly Advertiser*, April 10, 1855, 5. Epsom's case is discussed at length in chapter 3.

Chapter Three

1. Two older studies of boundaries in this period are Norton and Allworth, *Borough Boundaries*; Lipman, *Local Government Areas*.

2. Brock, *Great Reform Act*, 157–58; Gash, *Politics in the Age of Peel*, 66–77.

NOTES TO PP. 65–66 ❧ 177

3. A search for "boundary" at *Hansard* online (http://hansard.millbanksystems. com) generated only 134 hits before 1830. This is not to say that boundaries were not a concern of promoters of local acts, only that whatever concerns there were did not result in parliamentary debate. A search of the 1830s, in contrast, generated over six hundred hits (search conducted July 24, 2014).

4. The sense that the agricultural interest was shouldering an unfair burden lay at the root of the select committee hearings on county taxation in 1834: Select Committee on County Rates, PP 1834 (542); Select Committee of the House of Lords . . . into the Charges of the County Rates, PP 1835 (206).

5. By the 1880s, boundary making again acquired political significance as a result of further franchise reform and urban expansion: John Davis, "Central Government and the Towns," 261–86; Garrard, *Democratisation in Britain*, 95–96.

6. Gash, *Politics in the Age of Peel*, 67; Salmon, *Electoral Reform at Work*, 7. The making of poor-law union boundaries under the New Poor Law has received more attention. Anthony Brundage has shown how boundary making exposed the limits of central authority and the local politics of Poor Law reform. The New Poor Law permitted the formation of unions of parishes in order to achieve administrative and financial efficiencies. However, this reordering of the parochial landscape posed enormous challenges, requiring parishes to unite and cooperate on an unprecedented scale. Neither the Report of the Royal Commission on the Poor Laws nor the act itself provided instruction on how to do so. In order to provide some direction to the assistant commissioners responsible for forming unions, the Poor Law Commission developed guidelines suggesting that in rural areas, for example, unions would be most conveniently centered on the market town to which residents of surrounding parishes habitually resorted. In practice, as Brundage shows, the assistant commissioners had to take other factors into consideration, particularly the desire of local elites to manage union boundaries in accordance with their pattern of landholding. See Brundage, *Making of the New Poor Law*; Lipman, *Local Government Areas*, 42.

7. There was a lengthy Commons discussion of the boundary commissioners during the debate on the failed 1831 Reform Bill: *Hansard Parliamentary Debates*, 3rd ser., vol. 6 (September 1, 1831), cols. 982–1017. It was understood that enfranchisement required new boundaries, and boundary bills accompanied but were separate from the original reform bills. An appointed commission, including a small number of MPs, was created in 1832 to recommend borough boundaries.

8. Gash notes that the majority of new parliamentary borough boundaries were drawn for administrative convenience, but in order to ensure a sufficient number of electors, some boroughs encompassed very large tracts of suburban and surrounding land. Other boroughs that had very large electorates but small and overgrown boundaries often were not extended: Gash, *Politics in the Age of Peel*, 66–77.

9. Cannon, *Parliamentary Reform*, 256; Jupp, *Governing of Britain*, 222–23.

10. *Hansard Parliamentary Debates*, 3rd ser., vol. 28 (June 22, 1835), cols. 1020–1035; vol. 30 (August 13, 1835), cols. 464–66. Two kinds of boundaries engaged Parliament in 1835: the boundary of the municipal borough and the boundaries of wards within it, if it was large enough to need them. The Whigs initially were keen to have the boundaries determined by an order in council formed on the recommendation of another appointed boundary commission, but in the statute, ward boundaries were given to revising barristers, and municipal boundaries were set by the act. In both

cases, Parliament agreed to potential future revision, and the Whig-appointed boundary commission thus went about its work. The result of its labor was presented to
Parliament in 1838 in the shape of a boundary bill. It was rejected, and both ward and
municipal boundaries remained unchanged. Report of the Commissioners . . . upon
the Boundaries and Wards of Certain Boroughs and Corporate Towns, PP 1837 (238).

11. *Hansard Parliamentary Debates*, 3rd ser., vol. 28 (June 22, 1835), cols. 1020–
1035, especially 1026–27.

12. Norton and Allworth, *Borough Boundaries*, 2–7; *Hansard Parliamentary Debates*,
3rd ser., vol. 41 (March 14, 1838), cols. 891–98. As a result of the bill's failure, historical interest is even lower for this exercise. On the boundary commission's recommendations see Freeman, *Geography and Regional Administration*, 33–57.

13. *Hansard Parliamentary Debates*, 3rd ser., vol. 41 (March 14, 1838), cols. 891–98,
especially 891.

14. Carroll, "Medical Police."

15. Freeman noted that of 178 boroughs, the commissioners expanded 54,
reduced 71, left 33 untouched, and carried out minor revisions of 20: Freeman,
Geography and Regional Administration, 35.

16. Both of these models remained in circulation later in the century, when John
Stuart Mill invoked them in his treatise on representative government. Mill recognized that different towns might have different interests, but within a town all quar-
ters required the same things to be done, including paving, lighting, water supply,
drainage, and port and market regulations. Mill's model differed from that of the
1830s chiefly in the wider range of actions considered part of the police package:
Mill, *Considerations*, chap. 15; Waller, *Town, City, and Nation*, 254–55.

17. Lipman devotes two pages to boundaries for health authorities up to 1870:
Lipman, *Local Government Areas*, 55–56. Poor-law unions, in contrast, merited eighteen pages.

18. Local board of health areas were intended to coincide with natural drainage basins. That meant that parochial or other political or administrative boundaries could, in theory, be ignored in the formation of LBH districts. In reality, of
course, political considerations could not always or even frequently be ignored. The
boundaries of LBH districts were far too controversial to be left to engineers roam-
ing the countryside. Parliamentary opposition forced Lord Morpeth to introduce a
requirement for parliamentary scrutiny of the application of the act to any locality
whose boundaries were altered or where local acts were in force. According to the
1848 PHA, if the proposed local board district was coextensive with some existing
defined area, either a parish, a township, or a corporation, the act could be applied
by an order in council. If the proposed local board district was not coextensive with
any existing jurisdiction—that is, if it was larger (or smaller) than existing political
or administrative boundaries—parliamentary sanction was required before the act
could be applied. The Public Health Act also stipulated that no area beyond the
boundary of a corporate borough could be included in any LBH district containing
a part of a corporate borough, except for the purposes of drainage, unless a majority
of the inhabitants of that part agreed: 11 & 12 Vict., c. 63, ss. 20–21.

19. On the inspectors and their reports, see Hamlin, *Public Health and Social Justice*,
275–301; H. J. Smith, "Introduction," 3–14. The Harvester set is the most extensive
single collection of reports. It is not exhaustive: in some places a "Further Inquiry"

(such as at Aylesbury) exists in manuscript. Other reports (such as at Hertford) were published as parliamentary papers. Presumably there are a small number of other examples.

20. The GBH records indicate the degree to which boundary making and public health were intimately connected. Some places spent literally years fighting about the boundary before the act could even be applied. For one example, see the correspondence over Wrexham at MH/12/24, NA.

21. E. C. Hawtrey to E. Chadwick, November 10, 1842, file 964, Chadwick Correspondence, UCL Archives. The engineer they chose was one of Chadwick's favorites, John Roe of the Holborn and Finsbury Sewers Commission. See Roe, *To the Provost and Fellows.*

22. In consequence of the 1846 Nuisances Removal Act, the Guardians of the Union established a committee that apparently conducted some kind of sanitary survey of the town. The town sent a petition in favor of the 1847 Health of Towns Bill: W. J. Sanders to GBH, November 16, 1848, MH/13/71/1060/8, NA.

23. E. Cresy to GBH, March 12, 1849, p. 10, MH/13/71/1300/49, NA. Cresy, *Report to the General Board of Health . . . the Town of Eton,* 17.

24. According to a later document, the college was fighting this battle right from the start; Memorial from the Provost and College of Eton, May 1, 1851, MH/13/71/1594/51, NA.

25. W. J. Sanders to GBH, July 3, 1849, MH/13/71/2937/49, NA.

26. C. S. Voules to GBH, February 6, 1850, and draft reply, MH/13/71/339/50, NA.

27. C. S. Voules to GBH, December 2, 1850, MH/13/71/4211/50, NA; March 7, 1851, MH/13/71/891/51, NA.

28. Cresy, *Report to the General Board of Health on a Second Inquiry . . . the Town of Eton.*

29. Memorial from the Provost and College of Eton, May 1, 1851, MH/13/71/1594/51, NA; The Respectful Memorial of the Eton Local Board of Health, May 20, 1851, MH/13/71/2019/51, NA, plus MS notes of the LBH deputation held on July 25, 1851, MH/13/71/2536/51, NA. The college, of course, was not a monolith, and not all members opposed the extension. One of the masters sat on the LBH, and according to the deputation of the LBH he committed himself in writing to the justice of the LBH's argument.

30. The college still would have paid the parish but less than it would have in the past.

31. Webb and Webb, *Story of the King's Highway,* chap. 9, especially 207–10.

32. Memorial from the Provost and College of Eton, May 1, 1851, MH/13/71/1594/51, NA.

33. 11 & 12 Vict., c. 63, s. 20. Daunton noted that the plural franchise was in part invented to break the grip of lower-middle-class ratepayers on entrenchment: Daunton, *Trusting Leviathan,* 263–66. See also Redlich and Hirst, *History of Local Government,* 147.

34. A further ten of the properties were within the parish but outside the LBH district, which thus included only four valuable houses: J. Cleave to GBH, June 28, 1853, MH/13/71/1841/53, NA.

35. Local residents objected to this qualification, because it would likely severely restrict the pool of potential LBH members. In reply, the GBH suggested that the

qualification had been found to work well: W. J. Sanders to GBH, October 24, 1849, MH/13/71/8080/49, NA; J. Cleave to GBH, October 29, 1849, MH/13/71/8107/49, NA; draft GBH reply to Cleave, November 1, 1849, MH/13/71/8107/49, NA. Given that the Eton LBH was one of the first created in the entire country, the GBH's claim was without foundation, nor was it the whole truth. Cresy was clear that his intention was to keep owners of low-value housing off the local board for fear that they would oppose sanitary reform. He did not mention that the qualification had been found to work well: E. Cresy to GBH, November 1, 1849, MH/13/71/8107/49, NA. See Daunton, "Taxation and Representation."

36. The LBH also claimed that one part of the parish not included in the LBH district that students frequented was as yet unimproved and that the board would fix it: The Respectful Memorial of the Eton Local Board of Health, May 20, 1851, MH/13/71/2019/51, NA.

37. "Proposed Extension of the District of the Eton Board of Health," *Windsor and Eton Express*, February 8, 1851, 4; "Proposed Extension of the District of the Eton Board of Health," *Windsor and Eton Express*, February 15, 1851, 3.

38. F. D. Roberts, *Social Conscience*, 9–27.

39. This was not the old argument that sick people in the town would be a hazard to the college. The benefit for Eton College was not that the LBH protected it from diseased people in the town. Rather, a healthy town protected Etonians in their own right: The Respectful Memorial of the Eton Local Board of Health, May 20, 1851, MH/13/71/2019/51, NA.

40. According to the chair of the local board of health, the LBH district comprised about 439 ratepayers, and the rateable value of the district was £4,447. The college, meanwhile, comprised 162 ratepayers with an annual rateable value of £5,590. "The Respectful Memorial of the Eton Local Board of Health," May 20, 1851, MH/13/71/2019/51, NA; Account of a deputation of the LBH at the GBH held on July 25, 1851, MH/13/71/2536/51, NA.

41. J. Cleave to GBH, June 28, 1853, MH/13/71/1841/53, NA.

42. The college portrayed the LBH's request for extension as some kind of attempt at a tax grab, arguing that a comparatively wealthy and perfectly clean place like the college should not have to pay rates to a comparatively dirty and poor place like the LBH district. Memorial from the Provost and College of Eton, May 1, 1851, MH/13/71/1594/51, NA.

43. This dispute did not start in Eton with the Public Health Act. Disputes about the burdens cast on different species of property were of long standing and often revolved around real versus personal property. Those disputes partly reflected social divisions, real property representing landed wealth and personal property representing commercial, manufacturing, and trading wealth. However, that debate had been settled by 1840 for the Poor Law; Parliament had decided that poor rates, for example, were to be met with taxes on real property. An excellent discussion of these issues may be found in Daunton, *Trusting Leviathan*, 77–108.

44. Chairman LBH to GBH, December 31, 1855, MH/13/70/19/56, NA. The beneficial occupiers of Eton College—the Provost and Fellows—were apparently "extra-parochial" and thus escaped from some local burdens: J. Cleave to GBH, June 28, 1853, MH/13/71/1841/53, NA.

45. Draft GBH to LBH, February 10, 1852, MH/13/71/414/52, NA; LBH to GBH, October 22, 1852, MH/13/71/4446/52, NA; Cleave to GBH, June 28, 1853, MH/13/71/1841/53, NA; draft GBH to LBH, February 6, 1854, MH/13/71/351/54, NA.

46. Clerk to GBH, November 9, 1867, MH/13/71/3766, NA; Robert Morgan to Secretary of State, January 2, 1868, MH/13/71/17/68, NA.

47. In its 1851 response to the LBH deputation, the GBH claimed that it was too late in the session to apply to put Eton in the supplementary Public Health Bill. This claim rings hollow: Cresy had reported in May, and the session ended in August.

48. Draft GBH to LBH, February 6, 1854, MH/13/71/351/54, NA; LBH to GBH, March 14, 1854, MH/13/71/71025/54, NA.

49. Eton was in some senses atypical. Few places had the kind of elite institutional loyalty, and the power that flowed from it, that Eton College did. But in other places, the GBH met local concerns over the boundaries of health with a similar want of candor. For some examples, see the debates at Ware and Great Amwell, Llangollen, and Wrexham.

50. The Town and Franchise represented the area serviced by Swansea's 1809 local act: G. Roberts, *Municipal Development*, 33. See also Miskell, *Intelligent Town*, 91–92, 153–56; Miskell, "Urban Power," 21–36.

51. George Thomas Clark, *Preliminary Inquiry into . . . the Town and Borough of Swansea*, 3. The copper works were outside the old corporate borough as a result of earlier decisions to exile them from the town: Rees, "The South Wales Copper-Smoke Dispute." Swansea was one of the pre-1835 corporate towns that gained much larger boundaries in 1835, when it was granted the boundary of the parliamentary borough.

52. Clark's *Preliminary Inquiry into . . . the Town and Borough of Swansea*, 28, stated that "each district should bear its own charges by special district rates." See also "Health of Towns' Act," *Swansea and Glamorgan Herald*, May 23, 1849, 2; "Inquiry at Swansea Under the Health of Towns' Act," *Swansea and Glamorgan Herald*, May 30, 1849, p. 3; "Paving Commissioners' Meeting," *Swansea and Glamorgan Herald*, November 28, 1849, 2.

53. Clark, *Further Inquiry . . . the Borough of Swansea*. The newspaper report of the second inquiry noted that no one formally appeared against the proposed district: "Swansea and the Health of Towns Act," *Swansea and Glamorgan Herald*, January 16, 1850, 2. The report in the *Cambrian*, a political rival of the *Herald*, was not different.

54. Clark, *Report on . . . the Borough of Bangor*.

55. Rammell, *Report to . . . the Borough of Bangor*, 4.

56. P. Gaskell to GBH, January 18, 1853, MH/13/13/193/5, NA; P. Gaskell to GBH, February 8, 1853, 390/53.

57. T. W. Rammell to GBH, January 31, 1853, MH/13/13/309/53, NA. Rammell presumably saw advantage in wider terms than direct benefit, though he did not make his meaning clear.

58. GBH opportunism occasionally led to trouble. At Waltham Holy Cross the LBH found itself in front of the Queen's Bench in a case involving some shenanigans around boundary formation: see "Barber v. Jessop," *Justice of the Peace*, February 28, 1857, 136–37; *Barber v. Jessop, Clerk to the Local Board of Health for the Parish of Waltham Holy Cross*, 156 English Reports 1332–37.

59. Hanley, "Metropolitan Commissioners of Sewers."

60. A property was exempt if it was previously exempt in respect of purposes for which a general district rate or a special district rate could be levied under the PHA. The exemption was for those purposes only, and was only to be exempted to the same extent: 11 & 12 Vict., c. 63, s. 88.

61. Facts taken from report in *Archibald Campbell Tait, Appellant, against The Local Board of Health of the City of Carlisle, Respondents,* 118 English Reports 855–57. The Chelmsford case, *The Guardians of the Chelmsford Union v. The Local Board of Health for Chelmsford,* was decided on May 4, 1852. Unfortunately, no oral arguments were reported. The Chelmsford LBH was created in 1850 and the rate made in 1851.

62. In a series of cases in 1858 brought against the Plymouth LBH and decided in 1858, the judges again wrestled with this issue of exemption: *Robert Luscombe, Appellant, against The Local Board of Health for the Borough of Plymouth, Respondents. Elizabeth Shortland, Appellant, against the Same, Respondents. Alexander Pontey, Appellant, against the Same, Respondents,* 120 English Reports 668–70, and the next several cases. In Hull, the issue was rating small tenements: "Coates *v.* Local Board of Health of Kingston-Upon-Hull," *Justice of the Peace,* July 26, 1856, pp. 467–70.

63. *Archibald Campbell Tait, Appellant, against The Local Board of Health of the City of Carlisle, Respondents,* 118 English Reports 851–60. The LBH was created in 1850 and the rate assessed in 1851. The case was decided in 1853.

64. *The South Wales Railway Company, Appellants, against The Local Board of Health of the Borough of Swansea, Respondents,* 119 English Reports 73–77. The LBH was created in 1850 and the rate levied in 1853. The case was decided in 1854.

65. Where a local board did not fully and fairly rate all eligible parties, it could be challenged: *The Queen against the Newport Local Board of Health,* 122 English Reports 129–31.

66. *The Guardians of the Chelmsford Union v. The Local Board of Health for Chelmsford,* 118 English Reports 855–57, quotations on 855, 856.

67. *Archibald Campbell Tait, Appellant, against The Local Board of Health of the City of Carlisle, Respondents* 118 English Reports 859.

68. According to Justice Erle, there was no case law on rating railroad property for the relief of the poor, though practice appeared to support the Swansea LBH: *The South Wales Railway Company, Appellants against the Local Board of Health of the Borough of Swansea, Respondents,* 119 English Reports 77.

69. *The South Wales Railway Company, Appellants, against the Local Board of Health of the Borough of Swansea, Respondents,* 119 English Reports 76. Justice Erle, too, argued that the general principle of the PHA was that occupiers of property less benefited by expenditure paid the lower rate. The railroad property that the judges decided to rate fully thus fell into the category of highly benefited property.

70. 11 & 12 Vict., c. 63, s. 89.

71. For example, in the 1833 General Sewers Act (3 & 4 Will. 4, c. 22, s. 14), Lincoln's 1845 Health of Towns Bill [PP 1845 (574), s. 260], the 1847 Towns Improvement Clauses Act (10 & 11 Vict., c. 34, s. 162).

72. GBH Minutes, March 5, 1851, MH/5/4, NA; June 2, 1851, July 1, 1851, August 13, 1851, August 30, 1851, December 23, 1851, MH/5/5, NA; January 23, 1852, MH/5/6, NA; November 2, 1852, MH/5/7, NA. In extreme cases, the GBH

supported proposals to exclude formally parts of a district from any further operation of the act.

73. Johnson, *Acts for Promoting the Public Health*, 133, note *i*: "The General Board of Health . . . were of opinion that 'a local board has not a discretionary power to rate premises in a special district rate which are not benefited by the outlay of the rate.[']" He claimed they took a case on March 27, 1851. Johnson was a barrister, a former member of the Metropolitan Commission of Sewers, and the chair of the Croydon LBH: Finer, *Life and Times*, 364, 367, 447. In the 1850s, Johnson's work was an official favorite. I could not find this opinion in the GBH minutes, but see GBH Minutes, November 10, 1851, MH/5/5, NA for a reference to a related but distinct query from Croydon on which an opinion would be sought.

74. Draft GBH to LBH, November 3, 1852, MH/13/76/4584/52, NA. "Fairly" was a later interpolation.

75. Newport to GBH, November 22, 1853, and GBH to LBH draft reply, December 3, 1853, MH/13/133/5783/53, NA.

76. Instructions of the General Board of Health to the Superintending Inspectors, in Report of the General Board of Health on the Administration of the Public Health Act and the Nuisances Removal and Diseases Prevention Act from 1848 to 1854, PP 1854 (1768), 99–100.

77. Clark's *Preliminary Inquiry* at Swansea is an example.

78. The Bristol Town Council petitioned to adopt the PHA in 1849, and by 1851 the council had formed itself into a LBH under the act: Large, "Records of the Bristol Local Board of Health," 125.

79. Large, "Records of the Bristol Local Board of Health," 130. A nineteenth-century commentator in Bristol noted that the construction of the system "necessarily" took a long time, but one might wonder if it needed to take the same amount of time as Joseph Bazalgette took to build the main drainage scheme for London. See Latimer, *Annals of Bristol*, 3: 316. The GBH records a deputation from Bristol inquiring if the LBH district could be divided for the purposes of rating: GBH Minutes, August 4, 1851, MH/5/5, NA.

80. Thus, the same mode was adopted for the Bedminster drainage district in 1854: Large, "Proceedings of the Bristol Local Board of Health," 136–40.

81. Large, "Proceedings of the Bristol Local Board of Health," 146.

82. "Bristol Town Council," *Bristol Gazette*, September 3, 1857, 6. The districts themselves often contained more than one parish, and the Bristol Local Board of Health did not contemplate assessing parishes separately with a drainage district. That battle was fought and won in London in the 1830s and 1840s. See the discussion of the Avon Intercepting District, where several parishes were united to form a separate district in 1871: "Proceedings of the Bristol Local Board of Health," 196.

83. When Fishwick Township in 1851 petitioned to separate from the Preston LBH, after a lengthy investigation the GBH rejected the petition, again entering the rejection fully in its minutes. The GBH did not believe that the petitioners had demonstrated any harm as a result of being part of the district and noted that many houses in Preston were occupied by working people employed in Fishwick: GBH Minutes, July 1, 1851, MH/5/5, NA. See also Draft GBH to LBH, June 3, 1851, MH/13/148/1753/51, NA.

84. The Epsom LBH inquired about the liability of the tithe rent charges in LBH to GBH, January 11, 1851, MH/13/70/153/51, NA.

85. LBH to GBH, January 23, 1851, MH/13/70/316/51, NA; February 20, 1851, MH/13/70/470/51, NA.

86. 3 & 4 Will. 4, c. 90, s. 73 (1833). The General Lighting and Watching Act was in effect but dealt only with lighting. Epsom was within the jurisdiction of the Metropolitan Police Act, being only fifteen miles from London: William Lee, *Report to . . . Epsom*, 5.

87. A Bill to Repeal an Act of the Eleventh Year of His Late Majesty King George the Fourth, for the Lighting and Watching Parishes in England and Wales, and to Make Other Provisions in lieu thereof, PP 1833 (385), 33–34.

88. The LBH was confused about the purposes for which the general district rate and the special district rate were to be levied: see draft letter from GBH to LBH, August 15, 1851, MH/13/70/2803/51, NA.

89. GBH to LBH, draft, January 27, 1851, MH/13/70/316/51, NA; GBH to LBH, draft, February 11, 1851, MH/13/70/470/51, NA; GBH to LBH, draft, August 15, 1851, MH/13/2803/51, NA.

90. Neave may have been the same individual who was an assistant Poor Law commissioner in the 1830s. He and Chadwick may have had a history: Charlesworth, *Welfare's Forgotten Past*, 155.

91. This was an issue for other boards as well: see GBH Minutes, August 13, 1851 (Nuneaton LBH), August 30, 1851 (Luton LBH), MH/5/5, NA.

92. D. Neave to E. Chadwick, August 19, 1851, MH/13/70/2803/51, NA; GBH to D. Neave, August 23, 1851, MH/13/70/2803/51, NA. Note that the GBH always seemed to suggest that the district benefiting should pay the capital costs. This letter was apparently drafted by the GBH secretary, Henry Austin.

93. The Epsom Board Chair, Sir Richard Digby Neave, attended the GBH in October, presumably to express frustration with the GBH. The GBH immediately drafted a self-justifying letter to the LBH. See GBH to LBH, October 17, 1851, MH/13/2803/51, NA for Asst. Secretary Taylor's explanation.

94. Details in this paragraph taken from "Dorling *v.* the Local Board of Health of Epsom," *Justice of the Peace,* January 12, 1856, pp. 20–23.

95. Epsom's resort status probably explains this decision. But the racetrack, which apparently operated only one week a year, had its own water supply and sewerage disposal system. Local enthusiasm for the act also was also very general, as were complaints by citizens about ill-health caused by bad drainage: A. Holland et al. to GBH, June 23, 1851, plus enclosures, MH/13/2332/51, NA.

96. Initially, the works were estimated to cost £7,000, although the GBH whittled it down to £5,000. Both sums were well within the means of the LBH: GBH to LBH, draft letter, September 24, 1852, MH/13/3994/52, NA. Unfortunately, the site from which the LBH proposed to draw water required the agreement of the lord of the manor. Although he cooperated with some feasibility studies, he declined to give his final agreement, and for this and other reasons the LBH was forced to modify its plan: W. Lee to GBH, April 14, 1854, MH/13/1549/54, NA. The sums the LBH required increased considerably: H. Austin to GBH, February 21, 1854, MH/13/732/54, NA.

97. These facts are all derived from the case subsequently fought over the board's decision: *Dorling, Appellant, against the Local Board of Health for the District of Epsom*, 119 English Reports 557–59.

98. Local board minutes for the period before March 15, 1854, were unavailable for consultation in early 2006. Epsom did not have a local newspaper until 1856; Surrey papers circulating in the area do not discuss the local board's decision.

99. I base this claim on the two questions that the appellants and respondents decided to submit to quarter sessions for decision. The development of the case is discussed in "Epsom Local Board of Health: Case" found at MH/13/70/778/55, NA. The case is not dated but probably was prepared in July 1854: Minutes of Epsom LBH, July 31, 1854, 3554/1/2, SRO.

100. "Surrey Quarter Sessions," *County Chronicle, Surrey Herald, and Weekly Advertiser*, April 10, 1855, 5.

101. Certainly some residents of Epsom were concerned that under the Public Health Act, land was taxed at one fourth the rate of houses for highway purposes, a fact that town dwellers believed forced town to subsidize country: S. Hanson to GBH, February 13, 1855, MH/13/70/602/55, NA. See also H. Dorling to GBH, February 27, 1855, MH/13/70/808/55, NA.

102. "Surrey Midsummer Sessions," *County Chronicle, Surrey Herald, and Weekly Advertiser*, July 4, 1854, 4. The Epsom documents claim the case was argued at great length: "Epsom Local Board of Health: Case," MH/13/70/778/55, NA.

103. "Epsom Local Board of Health: Case," q. 11, MH/13/70/778/55, NA.

104. Epsom Local Board of Health Minutes, July 24, 1854; July 31, 1854, 3554/1/2, SRO.

105. The Epsom board asked the General Board of Health to solicit the law officers' opinion, which it duly did; GBH to LBH, draft letter, November 15, 1854, MH/13/70/5751/54, NA. Two of the questions the GBH proposed to the law officers concerned the local board's right to determine the area and the meaning of benefit. The opinion was sent in a draft letter from the GBH to LBH, December 5, 1854, MH/13/70, NA. A review of letters to and from the law officers from the Home Office failed to turn up any evidence of their opinion.

106. Epsom Local Board of Health Minutes, December 15, 1854, 3554/1/2, SRO. See also Select Committee on the Public Health Bill, PP 1854–55 (244), q. 1307.

107. Freshfield was a significant landowner in Surrey and the Conservative MP for Penryn: Jenkins, "Freshfield, James William."

108. "Surrey Quarter Sessions," *County Chronicle, Surrey Herald, and Weekly Advertiser*, April 10, 1855, 5; S. Hanson to General Board, April 5, 1855, MH/13/70/1446/55, NA.

109. *Dorling, Appellant, against the Local Board of Health for the District of Epsom* (1855), 119 English Reports 561.

110. *Dorling, Appellant, against the Local Board of Health for the District of Epsom* (1855), 119 English Reports 560.

111. The 1848 Public Health Act ran for only five years; in 1854 Parliament gave it a one-year extension. In the spring of 1855, the House of Commons held hearings on a proposed amendment to the act, along with amendments to the Nuisances Removal and Diseases Prevention Acts; PP 1854–55 (244).

112. Everest-Phillips, "William Everest of Epsom." Although Everest-Phillips does not discuss the case or Everest's involvement in public health in Epsom, this is probably the same Everest.

113. Everest's view was echoed in some written correspondence the GBH received in response to its draft bill. The GBH apparently circulated the 1855 Public Health Bill, printed in January, to the local boards of health for their comment. The Tenby LBH in Wales decided not to comment on the bill, yet one member felt sufficiently strongly about it to do so on his own. Mr. T. Wedgwood wished to see some "well defined protection" to houses outside town boundaries but within district boundaries "from being rated towards the sewerage of the Town and any other expenses they derive no benefit from." T. Wedgwood to GBH, February 20, 1855, in A. W. Williams, *Public Health in Mid-Victorian Wales*, 3: 1402–3.

114. White provided detailed comments to the GBH on the amending bill; White to GBH, February 19, 1855, MH/13/70/671/55, NA; February 24, 1855, MH/13/70/766/55, NA.

115. Select Committee on the Public Health Bill, PP 1854–55 (244), q. 1290.

116. Select Committee on the Public Health Bill, PP 1854–55 (244), q. 1291.

117. Select Committee on the Public Health Bill, PP 1854–55 (244), q. 1297. White's failure to elaborate and the select committee's failure to interview the medical officer deprives us of the ability to hear from Epsom's officers what they thought exactly constituted the medical benefit. White's testimony revealed that the condition of cottages owned by wealthy owners was a problem and that the board would drain them. But the fact that the Poor Law medical officer was put forward suggests that indirect benefit matched counsel's argument at the hearing.

118. In a case likely prepared sometime in July 1854, the Epsom LBH claimed it had decided on the district on the basis of health: "Epsom Local Board of Health: Case," p. 3, MH/13/70/778/55, NA.

119. Details in this paragraph taken from "Dorling *v.* the Local Board of Health of Epsom," *Justice of the Peace,* January 12, 1856, pp. 20–23. The opinion was delivered by John Coleridge, Samuel Taylor's nephew, although two other justices were present when the case was argued (William Wightman and the Liberal Charles Crompton).

120. *Dorling, Appellant, against the Local Board of Health for the District of Epsom* (1855), 119 English Reports 561; "Dorling *v.* the Local Board of Health of Epsom," *Justice of the Peace,* January 12, 1856, p. 23.

121. *Dorling, Appellant, against the Local Board of Health for the District of Epsom* (1855), 119 English Reports 561. The argument about lowered poor rates echoed Chadwick's claim and was probably the argument that the Epsom LBH advanced. The enhanced quality of the urban environment is self-explanatory. The increased value in land for an outlying ratepayer is a result of the general increase in property value in well-drained, desirable areas.

122. In the future, these benefits would be called positive externalities. It is worth noting that all resident landowners and occupiers of the parish received the indirect benefits that Coleridge identified; they were not specific to those outside the area drained. It is interesting that Coleridge chose to highlight shared indirect benefits rather than those not shared.

123. According to his biographer Lewis, Chadwick was barely involved in drafting either the 1847 Health of Towns Bill or the 1848 Public Health Act: Lewis, *Edwin*

Chadwick, 145, 160. Morpeth's biographer suggests, in contrast, that Morpeth worked closely with Chadwick on the Public Health Act: Olien, *Morpeth*, 318. Her view is supported by the Chadwick correspondence, which records several meetings between Chadwick and the solicitor drafting the Public Health Act, Edward Lawes: Chadwick Correspondence, UCL.

124. In an 1852 Queen's Bench case, *The Guardians of the Chelmsford Union v. The Local Board of Health for Chelmsford*, the Court noted the care with which the rating provisions of the Public Health Act were drafted: 118 English Reports 856.

125. The decision to rate agricultural and some other land at one quarter the net annual value reflects political compromise. In the overheated political environment of post-1846 England, any decision to make rural property owners share the burden for what was seen as primarily an urban benefit was a political nonstarter. See also Lewis, *Edwin Chadwick*, 146; 11 & 12 Vict., c. 63, s. 88. The 1833 Lighting and Watching Act was the first general act to introduce differential rating for agricultural land: Beckett, *Local Taxation*, 39.

126. The sewers rate was traditionally a landlord's charge. Chadwick did not believe that owners could be charged, but he was also skeptical that occupiers could bear the costs. As Hamlin notes, the 1848 Public Health Act was a compromise on this vexing issue: *Public Health and Social Justice*, 255. Lawes claimed that the drainage of property and the provision of a sufficient privy was largely the owner's expense: Lawes, *Act for Promoting the Public Health*, 82, note *f*; 88, note *m*. The ultimate incidence of urban rates as between owners and occupiers was controversial among national political leaders for the remainder of the century: Offer, *Property and Politics*.

127. Anxiety about debt took two forms. The first concerned the distribution of costs between present and future generations. A strong predisposition existed in favor of present generations paying for the costs of works from which they benefited and not sloughing the costs onto the future. But the reverse also held true. In 1852, the GBH rejected Superintending Inspector T. W. Rammell's plan for the drainage of Cardiff in part because they believed future beneficiaries would end up paying too little: GBH Minutes, February 17, 1852, MH/5/6, NA. In addition, observers worried that if local governments could defer their costs into the future, they would have little incentive to control spending in the present. The metropolitan sewers commissions had only limited ability to incur debt; the commissioners had to return to Parliament whenever they required new debt ceilings. For Gladstone's opposition to debt, see Daunton, *Trusting Leviathan*, 70, 115–17. The Public Health Act allowed local boards to finance capital improvement with long-term debt but capped the amount of debt.

128. Dicey, *Lectures*, 362 (quote), 370. According to conventional thinking, judges did not make law, not even the common law. Rather, they applied the law that already existed to new situations.

129. In delivering the judgment of the court in *Dorling v. Epsom*, Coleridge noted that his preliminary comments about benefit, "although not without their weight, *a priori*, do not decide the case, which must depend upon an examination of the sections [of the statute] before mentioned." See "Dorling *v.* the Local Board of Health of Epsom," *Justice of the Peace*, January 12, 1856, p. 23.

130. "Dorling *v.* the Local Board of Health of Epsom," *Justice of the Peace*, January 12, 1856, p. 23. Coleridge concluded his analysis by noting, "On the review, therefore,

of the sections of the act, as well as on the general grounds first stated, our judgment will be for the respondents."

131. On these various points, see Brenner, Nuisance Law"; Dingle, "The Monster Nuisance"; Kearns, "Cholera, Nuisances and Environmental Management"; McLaren, "Nuisance Law"; Mosley, *Chimney of the World*; Platt, *Shock Cities.*

132. Newport LBH to GBH, November 22, 1853; GBH to LBH draft reply, December 3, 1853, MH/13/133/5783/53, NA.

133. One of the members of the LBH, a man named Hanson, was upset that under a general district rate, certain lands escaped the full burden of taxation to which they had been subject under the 1835 Highway Act. In early 1855, Hanson wrote to Sir B. Hall protesting that fact when the Public Health Amendment Bill was under consideration. See S. Hanson to GBH, February 13, 1855, MH/13/70/602/55, NA.

134. *Hanson, Appellant, and the Local Board of Health for the District of Epsom, Respondents* (1855), 118 English Reports 603–6. In two previous highway rate cases, the Court had decided that the LBH must use a GDR, not a highway rate. See *John Elmer against the Local Board of Health of Norwich* (1854), 118 English Reports 1236–41; *Queen against the Trustees of the Worthing and Lancing Turnpike Road* (1854), 118 English Reports 1412–20. Parliament passed a short amending act on highways in 1854: 17 & 18 Vict., c. 69. All of these cases depended on the nature of the particular LBH district, and in particular the number of separate parishes in it.

135. In *Charles Moseley, Appellant, against the Local Board of Health of the District of the City of Ely, Respondents,* 119 English Reports 958–61, the Court appeared to reverse direction, again requiring the local board to pay for highway repairs with a general district rate rather than highway rates. See also Barber v. Jessop, in which a rate levied by a LBH according to the 1835 Highway Act was ruled illegal: "Barber v. Jessop," *Justice of the Peace*, February 28, 1857, pp. 136–37. In an 1857 case, counsel argued that *Moseley* virtually overruled *Hanson; Taff Vale Railway Company against the Local Board of Health for the District of Cardiff,* 120 English Reports 200. The Court did not explicitly respond to this claim. In the Moseley case, the Court took the time to infer what it believed might have been the legislature's intention. Chief Justice Lord Campbell argued that the LBH surveyors were meant to do more than mere highway surveyors under the 1835 act. The things that the LBH surveyors were meant to do, furthermore, were distinctly urban; although they would profit townsmen, they would be useless to "rustics" (961). The holding is odd because in *Dorling*, the Court sanctioned the rating of rural property not directly benefited at all, because it would benefit indirectly. Why that did not apply in the case of highways the Court did not make clear. In an 1864 case, the Court certainly recognized that improperly maintained streets were potentially unhealthy: *Caley, Appellant, The Local Board of Health for the Borough of Kingston upon Hull, Respondents,* 122 English Reports 1035.

136. The case was reported in newspapers around the country. Even from the limited selection in British Newspaper Archive online, I found "Court of Queen's Bench," *Carlisle Journal*, July 6, 1855, 6; "Law Intelligence," *Hampshire Advertiser*, July 7, 1855, 3; "Miscellaneous," *Reading Mercury*, July 14, 1855, 8; "Court of Queen's Bench," *London Daily News*, July 2, 1855, 6. The Epsom clerk reported that he had received several applications for copies of the decision: LBH to GBH, November 19, 1855, MH/13/70/4336/55, NA.

137. On Swansea's early political development, see Miskell, "Urban Power, Industrialisation and Political Reform."

138. Clark, *Preliminary Inquiry into . . . the Borough of Swansea*, 28. It is striking that many, including Clark, regarded special district rates as applying to special areas rather than special purposes. However, according to the PHA, the special district rates were to be used for works of permanent improvement such as water supplies or drainage projects, irrespective of the area to which they applied. Nevertheless, both special district rates and general district rates could be levied over any area, ranging from an entire district to some portion of it. Thus, there could be as many special district rates applying to as many different subareas as there were permanent improvement projects.

139. "Inquiry at Swansea Under the Health of Towns Act," *Swansea and Glamorgan Herald*, May 30, 1849, 3.

140. For public health purposes, Swansea borrowed over 17 percent of the total sums sanctioned in Wales for sewerage, drainage, and water supply from 1848 to 1871, and that within a span of fifteen years: I. G. Jones, "The People's Health," 128. The LBH had borrowed £170,000 by 1870, fifteen years after it was created: G. Roberts, *Municipal Development*, 47. But see Luckin, "Pollution in the City," 215.

141. "Swansea Local Board of Health," *Swansea and Glamorgan Herald*, September 27, 1854, 4. The LBH's decision to levy a water rate was one of the factors that triggered a ratepayers' movement in Swansea in late 1854. In the municipal elections that year (town councilors were automatically the members of the LBH), the water supply became one of the main issues. A former mayor who was running for reelection as a councillor was involved in a challenging and extensively reported discussion of the water issue at a ward meeting that fall. See "Meeting of the Electors of the Lower Ward," *Swansea and Glamorgan Herald*, October 11, 1854, 3.

142. See the discussion in "Special Meeting for Making Rates," *Swansea and Glamorgan Herald*, February 11, 1857, 4.

143. "Swansea Local Board of Health," *Swansea and Glamorgan Herald*, November 12, 1856, 4.

144. Swansea to GBH, December 23, 1856, minute, MH/13/178/15050/56, NA. The GBH's reply would have been read aloud at the meeting.

145. "Swansea Local Board of Health," *Swansea and Glamorgan Herald*, January 14, 1857, 4.

146. "Special Meeting for Making Rates," *Swansea and Glamorgan Herald*, February 11, 1857, 4.

147. R. Morgan recommended that the petition to split the district be dismissed: November 3, 1864, MH/13/178/3023/64, NA. A newspaper account of the inquiry into splitting the district follows his report. The socioeconomic diversity of Swansea was a problem in the early post-1835 period: Miskell, *Intelligent Town*, 143–50.

148. "The Sewerage of Swansea," *Swansea and Glamorgan Herald*, January 21, 1857, 2.

149. "Special Meeting for Making Rates," *Swansea and Glamorgan Herald*, February 11, 1857, 4. It is interesting that one member saw benefit and whole-district rating in mutually exclusive terms, because indirect benefit squared that circle or exposed the false dichotomy.

150. For the Queen's Bench, see *Pew and Others, Appellants, The Metropolitan Board of Works, and Collins and Another, Respondents*, 122 English Reports 1188. This case is discussed in chapter 4.

151. At the very least, the *Dorling* decision provided the Swansea LBH with solid legal cover; indeed, the mayor (erroneously) believed that a rate on less than the entire district was actually illegal: "Special Meeting for Making Rates," *Swansea and Glamorgan Herald*, February 11, 1857, 4.

152. "The Sewerage of Swansea," *Swansea and Glamorgan Herald*, January 21, 1857, 2.

153. Select Committee on Cheltenham Improvement Bill (Lords), May 12, 1852, pp. 33–34 (Charles Paul), HL/PO/PB/5/18/1, PA; Select Committee on Cheltenham Improvement Bill (Commons), March 17, 1852, p. 208 (W. Newman), HC/CL/PB/2/20/5, PA. On one of the private estates, see S. Blake, *Pittville*.

154. C. W. Jones, "The Sewers Company and the Commissioners," letter to the editor, *Cheltenham Examiner*, November 1, 1854, 8. By his own account, Jones "loathed" the "monstrosity" of a corporation, so presumably his testimony is reliable.

155. Cheltenham's drainage had two main problems. First, not enough people had access to it; only one ninth of Cheltenham's houses drained into company sewers: Cresy, *Report on . . . the Town of Cheltenham*, 20. And only half of the houses that could connect to the company did so: "The Sewers Question," *Cheltenham Examiner*, October 11, 1854, 4. Second, the existing drains emptied into one of the three open brooks or rivers that ran through the town, rendering them intolerable nuisances: Select Committee on Cheltenham Improvement Bill (Lords), May 12, 1852, pp. 13–22 (Charles Paul), HL/PO/PB/5/18/1, PA. According to Paul (p. 58), the drainage on the private estates was very good.

156. Circumstances at Cheltenham were believed to require the alteration of some of the clauses of the PHA. Although the GBH was not opposed to the idea, the Attorney General and Edward Lawes, the solicitor who drafted the PHA, recommended against it. Cheltenham's elites then sought a local act incorporating large parts of the PHA with the GBH's blessing. For a history of proceedings at Cheltenham, see Select Committee on Cheltenham Improvement Bill (Commons), March 17, 1852, pp. 3–75 (G. Williams), HC/CL/PB/2/20/5, PA.

157. Clauses permitting the compulsory purchase of the sewer company contributed to the defeat of the 1851 bill, because the Lords believed that the purchase price was too high. See Select Committee on Cheltenham Improvement Bill (Lords), July 18, 1851, pp. 10–13, HL/PO/PB/5/17/8, PA. In 1852, the town committee voted to renew the application for a local act, including the compulsory purchase clauses, but opposition from the company and the GBH led the committee to abandon the purchase clauses. The 1852 bill passed; in 1857, the commissioners negotiated a purchase of the company, with the GBH's blessing, for £9,000, well above the £6,820 it was appraised at in 1857 but well below £12,700 offered in 1851. The original capital was £7,600. See W. Ranger to GBH, August 11, 1857, MH/13/149, NA for approval of purchase. The 1852 bill elicited much more local objection to the sewerage scheme: Select Committee on Cheltenham Improvement Bill (Lords), May 12, 1852, HL/PO/PB/5/18/1, PA.

158. A memorial from one of the private estates specifically drew attention to this point, a point with which some members of the ad hoc committee promoting the bill

were in agreement: Select Committee on Cheltenham Improvement Bill (Lords), May 11, 1852, pp. 36–38 (Landsdowne memorial), HL/PO/PB/5/18/1, PA. For a committee member, see Select Committee on Cheltenham Improvement Bill (Commons), March 17, 1852, p. 273 (J. Bubb), HC/CL/PB/2/20/5, PA.

159. Select Committee on Cheltenham Improvement Bill (Lords), May 11, 1852, pp. 21–25 (G. Williams) HL/PO/PB/5/18/1, PA; Select Committee on Cheltenham Improvement Bill (Commons), March 17, 1852, pp. 296–300 (J. Bubb), March 18, 1852, pp. 135–36 (Charles Paul), HC/CL/PB/2/20/5, PA.

160. Select Committee on Cheltenham Improvement Bill (Lords), May 12, 1852, pp. 138–40 (Admiral Lloyd); p. 162 (Charles Jones), HL/PO/PB/5/18/1, PA. Williams defended the decision in 1852; Select Committee on Cheltenham Improvement Bill (Lords), May 11, 1852, pp. 101–2 (G. Williams), HL/PO/PB/5/18/1, PA.

161. "Cheltenham Town Commissioners," *Cheltenham Examiner*, October 11, 1854, 3.

162. Williams to GBH, and Tom Taylor minute, April 14, 1857, MH/13/49/1143/57, NA.

163. The hearings repeatedly state that the worst houses had no drainage and that the company had only drained well-to-do areas. Select Committee on Cheltenham Improvement Bill (Commons) May 19, 1851, (C. Paul), p. 52; May 27, 1851, p. 42 (C. Paul), HC/CL/PB/2/19/42, PA; Select Committee on Cheltenham Improvement Bill (Lords), 12 May 1852, p. 11 (Dr. W. Brooks); p. 17 (Charles Paul). HL/PO/PB/5/18/1, PA,

164. *The King against the Commissioners of Sewers for the Tower Hamlets*, 109 English Reports 195.

165. "Local Board of Health," *Kentish and Surrey Mercury*, January 15, 1859, 5.

166. "Local Board of Health," *Kentish and Surrey Mercury*, January 29, 1859, 5. An arrangement with Mr. Cheffins ensured that he would not protest again; "Local Board of Health," *Kentish and Surrey Mercury*, May 12, 1859, 5.

167. I do not want, however, to overcredit the Epsom LBH. The Epsom board's rationale for rating as it did was the culmination of several decades' worth of argument about indirect benefit, mainly by metropolitan sewers commissions. The language of health and indirect benefit, as I argued in chapter 2, had been developed for nearly forty years prior to this case, though for most of that time it had little traction.

168. Simon Szreter's observation about the "dogged campaign of a million Minutes" is apt; Szreter, "Importance of Social Intervention," 25.

169. Parliament's first attempt to extend the benefits of sanitary legislation to all districts was the 1865 Sewage Utilisation Act (28 & 29 Vict., c. 75), which permitted all corporate boroughs, local act authorities, and parishes not under the PHA/LGA to carry out drainage works as if they were. In the 1866 Sanitary Act, Parliament amended the 1865 SUA and permitted the newly constituted sewer authorities to subdivide their districts: 29 & 30 Vict., c. 90, s. 5. Parliament in 1867 passed another SUA, permitting an even more diverse range of potential sewer authorities and subdivided districts: 30 & 31 Vict., c. 113 ss. 2, 6.

170. Royal Sanitary Commission, 2nd Report, vol. III, Minutes of Evidence, PP 1871 (281-II), R Latter, q. 11377; C. F. Devas, q. 11368.

171. See LBH to LGAO, November 30, 1870 (emphasis in original), plus minute, MH/13/2/4717/70, NA. The GBH could have made the same case with respect to Eton College in the early 1850s but did not.

172. Briggs, *Victorian Cities*, 333.

173. Insofar as drainage was the preferred means to health in the Public Health Act, watersheds would have been a boundary option. However, even if these local authorities tried to forge boundaries that were in some sense organically connected to the purposes of the PHA, that would not have changed the decisions they had to reach regarding financing.

174. Of course, other processes were involved in this difference, most notably changing conceptions of poor relief: Lees, *Solidarities of Strangers*. The post-1867 Metropolitan Poor Act, permitting as it did shared (Union) costs of medical treatment for paupers, echoes in interesting ways the debate over the cost of preventive medicine under the PHA.

175. Gilbert, *Cholera and Nation*; Hamlin, *Cholera*; Hamlin, "Nuisances and Community," 371; Jenson, "Getting to Sewers."

176. Historians draw attention to the active character of late-nineteenth-century ideas of citizenship: Beavan and Griffiths, "Creating the Exemplary Citizen"; Meller, "Urban Renewal and Citizenship." For the diversity of local citizenship ideals, see Beavan and Griffiths, "Urban Elites"; D. Gilbert, "Community and Municipalism"; O'Reilly, "From 'the People.'"

Chapter Four

1. Halliday, *Great Stink*; Owen, *Government of Victorian London*, 47–73. For the related embankment, see D. H. Porter, *Thames Embankment*.

2. Dennis, "Modern London," 95–102; Halliday, *Great Stink*, 58–61; Sheppard, "Crisis of London's Government," 25.

3. The metropolitan census district was based on the old bills of mortality district, which had been substantially expanded in the 1830s: Freeman, *Geography and Regional Administration*, 153–54.

4. John Davis, *Reforming London*, app. 1; Sheppard, "Crisis of London's Government," 23–30; Webb and Webb, *Statutory Authorities*.

5. The separate commissions are explored in Hanley, "Metropolitan Commissioners"; P. J. Smith, "Before Bazalgette"; Sunderland, "Monument to Defective Administration?"; Webb and Webb, *Statutory Authorities*, 57–102.

6. Briggs, *Victorian Cities*, 332.

7. The principal reformations were the remaking of vestries under Hobhouse's act and the creation of twenty-eight metropolitan Poor Law unions: Green, *Pauper Capital*, 81–113.

8. Sheppard, "Crisis of London's Government," 24.

9. Finer, *Life and Times*, 306.

10. On cholera's role, see Dennis, "Modern London," 101; Owen, *Government of Victorian London*, 31; D. H. Porter, *Thames Embankment*, 62–63; Sheppard, *London, 1808–1870*, 247–96.

11. Parliament gave this body statutory sanction in 1848 (11 & 12 Vict., c. 112). Its boundary was the London death-registration district: Freeman, *Geography and Regional Administration*, 153–54. On the Metropolitan Commission of Sewers, see Dobraszczyk, *Into the Belly of the Beast*; Finer, *Life and Times*, 301–18, 326–31, 355–78; Halliday, *Great Stink*, 32–57; Hamlin, "Edwin Chadwick and the Engineers"; Sheppard, "Crisis of London's Government," 27–28.

12. Plagued with a dysfunctional membership from its inception, the Metropolitan Commission of Sewers struggled to implement its mandate to drain London. The work for which the commission is most remembered is the defective Victoria Street sewer, built at a high cost and prone to failure from the word go. The Metropolitan Board of Works' accountant, G. S. Hatton, said it cost about £90,000: Select Committee on the MMA (Commons), June 25, 1860, p. 24, HC/CL/PB/2/28/82, PA. Yet the commission did and planned to do more than is sometimes remembered. For the commission's work on mapping, see Dobraszczyk, *Into the Belly of the Beast*, 23–55; Hamlin, "Edwin Chadwick and the Engineers."

13. Report Presented to the Metropolitan Board of Works by Messrs. Hawksley, Bidder and Bazalgette, 1858, PP 1857–58 (419), 4–5.

14. T. Hunt, *Building Jerusalem*, 259–312. Joshua Toulmin Smith was one of the proponents of this view. On Smith see Claus, "Languages of Citizenship"; Weinstein, "Local Self-Government."

15. Briggs, *Victorian Cities*, 332–33; Owen, *Government of Victorian London*, 32.

16. 18 & 19 Vict., c. 120. Owen, *Government of Victorian London*, 31–46. The MMA determined the structure of metropolitan government until 1889.

17. Hall used parishes as the second tier. Thus, parochial boundaries determined the boundary of his new district. He had to end it somewhere and chose the recently developed metropolitan census district: Dennis, "Modern London," 102.

18. On these bodies see John Davis, *Reforming London*; Halliday, *Great Stink*; Owen, *Government of Victorian London*; D. H. Porter, *Thames Embankment*, 50–76; Young and Garside, *Metropolitan London*.

19. Historians have already documented another well-known financial crisis: the MBW was not authorized to borrow enough money to allow it to complete the works it was expected to do. In 1858, Parliament gave the MBW the financial authority it needed: Owen, *Government of Victorian London*, 39, 53–55, 165. Halliday, *Great Stink*, 58–76 is an excellent synopsis of the MBW's problems in this light. Martin Daunton highlights the key issue discussed in the present chapter in *Trusting Leviathan*, 275–76.

20. Daunton, "Taxation and Representation," 110.

21. *Hansard Parliamentary Debates*, 3rd ser., vol. 160 (August 1, 1860), col. 460.

22. For Poor Law rates, see Green, *Pauper Capital*, 189–246. John Davis, who deals with the MBW, argues that vestries were unequalized before the 1894 London Equalization of Rates Act: see *Reforming London*, 35–37, 168–71. I have been strongly influenced by Davis's argument that social differentiation in London and thus unequal access to resources for vestries and district boards was the major structural problem with metropolitan government under the 1855 Metropolis Local Management Act (10–50). Yet I am impressed with the possibility for equalization within the district boards before 1894 which, though discretionary, required particular ideological, legal,

and political strategies. In addition, although Davis is correct in stating that first-tier charges (metropoliswide MBW rates, which were levied according to rateable value) were not a direct transfer to poor parishes and that the resulting expenditure benefited wealthy parishes (174), it was a real struggle to get drainage classed as a standard first-tier charge. The present chapter thus complements Davis's work on metropolitan equalization. See also Offer, *Property and Politics*, 161–76.

23. I include a bill prepared but not submitted in 1858.

24. On the Poor Law and public health, see Hamlin, *Public Health and Social Justice*.

25. "The Metropolitan Board of Works *v.* the Vauxhall Bridge Company," *Justice of the Peace*, July 25, 1857, pp. 469–70; *The Metropolitan Board of Works against The Vauxhall Bridge Company*, 119 English Reports 1505–12. This latter case was an action to recover rates going back to the Surrey and Kent Commissioners of Sewers and the Metropolitan Commission of Sewers. The MBW was responsible for them under the 1855 MMA, and the outcome would of course determine the MBW's future behavior.

26. This case was one of the very many cases brought before the courts by companies of one sort or another. At the Middlesex Quarter Sessions in July 1859, twenty-five different cases (out of ninety) concerned rate appeals by various companies, quite a number of them being appeals against rates levied under the 1855 MMA: St. George in the East Vestry, L/SGE/A/5/25, THLHLA. The greater financial resources of waterworks, dock, gas, railway, and bridge companies ensured that if anyone was going to appeal, chances were that those companies would be among them. In another case, the Vestry of St. George Parish tried to raise the amount it assessed the London Dock Company from £17,000 to £73,000: *Howell . . . against The London Dock Company*, 120 English Reports 79–86, especially 85–86. Hanley, "Metropolitan Commissioners."

27. *The Metropolitan Board of Works against The Vauxhall Bridge Company*, 119 English Reports 1509–10. Counsel for the company argued, in contrast, that sewers had always served "sanatory" purposes (1511). The *Justice of the Peace* did not report this claim, from which counsel quickly moved on.

28. The decision by Queen's Bench to comment on the "great question" was itself interesting. Although this was always at the court's discretion, and although it was asked to do so by both parties in this case, the Court did not always answer questions not required to be answered because it had reached its conclusion on other grounds. *The Metropolitan Board of Works against The Vauxhall Bridge Company*, 119 English Reports 1512.

29. *The Metropolitan Board of Works against The Vauxhall Bridge Company*, 119 English Reports 1511.

30. *The Metropolitan Board of Works against The Vauxhall Bridge Company*, 119 English Reports 1512.

31. *Howell . . . against the London Dock Company*, 120 English Reports 79–86.

32. *Howell . . . against the London Dock Company*, 120 English Reports 85. Some indication of the flawed character of this ruling came less than a year later. The Wandsworth DBW, a very frequent early litigant, rated property of the West Middlesex Waterworks Company within its area. In one of the quirks of English parochial organization, the company had property in Putney, a parish within the Wandsworth DBW, but some of that property was detached from the parish and was an island within the parish of Barnes. Barnes, however, was not within the Wandsworth DBW;

thus, the DBW would do no work in Barnes or, by extension, in the detached part of Putney surrounded by Barnes. The waterworks company argued, not unreasonably, that its land in the detached part of Putney could not possibly be benefited by the work of the DBW; under the 159th section, the DBW was bound to order the property exempt from rating. The court ruled against the company, basing its ruling on the fact that the DBW was not required to order an exemption. The board was required to consider it, but the final decision was the DBW's alone. In the ruling, the court made no reference to the *Howell* decision, although counsel for the waterworks stressed it in oral argument. It is telling that the court noted that it would not rule on whether the Wandsworth DBW's decision was right or wrong, but given the judges' comments both before and after this case on benefit and the need to consider it, this claim of neutrality functioned rhetorically to undermine the Wandsworth DBW's decision: "The West Middlesex Waterworks Company *v.* the Wandsworth District Board," *Justice of the Peace*, May 29, 1858, pp. 336–37. The court would revisit this section in *St. Botolph's* case, discussed below.

33. *Howell against the London Dock Company*, 120 English Reports 85.

34. *Howell against the London Dock Company*, 120 English Reports 86. Although the judges acknowledged that under the old dispensation, property could be rated for paving only if it fell within a certain distance of a street, and that the MMA had no such limitation, implying that the principle had changed, they nonetheless believed that Parliament had not altered the principle on which rates should be based.

35. See "The West Middlesex Waterworks Company *v.* the Wandsworth District Board," *Justice of the Peace*, May 29, 1858, pp. 336–37; *The Queen, on the prosecution of the Vestry of Paddington, v. the Great Western Railway Company* (1858), 28 LJ (MC) 59–64; *The Queen, on the prosecution of the Trustees of the Poor of and within the Parish of St. John, at Hackney, respondents, v. Thomas Oliver Goodchild, clerk, appellant;* and *The Queen, on the Prosecution of the same respondents, v. Thomas Davis Lamb, clerk, appellant* (1858), 27 LJ (MC) 233–54. When it applied to amend the 1855 MMA, the MBW itself twice cited the court's "Decision" in the case of *Vauxhall:* Report of the Main Drainage Committee on the Draft Bill for Amending the Metropolis Local Management Act, March 18, 1860, pp. 9, 12, MBW/2410/0103, LMA.

36. "The West Middlesex Waterworks Company *v.* the Wandsworth District Board," *Justice of the Peace*, May 29, 1858, pp. 336–37; *The Queen, on the prosecution of the Vestry of Paddington, v. the Great Western Railway Company* (1858), 28 LJ (MC) 59–64.

37. See *The Queen, on the prosecution of the Trustees of the Poor of and within the Parish of St. John, at Hackney, respondents, v. Thomas Oliver Goodchild, clerk, appellant;* and *The Queen, on the Prosecution of the same respondents, v. Thomas Davis Lamb, clerk, appellant* (1858), 27 LJ (MC) 241. This was the tithe rent-charge exemption: Report of the Building Act and General Purposes Committee on the Amendment of the Metropolis Local Management Act, May 27, 1858, p. 5, MBW/2405, LMA.

38. At least three different sources of funds were involved: the Rock Loan (£200,000), the Clergy Mutual Assurance Fund Loan (£140,000), and various other debts of the old commissioners (£95, 689, including additional money owed to the Rock Insurance Company). Owen's discussion of this episode is in *Government of Victorian London*, 45.

39. Select Committee on the MMA, 27 June 60, pp. 151–52 (Bazalgette), HC/CL/PB/2/28/82, PA; June 29, 1860, p. 211, 216 (Hatton).

40. St. Luke, Chelsea Vestry, MBW/2409/030, LMA; St. Mary Abbots, Kensington Vestry, MBW/2409/031, LMA; Fulham DBW, MBW/2409/032, LMA.

41. This position had some parliamentary support. In 1860, John Hubbard, MP maintained that there was no other way of establishing benefit than the amount of work done in the parish: *Hansard Parliamentary Debate*, 3rd ser., vol. 160 (August 1, 1860), col. 464.

42. "Greenwich and Deptford District Board of Works," *Kentish and Surrey Mercury*, October 18, 1856, 4; "Greenwich and Deptford District Board of Works," *Kentish and Surrey Mercury*, December 13, 1856, 6; "Greenwich and Deptford District Board of Works," *Kentish and Surrey Mercury*, January 24, 1857, 5. The MCS had trouble with Greenwich at the end of its existence: "Metropolitan Commissioners of Sewers," *Times*, September 28, 1855, 10; "Metropolitan Commissioners of Sewers," *Morning Chronicle*, September 29, 1855, 3. For another example, see the discussion on Camberwell in "Metropolitan Board of Works," *Times*, November 26, 1856, 4.

43. Greenwich accepted that under the Metropolitan Commission of Sewers, all parishes within a separate sewerage district paid for all works within that district. However, Greenwich believed that the Metropolitan Commission of Sewers system came to a close before its parish had a chance to get works done that would have benefit it more directly.

44. "Greenwich and Deptford District Board of Works," *Kentish and Surrey Mercury*, October 18, 1856, 4; "Metropolitan Board of Works," *Kentish and Surrey Mercury*, March 7, 1857, 4. Greenwich also was unsuccessful in trying to overturn the precept based on the fact that the wrong assessment was used: "The Precept of the Metropolitan Board of Works," *Kentish and Surrey Mercury*, May 8, 1858, 4, "Greenwich and Deptford District Board of Works," *Kentish and Surrey Mercury*, June 12, 1858, 4. On the county rate, see Owen, *Government of Victorian London*, 163–64.

45. The DBW attempted to obtain a loan for the sums but was unsuccessful and as a result washed its hands of the matter: "The Metropolitan Board of Works and the Greenwich Ratepayers," *Kentish and Surrey Mercury*, October 15, 1859, 4.

46. "The Ratepayers and the Claims of the Metropolitan Board of Works," *Kentish and Surrey Mercury*, 25 February 1860, 4–5. A case on these rates appeared at Queen's Bench in 1861; the appeal against the rate was dismissed on technical grounds: "Empson (Appellant) v. the Metropolitan Board of Works (Respondents)," *Times*, January 17, 1861, 11.

47. An early, unsuccessful appeal came out of St. Luke, Chelsea in February 1858: *Christie, appellant, v. the Guardians of the Poor of St. Luke, Chelsea, respondents* (1858), 27 LJ (MC) 153–60.

48. Part of the parish was within the Western Division of Westminster, a separate sewerage district under the 1848 act; the MBW assessed that part with more than £1,500 for the work. "Ex Parte the Vestry of St. Marylebone, in the County of Middlesex," *Justice of the Peace*, December 18, 1858, pp. 799–800.

49. Finance Committee Minutes, November 29, 1858, MBW/831, LMA.

50. For Edmund Humphrey Woolrych's October 28, 1856, reply to the memorials against the apportionment, see MBW/2409/029, LMA. The Report of the Building Act and General Purposes Committee on the Amendment of the MMA, May 27, 1858, p. 13, declined to reapportion the debt apart from Counter's Creek: MBW/2405, LMA.

51. St. Pancras apparently had refused to pay all but one of the precepts charged on it for the debts: Select Committee on the MMA (Commons), July 2, 1860, pp. 14–15 (William Durrant Cooper), HC/CL/PB/2/28/83, PA. Owen claims that only in St. George's, Hanover Square did reluctance to pay reach open resistance: Owen, *Government of Victorian London*, 45.

52. MBW Printed Minutes, October 22, 1858, LMA; MBW Printed Minutes, December 31, 1858, LMA.

53. The reapportionment was done by the Works and General Purposes Committee, which was a committee of the whole board: Clifton, *Professionalism, Patronage and Public Service*, 20. Two further reapportionments were prepared. The second apportionment may be found at MBW/2409/084, LMA. The third apportionment is found in MBW Printed Minutes, July 1, 1859, LMA.

54. In the preliminary inquiry held on the occasion of the Surrey and Kent Commission of Sewers Bill in 1847, the riverfront parishes opposed rateable value, because their vastly more densely populated parishes had more rateable value simply by virtue of the greater number of houses. Unimproved land was rated at one quarter: Copies of Reports for the Commissioners of Woods and Forests relative to Applications for Local Acts, PP 1847 (124–61), 266–67. (The Surrey and Kent Report is number 61 of the eighty-six reports in Parliamentary Paper no. 124.) In other situations, however, rating on the basis of area instead of rateable value tended to equalize the costs between equally built-up areas with different-quality housing; thus, a wealthy area benefited more than a poor area. MBW Printed Minutes, April 29, 1859, LMA prints a memorial from Lewisham indicating the kind of frustration that could result.

55. The criteria were rateable value within separate sewerage districts (the original Metropolitan Commission of Sewers method), work actually done within the parish, area benefited by the work, and rateable value of the area benefited by the work. In the case of a contract for one sewer, Greenwich profited from the exercise in reapportionment, seeing its cost fall from nearly £5,000 under the original apportionment to about £50: Works and General Purposes Committee Papers, June 13, 1859, MBW/699, LMA.

56. As a result of the final reapportionment, West End parishes on the north side of the river had the entire cost of the Counter's Creek sewer (some £43,000) thrown onto the main drainage rate. Lewisham and Greenwich managed to have a considerable portion of the costs of the Ravensbourne sewer (£10,000) thrown onto the main drainage rate and shifted other costs onto St. Paul Deptford, a poor parish within the Greenwich DBW that saw its portion rise from £5,000 to £6,300 to £8,100. Riverside parishes in the old Surrey and Kent Commission of Sewers, too, assumed a greater burden than their wealthier upland neighbors, replicating the 1847 situation described in chapter 2.

57. On the MMA, see John Davis, *Reforming London*, 10–16; Sheppard, "Crisis of London's Government," 23–39. For an overview of London's nineteenth-century government, see R. Porter, *London: A Social History*, 288–311.

58. 19 & 20 Vict., c. 112.

59. Report of the Building Act and General Purposes Committee on the Amendment of the Metropolis Local management Act, May 27, 1858, MBW/2405, LMA.

60. Report of the Building Act and General Purposes Committee on the Amendment of the Metropolis Local Management Act, May 27, 1858, pp. 4–5, MBW/2405, LMA. Section 164 of the MMA stipulated that any land exempt from the sewers rate under 11 & 12 Vict., c. 112 (the act governing the Metropolitan Commission of Sewers) should remain so under the 1855 MMA; 18 & 19 Vict., c. 120, s. 164. The MBW believed that the exemption was without merit, but if it was to continue, the kinds of property exempt should be specifically listed. Section 175 offered an exemption to certain extraparochial places. The MBW declined to tackle the lower rating on agricultural land, presumably because the MBW did not want the bill to get bogged down by opposition. Rating agricultural land was politically contentious into the twentieth century: Keith-Lucas and Richards, *History of Local Government*, 135–41.

61. A Bill for the Better Local Management of the Metropolis, PP 1854–55 (60), s. 131.

62. This seems to be the case on the basis of the reported debate in *Hansard Parliamentary Debate*, 3rd ser., vol. 138 (June 12, 1855), cols. 1864–65 and (June 21, 1855), col. 2308.

63. A Bill . . . for the Better Local Management of the Metropolis, PP 1854–55 (234), s. 162. See 18 & 19 Vict., c. 120, s. 170 for similar wording.

64. *Hansard Parliamentary Debate*, 3rd ser., vol. 138 (June 21, 1855), col. 2308.

65. Report of the Building Act and General Purposes Committee on the Amendment of the Metropolis Local Management Act, May 27, 1858, p. 11, MBW/2405, LMA. Historians have noted that the bill attracted little parliamentary attention. Owen suggests that the amendments that were made were mostly insignificant: see Owen, *Government of Victorian London*, 37. The MBW would have disagreed.

66. Select Committee on the MMA (Commons), July 2, 1860, p. 118–20, HC/CL/PB/2/28/83, PA. The witness was William Durrant Cooper, a solicitor to the St. Pancras Vestry. According to Farrant, he was a "zealous liberal" and secretary of the Reform Club. Possibly Hall knew him through this connection: Farrant, "Cooper, William Durrant."

67. Report of the Building Act and General Purposes Committee on the Amendment of the Metropolis Local Management Act, May 27, 1858, pp. 11–12, MBW/2405, LMA.

68. For a list of Metropolitan Commission of Sewers districts, see Papers relating to Metropolitan Drainage, PP 1854 (180), 34. These separate sewerage districts were generally formed out of the even older separate commissions of sewers for the metropolis. The relationship between these separate sewerage districts and the vestries and districts of the MBW was not exact: the MMA was based on parochial boundaries, which the Metropolitan Commission of Sewers' separate sewerage districts occasionally traversed.

69. Papers Relating to Metropolitan Drainage, PP 1854 (180), 24–25.

70. Select Committee on the Great London Drainage Bill, PP 1852–53 (629), q. 3237. Stephenson argued that Bermondsey, for example, would never be able to pay for its own drainage.

71. A bill creating a new body to complete London's drainage was introduced at the end of 1853, primarily for discussion. This bill made no reference to the two divisions Jebb proposed: A Bill to Establish a Metropolitan Board of Sewers, PP 1852–53 (905).

72. This was a concern for at least one vestry: Hanley, "Public Health, London's Levels," 33.

73. For the circumstances associated with this, see Halliday, *Great Stink*, 62–70; Owen, *Government of Victorian London*, 39, 53–55.

74. Halliday, *Great Stink*, 71–76. MBW Special Committee minutes, July 2, 1858, MBW 675, LMA. The Report of the Proceedings of the MBW for the Year 1858–59 suggested that the 1858 amending act was prepared in consultation with the MBW and the government: PP 1859 (sess. 2), (178), 1. The MBW reviewed a copy of the amending bill on July 19, 1858: MBW Printed Minutes, LMA.

75. For the bill, see PP 1857–58 (216), s. 15. For the statute, see 21 & 22 Vict., c. 104, s. 12. According to Joseph Bazalgette, difficulties with the working of the 1855 act led to this clause: Select Committee on the MMA (Commons), June 29, 1860, pp. 33–34, HC/CL/PB/2/28/82, PA.

76. *The Metropolitan Board of Works against The Vauxhall Bridge Company*, 119 English Reports 1512.

77. The fact that this was at best a partial attempt to prevent disease, and that many of the MBW's other actions actually increased disease, does not change the character of this development. On the MBW's exacerbation of overcrowding and its misguided attempts at fixing the problem, see Stedman Jones, *Outcast London*, 151–96. On typhus and overcrowding in London and the work of the London medical officers of health (MOH), see Hardy, *Epidemic Streets*, 191–210; Hardy, "Urban Famine"; Wohl, "Unfit for Habitation."

78. It could be argued that the MBW's first-tier duties and charges had already defined a new community. That is true, but the 1855 statute gave the MBW very few specific duties compared with those of the vestries and the district boards. The MBW's two-page list of duties (18 & 19 Vict., c. 120, ss. 135–44) included mainly drainage-related powers, street naming and house numbering, and, finally, traffic improvements. This last was a large power, allied with the power to obtain land by voluntary or forced sale (ss. 139–44). The MBW would use it destructively, but it was hedged in by financial limits. In 1855, the main drainage was the most important metropolitan duty of the MBW: Owen, *Government of Victorian London*, 37–38. In contrast, the V/DBW list of duties (ss. 67–134) was twelve pages long.

79. The 1858 act strengthened the MBW's hand for future amendments. The board could now argue that the charges for what the 1855 statute called intercepting and main sewers were inconsistent, the intercepting a metropolitan charge as sanctioned by the 1858 amending act, the main a local charge assessed according to benefit as sanctioned by the original 1855 act. See Report of the Committee of Works and Improvements, July 11, 1859, MBW/2410/093, LMA.

80. MBW Special Committee Minutes, July 2, 1858, MBW 675, LMA. Owen sees Thwaites's tenure as chair (1856–70) as crucial: Owen, *Government of Victorian London*, 40–41. The notorious Great Stink was obviously important in focusing parliamentary attention, but the Stink by itself does not explain the character of this change. Something about the MBW's powers also was going to have to change.

81. The MBW directed the Committee of Works and Improvements to prepare a bill to reapportion the Metropolitan Commission of Sewers debt and amend the MBW's powers in the 1859 session: MBW Printed Minutes, December 31, 1858, February 11, 1859, LMA. The principal objects of the 1859 bill were the

reapportionment of the Metropolitan Commission of Sewers debt and the enactment of a new benefit clause (effectively repealing s. 170): see Works and General Purposes Committee Minutes, April 4, 1859, MBW/730, LMA; Report of the Committee of Works and Improvement, July 11, 1859, p. 1, MBW/2410/093, LMA. For the bill, see PP 1859 (sess. 2), (128). The bill was not settled in committee until July 11, 1859, and was not introduced to the House of Commons until August 13, 1859, far too late for passage. For the chronology, see Report of the Main Drainage Committee on the Draft Bill for Amending the Metropolis Local Management Act, March 18, 1860, p. 5, MBW/2410/0103, LMA. In October 1859, the MBW directed the committee to return to the task of an amending bill and to include all desired amendments, not just those pertaining to the powers of the MBW. This new bill, a major amending act touching on a very wide range of MBW and V/DBW powers, was presented to the MBW on March 18, 1860.

82. Report of the Main Drainage Committee on the Draft Bill for Amending the Metropolis Local Management Act, March 18, 1860, pp. 7–9, and 11–13 (clauses 8 and 19), MBW/2410/0103, LMA. For the bill, see PP 1860 (122). In the bill, these two clauses were numbered 7 and 20. The bill was brought in on April 3, 1860. In it, the MBW made three changes regarding debts and rates. In the first place, the MBW applied for statutory sanction for reapportioning the old Metropolitan Commission of Sewers debts. In addition, the board proposed that all expenses after January 1, 1856, on the Victoria Street sewer be considered a metropolitan charge. The MBW endorsed its third apportionment on December 23, 1859: MBW, Printed Minutes, LMA. Second, the board emphatically rejected benefit as a criterion of rateability. Going beyond the relevant section in the 1858 amending act, the bill stipulated that rates should be raised on the basis of annual rateable value "and according to no other Principle or Criterion whatever": Report of the Main Drainage Committee on the Draft Bill for Amending the Metropolis Local Management Act, 18 March 1860, p. 8, MBW/2410/0103, LMA. For the bill, see PP 1860 (122), s. 7. Finally, the board repealed section 164 (authorizing certain exemptions). The rationale for the repeal provided the clearest and strongest indication of the MBW's thinking about health, justice, and property: Report of the Main Drainage Committee on the Draft Bill for Amending the Metropolis Local Management Act, March 18, 1860, pp. 12–13, MBW/2410/0103, LMA. This repeal article, present in the 1858 draft amending bill but abandoned in the 1859 bill, likely for strategic reasons, explicitly removed all preexisting exemptions to contribution.

83. The sewers rate could be spent on public conveniences and the suppression of nuisances, to name only two examples: Report . . . on the Draft Bill, pp. 11–13, MBW/2410/0103, LMA.

84. It was not always clear why some petitioners opposed the bill, because they did not always show up at the hearings. See MBW Printed Minutes, July 13, 1860, LMA, for list of petitioners.

85. The select committee completely rewrote the MBW's suggested clause to grant the MBW discretion in assessing rates on the entire metropolis or parts of it as they saw fit, having regard only to the annual rateable value: Select Committee on the MMA (Commons), July 3, 1860, pp. 62–64, HC/CL/PB/2/28/83, PA. The select committee returned to this amended clause after passing it, almost certainly at the MBW's instigation, clarifying the wording by making the repeal of section 170

of the 1855 act explicit: Select Committee on the MMA (Commons), July 4, 1860, pp. 2–3, HC/CL/PB/2/28/83, PA. The 1860 bill did not pass, but the 1860 Select Committee's language reappeared in the (failed) 1861 bill. Slightly different language in the 1862 bill raised alarms at the MBW: see Special Committee Minutes, March 11, 1862, pp. 12–14, MBW/676, LMA. For the 1862 Act see 25 & 26 Vict., c. 102, s. 5.

86. The select committee possibly found the 1860 bill's provisions contradictory. The bill claimed both that benefit could be apportioned (in the Rock Loan clauses) and that it could not (in the repeal of s. 170). The chairman certainly drew attention to the contradiction: Select Committee on the MMA (Commons), June 27, 1860, pp. 24–25, HC/CL/PB/2/28/82, PA. The select committee accepted that some of the debt from the Metropolitan Commission of Sewers could be thrown onto the metropolis as a whole. The fact that Parliament had already sanctioned a metropoliswide charge for the intercepting sewers scheme in 1858 must have helped the select committee make this decision, which involved no new principle but only the application of the principle settled in the 1858 act—that parts of the main drainage were paid for by the whole metropolis—to a new situation. The MBW floated the reapportionment as a separate bill in 1861, but that bill was withdrawn by the member who had introduced it. There was no reference to reapportionment of the Rock Loan in the 1862 amending bill, although during the Lords hearings, some parishes tried unsuccessfully to get amendments reapportioning some of the debt: Select Committee on the MMA (Lords), July 22, 1862, p. 21, HL/PO/PB/5/28/22, PA.

87. The select committee decided to strike clause 20, which removed the exemption from taxation that section 164 of the 1855 MMA had conferred. This was not a disaster for the MBW. The only exemptions explicitly in force on January 1, 1856, applied to tithe rent-charge exemptions and a small amount of property in Hackney: Report . . . on the Draft Bill, March 18, 1860, pp. 12–13, MBW/2410/0103, LMA. The MBW was probably less afraid of those exemptions continuing than of other parties claiming that the section should apply to them as well. The select committee may have trusted to the courts to police this clause; at all events, they explicitly refused to give mainly dock companies the statutory exemption they wanted: Select Committee on the MMA (Commons), July 4, 1860, pp. 2–5, July 5, 1860, pp. 1–2, HC/CL/PB/2/28/83, PA.

88. The committee room was cleared of observers and shorthand note takers during votes on clauses.

89. Select Committee on the MMA (Commons), July 3, 1860, p. 11, HC/CL/PB/2/28/83, PA. Hawksley correctly noted under examination by the MBW's attorney that this kind of division was exactly what the 1848 Public Health Act permitted (p. 14). But he ignored, or was unaware of, the recent case in which the Epsom LBH did not divide but instead threw the expense on the whole district. The decision in Queen's Bench undermined his notion of benefit. See also Bazalgette's discussion of the politics of this sewer: Select Committee on the MMA (Commons), June 29, 1860, pp. 14–20, HC/CL/PB/2/28/82, PA.

90. Select Committee on the MMA (Commons), July 3, 1860, p. 17, HC/CL/PB/2/28/83, PA.

91. Select Committee on the MMA (Commons), June 29, 1860, p. 74, HC/CL/PB/2/28/82, PA.

92. Select Committee on the MMA (Commons), June 29, 1860, pp. 81–83, HC/CL/PB/2/28/82, PA. Bazalgette did not volunteer the fact that Rotherhithe was very poor, and would probably not get drained unless St. George's Hanover-square (as referred to by the shorthand writer) helped pay for it. Opposing counsel certainly did not raise the issue.

93. Select Committee on the MMA (Commons), July 3, 1860, p. 23, HC/CL/PB/2/28/83, PA.

94. No medical witnesses testified at these hearings. Medical witnesses often testified at select committee hearings on public bills dealing with public health (such as the 1855 hearings on the Nuisance Act), and at the preliminary inquiry local act hearings in 1847 (discussed in chap. 2). Given the MBW's emphasis on the sanitary benefits of its work, the lack of a medical witness is noteworthy. The MBW did not itself have medical officers, and there was no medical man to whom it could obviously turn. The board also might not have wanted to risk controversy over disease causation, as when John Snow testified in 1855. However, if the significance of miasma for health was controversial, one would expect opposed counsel to have called medical witnesses, but they did not. The consequence of having no medical witnesses, however, was that the issue of benefit at the hearings tended to be discussed in engineering terms, or at least by engineers (and surveyors). The MBW's sanitary arguments as advanced in court and in internal documents were not aired. In 1862, Bazalgette had to be prompted even to allude to them: July 22, 1862, pp. 13–14, 18–19, HL/PO/PB/2/28/22, PA.

95. Select Committee on the MMA (Commons), July 3, 1860, p. 23, HC/CL/PB/2/28/83, PA.

96. *Hansard Parliamentary Debates*, 3rd ser., vol. 160 (August 1, 1860), col. 460; "Metropolis Local Management Act Amendment Bill," *Times*, August 2, 1860, 7. Opposition to the bill continued, however, and it was eventually withdrawn: *Hansard Parliamentary Debate*, 3rd ser., vol. 160 (August 22, 1860), cols. 1709–11. In 1861, the MBW tried again, hiving off the reapportionment clauses into a separate bill, entirely at the expense of some vestries and district boards that wanted it. Although the main bill passed the Commons, it did not survive the Lords. In 1862, five years after deciding to seek an amending act, the MBW finally obtained largely satisfactory rating clauses. The bill passed through the Commons with some difficulty. At one point it was feared it would fail, largely as a result of a new debate over the constitution of the MBW. The battle for benefit was fought even in 1862, although that one-day select committee hearing in the Lords was a far cry from the ten-day trial in 1860. Bazalgette was again called to the stand to testify that benefit could not be the basis of the MBW's assessments. Challenged by a Lord that "these new [rating] principles" in the bill could be "extremely arbitrary and tyrannical," Bazalgette at first pulled his punches, claiming that any rate levied according to benefit would be "more or less unjust." Pressed by the lord to admit that the new principles were unjust and arbitrary, Bazalgette fought back, testily noting that he was "hardly prepared to say that" until somebody showed him a better method. The lord abandoned this line of questioning, and the clauses passed: July 22, 1860, p. 16, HL/PO/PB/5/28/22, PA.

97. This generally was thought to result from an undervaluation of urban property relative to agricultural property. Parliament was not so concerned with this that it solved the problem, which lingered until the end of the century and beyond. But

it did, beginning in 1833 and increasingly thereafter, grant rate reductions to agricultural property for specific purposes such as urban drainage. Select Committee on County Rates, PP 1834 (542); Select Committee of the House of Lords . . . into the Charges of the County Rates, PP 1835 (206).

98. Counties collected rates not from individuals but from parishes, which collected them as property taxes.

99. The 1834 select committee agreed with this conviction but was uncertain about the implications of it, and it did not propose any radical redefinition of rating responsibility: Select Committee on County Rates, PP 1834 (542), iv–v.

100. Brundage, *Making of the New Poor Law*, 25; Green, *Pauper Capital*, 78–79; Poynter, *Society and Pauperism*, 218, 287–88, 298. I do not discuss here the very controversial issue of the taxation of real versus personal property in the funding of local services.

101. The history of settlement is thoroughly discussed in Charlesworth, *Welfare's Forgotten Past*. The law of settlement was complex and changing, but the importance of settlement persisted in the early nineteenth century and beyond.

102. This could of course arise in rural settings as well and was exacerbated by the practice of failing to provide housing for laborers within the parish in which they worked, forcing them to keep a settlement in their home parish. This is fully discussed in Caplan, "The New Poor Law."

103. An individual may well have moved to a new parish of employment, yet if he or she needed relief and had not acquired a fresh settlement, the new parish of residence could "remove" him or her to the settled parish. After 1819, Irish relief claimants could be removed back to Ireland. Indeed, some sixty thousand Irish were removed in the aftermath of the famine: Charlesworth, *Welfare's Forgotten Past*, 175–78; Green, *Pauper Capital*, 37, 43; MacRaild, *Irish Diaspora*, 51. In the mid-nineteenth century, the new legal category of irremovable poor allowed individuals who had migrated in search of work some security: Charlesworth, *Welfare's Forgotten Past*, 62–65.

104. The literature on the 1834 Poor Law is vast. I have used Brundage, *English Poor Laws*; Brundage, *Making of the New Poor Law*; Green, *Pauper Capital*; Hodgkinson, *Origins of the National Health Service*; and Lees, *Solidarities of Strangers*. Parishes were financially responsible for their settled poor even when a parish was in a Poor Law union, thus perpetuating the unequal burden of poor relief among parishes. Union expenses were themselves calculated on the basis of each parish's expenditure for poor relief. Prior to the 1834 act, some cities had formed unions of parishes with equal rating: see Webb and Webb, *Statutory Authorities*, 110–15.

105. Clerk to C. S. Butler, MP, August 1, 1860, Whitechapel DBW, Clerk's Out-Letters, L/WBW/10/1, THLHLA. Similar letters were sent to A. S. Ayrton, MP, R. Hanbury, MP, and G. H. C. Byng, MP.

106. Caplan, "The New Poor Law," 268–69, 276–78.

107. London's Poor Law history was distinctive; see Green, *Pauper Capital*, 201–8 for a discussion of the crisis of the 1850s. See also Ashbridge, "Paying for the Poor," 107–22.

108. The *East London Observer*, founded in 1857, also editorialized in favor of it: "Equal Poor Rates," *East London Observer*, October 3, 1857, 2; "Equalization of Poor Rates," *East London Observer*, June 9, 1860, 2.

109. Caplan, "New Poor Law," 282–84.

110. Poor-rate equalization was also debated in the medical press: Hodgkinson, *Origins of the National Health Service*, 456.

111. Papers Relating to Drainage, PP 1854 (180), 24–25.

112. In cases where the Poor Law had been introduced into London and Poor Law unions formed, Parliament could fall back on these preexisting unions and make the newly created DBWs coterminous with them. See Schedules A and B of the Act 18 & 19 Vict., c. 120 for the original list of vestries and district boards and the district board memberships. The arrangement of parishes into vestries and district boards changed somewhat over time as the population changed: see John Davis, *Reforming London*, app. 1 for a list of these changes.

113. 18 & 19 Vict., c. 120, s. 159. See John Davis, *Reforming London*, 35.

114. *Howell . . . against the London Dock Company*, 120 English Reports 79–86; "The West Middlesex Waterworks Company *v.* the Wandsworth District Board," *Justice of the Peace*, May 29, 1858, pp. 336–37.

115. The Whitechapel DBW had the same composition as the Whitechapel Union.

116. Whitechapel DBW Finance Committee minutes, February 13, 1856, February 21, 1856, and February 29, 1856, L/WBW/3/1, THLHLA.

117. Whitechapel District Board of Works, Minutes, March 3, 1856, L/WBW/1, THLHLA. The DBW referred the matter back to the Finance Committee, which in late May reiterated its support for a rate based on rateable value. The DBW again approved this decision shortly thereafter. Whitechapel District Board of Works, Finance Committee Minutes, May 30, 1856, L/WBW/3/1; DBW Minutes, June 2, 1856, L/WBW/1, THLHLA.

118. Whitechapel District Board of Works Minutes, August 4, 1856, L/WBW/1, THLHLA. Unfortunately, the records of the DBW do not provide any further information about the decision, and the district had no local newspaper until the establishment of the *East London Observer* in September 1857. However, the Whitechapel DBW's decision makes sense in light of the debate over equalization.

119. Return of the Rateable Value, PP 1864 (379), 1. For absolute rateable value in 1860, see THLHLA, L/WBW/10/1, Clerk's Out-Letters, February 8, 1860.

120. "Holy Trinity, Minories," *East London Observer*, January 30, 1858, 3.

121. Select Committee on the MMA Amendment Bill (Commons), July 3, 1860, pp. 59–60, HC/CL/PB/2/28/83, PA.

122. Whitechapel DBW, Clerk's Out-Letters, March 19, 1857, L/WBW/10/1, THLHLA.

123. Details of the case may be found in "The Overseers of the Poor of St. Botolph Without, Aldgate, Appellants, v. Whitechapel District Board of Works, Respondents," *Justice of the Peace*, September 8, 1860, pp. 564–67; *The Overseers of the Poor of the Parish of St. Botolph Without Aldgate, Appellants, against The Board of Works for the Whitechapel District, Respondents*, 121 English Reports 377–84; "The Whitechapel v. Aldgate Law Suit," *East London Observer*, June 9, 1860, 2; "The Whitechapel v. Aldgate Law Suit," *East London Observer*, June 16, 1860, 2. Note that the details provided in each source vary slightly, as do the observations of the justices. The transcripts cannot be considered verbatim records. The report in the *East London Observer* has the most information from the hearing; the legal reports have more information on the facts. The other defaulting parishes or places were Holy Trinity, Minories and the Precinct of Saint Katherine.

124. St. Pancras Vestry Minutes, December 31, 1856, January 8, 1857, P/ PN2/M/1/1, Camden Local Studies Library.

125. The MBW's 1858 report on amending the MMA claimed that vestries and district boards complained loudly about apportioning benefit: Report of the Building Act and General Purposes Committee, May 27, 1858, p. 11, MBW/2405, LMA.

126. Select Committee on the MMA (Commons), July 2, 1860, pp. 80–83, HC/ CL/PB/2/28/83, PA.

127. Select Committee on the MMA (Commons), July 2, 1860, p. 83, HC/CL/ PB/2/28/83, PA.

128. Select Committee on the MMA (Commons), July 2, 1860, p. 93, HC/CL/ PB/2/28/83, PA.

129. Select Committee on the MMA (Commons), July 2, 1860, p. 81, HC/CL/ PB/2/28/83, PA.

130. Clerk to C. S. Butler, MP, August 1, 1860, Whitechapel DBW, Clerk's Out-Letters, L/WBW/10/1, THLHLA. Similar letters were sent to A. S. Ayrton, MP; R. Hanbury, MP; and G. H. C. Byng, MP. The Whitechapel DBW Finance Committee records payment to Dyson & Co., Parliamentary Agents, for work on behalf of the 1860 amending bill: Whitechapel DBW Finance Committee minutes, August 31, 1860, L/WBW/3/1, THLHLA. The Docks Company hoped to attain its objective with an amendment to section 159, but failing that tried to get a specific exemption for its property. This exemption failed in committee and on the floor of the House.

131. East End labor markets are the subject of Stedman Jones, *Outcast London*.

132. Some MPs certainly did not see the justice of Turner's position. Speaking in support of the dock companies, John Hubbard wondered, Why "should those properties be taxed for the advantage of districts lying outside their barriers?" *Hansard Parliamentary Debate*, 3rd ser., vol. 160 (August 1, 1860), col. 456.

133. "Metropolis Local Management Act Amendment Bill," *Times*, August 2, 1860, 7.

134. Digby, *Pauper Palaces*, 96. Approximately 51 percent of poor relief was now a union charge as a result of this bill: Caplan, "New Poor Law," 290. Peter Wood also sees 1861 and 1862 (when the Union Assessment Committee Act was passed) as key: Wood, "Finance and the Urban Poor Law," 38. The year 1860 marks the revision of residualism for Lees, *Solidarities of Strangers*, 231–32.

135. In 1864, the temporary Poor Relief (Metropolis) Act (27 & 28 Vict., c. 116) made the cost of the houseless poor a metropoliswide charge based on rateable value: Caplan, "New Poor Law," 296. It was made permanent the following year: 28 & 29 Vict., c. 34. This involved a small amount of money, comparatively speaking, but an important principle: Green, *Pauper Capital*, 233–35.

136. 30 Vict., c. 6. This act made numerous changes in the organization of metropolitan relief. All parts of the metropolis were placed under the Poor Law Board. The newly created Metropolitan Asylums Board also took over paying for the houseless poor, built institutions, and paid for "lunatic," smallpox, and fever cases (other conditions were added over time) out of the Metropolitan Common Poor Fund. The board also could use this fund for a variety of other medical purposes including salaries, medicines, and dispensaries. See Hodgkinson, *Origins of the National Health Service*, 306–12, 500–3, 513–22 for the various medical provisions. Ayers calls these the first state hospitals: Ayers, *England's First State Hospitals*.

137. Ayers sees the 1867 act as a "significant step towards the socialization of medical care" in England in that the burden was distributed collectively on more equitable lines: Ayers, *England's First State Hospitals*, 28. This act did not necessarily address the most glaring inequities; Whitechapel, for example, remained a solo union, ordered to upgrade on its own: Hodgkinson, *Origins of the National Health Service*, 504. Waddington describes the various revenue strategies taken by the Whitechapel Union: "Paying for the Sick Poor."

138. For historians of medicine, the 1867 act is the outcome of a series of scandals and inquiries around metropolitan workhouse infirmary medical care, carried out by physicians and publicized by the *Lancet*. See Ayers, *England's First State Hospitals*, 14; Hodgkinson, *Origins of the National Health Service*, 429–50; Richardson and Hurwitz, "Joseph Rogers." Poor Law historians see the 1867 act in the context of a crisis in metropolitan relief. Green claims that equalization was accompanied by, and was intended to promote, a renewed attack on outdoor relief. See Green, *Pauper Capital*, 239–44; Daunton, *Trusting Leviathan*, 281–82. On the campaign against outdoor relief, see Lees, *Solidarities of Strangers*, 259–68.

139. These approaches to poor rate equalization were limited in the sense that although unions were often larger administrative units than parishes, they were frequently just as incapable of meeting the costs of their own poor as single parishes. The defect of this system was the root of the controversy in Poplar: Keith-Lucas and Richards, *History of Local Government*, 65–91. On local government finances in the twentieth century, see ibid., 127–58.

140. Referring to the 1860 *St. Botolph* case, Kelly claimed, "The court of law thus held that that was to be done which Parliament had determined ought not to be done." See "Metropolis Local Management Act Amendment Bill," *Times*, August 2, 1860, 7.

141. One case involved DBW discretion in allocating expenses among constituent parishes, one involved the liability of property to rating, and one involved the Rock Loan. There were, of course, other rates cases.

142. Details of the case may be found in "The Overseers of the Poor of St. Botolph Without, Aldgate, Appellants, v. Whitechapel District Board of Works, Respondents," *Justice of the Peace*, September 8, 1860, pp. 564–67; *The Overseers of the Poor of the Parish of St. Botolph Without Aldgate, Appellants, against The Board of Works for the Whitechapel District, Respondents*, 121 English Reports 377–84.

143. "The Whitechapel *v.* Aldgate Law Suit," *East London Observer*, June 9, 1860, 2.

144. "The Whitechapel *v.* Aldgate Law Suit," *East London Observer*, June 9, 1860, 2. "The Whitechapel *v.* Aldgate Lawsuit," *East London Observer*, June 16, 1860, 3. Notwithstanding the unanimous verdict, the justices apparently were not entirely comfortable with the outcome of this decision. Chief Justice Alexander Cockburn admitted that unfairness and injustice might be done where large parishes were united with small ones, but the Court was obliged to assume that Parliament had foreseen that possibility when it passed the law. Cockburn's claim that Parliament had with due deliberation passed an unjust law is remarkable. This claim appears in three otherwise very different accounts of the judgment and probably cannot be attributed to a shorthand writer's overactive imagination. Cockburn's comment foreshadowed the comment made to Joseph Bazalgette in the 1862 hearings in the Lords, where one lord argued that "these new principles" of rating in London were unjust, arbitrary, and tyrannical.

145. *The Metropolitan Board of Works against The Vauxhall Bridge Company*, 119 English Reports 1512.

146. *The Overseers of the Poor of the Parish of St. Botolph Without Aldgate, Appellants, against The Board of Works for the Whitechapel District, Respondents*, 121 English Reports 383. Unfortunately, neither Charles Crompton nor any of the other judges gave their opinion of the nature of indirect benefit in the *Whitechapel* case. Crompton, however, had heard the *Dorling v. Epsom* case, in which the verdict was unanimous, so his reference to indirect benefits in the Whitechapel case could be a reference to *Dorling v. Epsom*. In any event, this decision was a novel reading of benefit in the metropolis, and it is nearly unthinkable that a similar judgment would have been rendered in 1830 or even 1845, as cases from the time make clear: Hanley, "Metropolitan Commissioners of Sewers." To be sure, indirect benefit had already effectively made headway even before 1845. The criterion of individual benefit was not strictly applied in London by the 1830s, and rating by level generally implied that not everyone would benefit in the same way or to the same degree. Yet judges continued to voice support for individual benefit even as they permitted its erosion. Even when supporting level rating, judges did not support indirect benefits. Had the principle of indirect benefit been accepted from the time the commissioners first mooted it in the 1820s, the history of the metropolitan commissions of sewers would have been very different.

147. Chief Justice Cockburn asked Sir Fitzroy Kelly if he believed that under the old system, an individual could appeal a sewers rate if he received no benefit. When Kelly replied that the individual could, Cockburn fired back that "you would not have much chance of success." "The Whitechapel *v.* Aldgate Lawsuit," *East London Observer*, June 9, 1860, 2.

148. *The Queen against Head and the Metropolitan Board of Works*, 122 English Reports 158–63.

149. *The Queen against Head and the Metropolitan Board of Works*, 122 English Reports 160.

150. *The Queen, on the prosecution of the Imperial Gas-Light Company, appellants, v. Head and the Metropolitan Board of Works, respondents*, 32 LJ (MC) 115–20, especially 119.

151. In order to reconcile the MMA with the Court's previous opinions, however, the judges engaged in a substantial piece of legal gymnastics. In the first place, the Court argued that the use to which any property was put could not govern the rate, because the rapid development of London meant that property used for one purpose one day might be used for another some short time later, and the rates could not fluctuate up and down. The Court reconciled this with the statutory exemptions based on use, such as the one-quarter rating for agricultural and other land, by noting that gas pipes were not mentioned in the section: *The Queen against Head and the Metropolitan Board of Works*, 122 English Reports 158–63, especially 161–63.

152. It is not clear how the Court's reasoning in *R. v. Head*, where the test was drainage, was consistent with that in *Whitechapel* or in *Dorling*, where the test was indirect benefit. The Court can only have squirmed when counsel for the MBW began to expound on the ruling in *Dorling*. At this point, according to the reports, he was stopped by the Court: *The Queen against Head and the Metropolitan Board of Works*, 122 English Reports 158–63, 161.

153. *Pew and Others, Appellants, The Metropolitan Board of Works, and Collins and Another, Respondents,* 122 English Reports 1183–88.

154. *Empson v. MBW* in 1861 dealt with the same issue, but Epsom lost on a technicality. "Empson (Appellant) *v.* the Metropolitan Board of Works (Respondents)," *Times,* January 17, 1861, 11.

155. In oral argument, the Chief Justice suggested that the crucial issue was the old sewers law. "Pew and others *v.* The Metropolitan Board of Works," *Times,* January 19, 1865, 11.

156. The fact that Parliament rejected the MBW's attempt to reapportion according to benefit was not a factor in the decision. The Court was not allowed to review *Hansard* or early versions of bills in an attempt to determine legislative intent: Stebbings, *Victorian Taxpayer,* 117.

157. Copy of Short-Hand Writer's Notes of Judgment, Pew *v.* The Metropolitan Board of Works, p. 8, February 25, 1865, MBW, 2370, LMA.

158. "Pew and others *v.* The Metropolitan Board of Works," *Times,* January 19, 1865, 11.

159. Copy of Short-Hand Writer's Notes, MBW, 2370, LMA.

160. F. H. W. Sheppard, *London 1808–1870,* 247–96; Owen, *Government of Victorian London,* 169–92. On the Surrey and Kent Commission of Sewers, see Dyos, *Victorian Suburb,* 140. Gareth Stedman Jones delivers a scathing indictment of the MBW and second-tier sanitary administration in regard to slum clearances and housing in *Outcast London,* especially chapters 9 and 10. For another view of the disease-prevention work of metropolitan medical officers of health, see Hardy, *Epidemic Streets.*

161. See, Hanley, "Metropolitan Commissioners"; P. J. Smith, "Before Bazalgette"; and Sunderland, "Monument to Defective Administration?" for some recent evaluations of the separate commissions of sewers. On the MBW and V/DBW, see John Davis's structural account of the limitations of metropolitan government; Davis, *Reforming London,* 33, 50. See also Luckin, "Metropolitan and Municipal." For a study of the MBW's internal structure, see Clifton, *Professionalism, Patronage.*

162. The officers most involved were the surveyors of the old commissioners and the engineer of the MBW, Joseph Bazalgette. These men undoubtedly worked in conjunction with their political superiors, and it is difficult to know who was more important in formulating what would become the official position. Drawing on the "growth of government literature," Clifton stressed the role of the MBW's paid staff on policy formation: see Clifton, *Professionalism, Patronage,* x, 163. The role of the paid staff is difficult to detect in this case, and in any event the unpaid members were the ones who had to vote on every case and every clause.

163. Halliday, *Great Stink,* 65; Lancaster, "Thwaites, Sir John (1815–1870)." John Leslie served even longer, even if he was largely obstructionist. He began with the Westminster Commission of Sewers, moved to the Metropolitan Commission of Sewers, and ended up on the MBW: Clifton, *Professionalism, Patronage,* 172; Finer, *Life and Times,* 356–80. Richard Dennis is less impressed with the benefits of longevity: Dennis, "Modern London," 102.

164. Papers Relating to Drainage, PP 1854 (180), 25.

165. Daunton, *Trusting Leviathan,* 275–76 describes the shifting conception of the taxpayer from an individual consumer who paid for a charge for a service to an individual consumer who made a collective investment for health.

166. John Davis, *Reforming London*, 168.

167. As John Davis noted, the 1860 decision could just as easily be seen as permitting district boards to rate parishes according to parochial expenditure. It is perhaps not surprising that the Greenwich DBW remained largely unequalized in the 1890s: John Davis, *Reforming London*, 35n93. It is also true that even those district boards that did choose to equalize expenses according to the 1860 decision still remained constrained under the larger unequalized vestry system that Davis analyzed.

168. Owen, *Government of Victorian London*, 55–60. Camberwell Vestry, for example, only began to construct drainage works once the Metropolitan Board of Works' main drainage was available in 1864: Dyos, *Victorian Suburb*, 146. St. Leonard, Shoreditch, in contrast, was much more forward. It spent £30,000 between 1858 and 1863 for sewage and paving: Sheppard, "St. Leonard, Shoreditch," 341–42. Vestries and district boards spent substantial though widely varying amounts on improvements from 1855 to 1870, but vestry and district board spending escalated rapidly after about 1885: Clinton and Murray, "Reassessing the Vestries"; Halliday, *Great Stink*, 99; Owen, *Government of Victorian London*, 223.

169. As Simon Szreter pointed out, these principles can be recovered only through an analysis of a "million Minutes": "The Importance of Social Intervention," 25.

Chapter Five

1. A significant shift not made at this time was the one that permitted local authorities to build public housing. See, for example, Daunton, *House and Home*; Gauldie, *Cruel Habitations*; Rodger, "Political Economy."

2. Multiple practices of domestic privacy are discussed in Vickery, *Behind Closed Doors*, 25–48. See also Burnett, *Social History of Housing*, 74. On the late-century overlap of public and private spheres, see Adams, *Architecture in the Family Way*.

3. Mooney saw the control of common lodging houses in the mid-nineteenth century as one of the first steps in the control of individuals with contagious diseases: Mooney, "Public Health versus Private Practice," 239, 241. His study of infectious-disease notification after ca. 1870 tracks the state's ongoing concern with domestic relations and maps the changing contours of belonging and citizenship that arose from it: Mooney, *Intrusive Interventions*.

4. There were other objections to local control of domestic drainage, including the ill-health that many believed that household pipe drainage caused: Adams, *Architecture in the Family Way*, 36–72.

5. At the beginning of the nineteenth century, all drainage was a private benefit; that was the basis for taxing under the sewer rate. The movement to make main sewers, and only main sewers, a public benefit occupied metropolitan and provincial authorities, as we have seen, for several decades. One of the legacies of the traditional benefit principle was the persistence of individual drainage as a private benefit after the abstraction of main sewers from the category.

6. The House of Lords first defined the terms *drain* and *sewer* statutorily during the passage of the Public Health Act (PHA): Lawes, *Act for Promoting the Public Health*, 11, note *p*.

7. There was nothing inherent in the direct drainage of private property that determined its status as a private improvement. Some Victorian local authorities tried to destabilize the boundary between public and private drainage altogether. Indeed, this boundary has continued to shift over time. In 2011, for customers of Thames Water, the boundary literally moved. (The link to this development is now broken, but the author has the leaflet describing it.) This boundary is also permeable. The city in which I live recently adopted a program subsidizing homeowners who purchase low-flush toilets. In the mid-nineteenth century, the idea that the local authority would subsidize the purchase of a water closet would have been seen as using public money to improve private property. Today, we have decided that this essentially private improvement is enough of a public good that it should be subsidized: Winnipeg, "Water Conservation." The Province of Manitoba's public energy utility also subsidizes certain home improvements: Manitoba Hydro, "Find Ways to Save Energy."

8. The classic study is Mort, *Dangerous Sexualities*. See also Poovey, "Domesticity and Class Formation," 122–23. Poovey saw Chadwick's attack on common lodging houses in *Report on the Sanitary Condition* as part of his attempt to infuse working-class life with middle-class notions of domesticity. Mort (especially 13–22) drew attention to the way in which sexuality was integral to the public health movement from its earliest incarnation. Alan Hunt, *Governing Morals*, 80 also stresses the link between sex and moral reform.

9. For surveys of sanitary arrangements over the second half of the century, see Burnett, *Social History*, 214; Daunton, *House and Home*, 246–62; Luckin, "Pollution in the City"; Wohl, *Endangered Lives*, 89–110. Sanitary modernity, of course, is not a purely progressive development. Benidickson highlights the problematic environmental consequences in *Culture of Flushing*. See also the essays by Bernhardt and Stippak in Massard-Guilbaud and Rodger, *Environmental and Social Justice*.

10. The courts took these matters seriously. An 1858 case involving conversion to water closets (*Tinkler v. The Board of Works for the Wandsworth District*, 44 English Reports 989–94) went to the Court of Appeal in Chancery. An 1863 drainage case (*Cooper v. The Board of Works for the Wandsworth District*, 143 English Reports 414–21) yielded a legal principle that Justice Steven Rares of the Federal Court of Australia cited as a crucial case for the "fair hearing rule" in a 2006 speech (see "Blind Justice," 1). Benidickson describes the legal difficulties associated with the water-closet revolution in *Culture of Flushing*, 78–97.

11. In the 1851 (14 & 15 Vict., c. 28, s. 16) and 1853 acts, local authorities were exempt from the restrictions on time of inspection imposed by the 1848 Public Health Act. This provision was added as the bill passed through Parliament.

12. J. T. Smith, *Laws of England*, 44, note *n*, vigorously rejected domiciliary inspection, except with respect to lodging houses.

13. According to Shaftesbury, in 1857, after just over five years of operation, the police had made over seven hundred thousand lodging-house inspections. Assuming that these numbers are correct—and they suggest an astonishing level of activity—and that the police saw only ten people per visit, it is possible that they saw over 7 million people: *Hansard Parliamentary Debates*, 3rd ser., vol. 146 (July 16, 1857), col. 1544.

14. Crook, "Accommodating the Outcast."

15. On the taxonomy of the poor, see Himmelfarb, *Idea of Poverty*, 312–400; Luckin, "Revisiting the Idea." See also Jennifer Davis, "Jennings' Buildings."

16. Eastwood, *Government and Community*, 160–62.

17. Of course, much of this work was also authorized by local acts. For provincial cities, see the various locations described in D. Fraser, *Power and Authority*. For London, see Halliday, *Great Stink*; Owen, *Government of Victorian London*, 47–73.

18. The PHA (11 & 12 Vict., c. 63, s. 49) permitted local boards of health to order the compulsory drainage of property within one hundred feet of a sewer. See Johnson, *Acts for Promoting*; Lawes, *Act for Promoting the Public Health*. For similar powers in London, see the 1848 Metropolis Sewers Act, 11 & 12 Vict., c. 112, s. 46.

19. 11 & 12 Vict., c. 63, s. 51 (1848 Public Health Act); 11 & 12 Vict., c. 112, s. 48 (1848 Metropolis Sewers Act); 18 & 19 Vict., c. 120, s. 81 (1855 Metropolis Local Management Act).

20. Although indoor plumbing is regarded as the standard today, even in the period leading up to World War I, fewer than half of the houses in major British cities were equipped with indoor water closets. Wohl explained the delay, if such it can be called, as a result of a variety of factors: Wohl, *Endangered Lives*, 101–7, 166–73. On the technical and legal complexity of some sanitary schemes, see Burn, *Age of Equipoise*, 137; D. Fraser, *Power and Authority*, 64–65; Hamlin, "Muddling in Bumbledom"; Luckin, "Pollution in the City," 213–17. On the water-closet revolution, see Benidickson, *Culture of Flushing*, 78–97.

21. Property owners in the pre-1840 period were, it is true, not completely free of government oversight. See Hennock, "Urban Sanitary Reform," 113; Jones and Falkus, "Urban Improvement."

22. Wohl, *Endangered Lives*, 198, 310–13.

23. HOTC, First Report, PP 1844 (572), q. 1560 (James Beck), q. 1674 (John Newman), q. 1875 (Samuel Mills), q. 2321 (Lewis Hertslet).

24. HOTC, First Report, q. 3168. Most metropolitan sewer authorities were comfortable with the notion that compulsory powers should be granted: James Beek, surveyor to Tower Hamlets, q. 1564; Thomas Donaldson, Chairman of the Westminster Commission of Sewers, q. 4064–7; Col. Grant, Chairman of the Tower Hamlets Commission, q. 3007.

25. HOTC, First Report, q. 3524.

26. "The Health of Towns' Bill," *Hertford Mercury and Reformer*, January 27, 1849, 2.

27. "Preservation of the Rights of Property," *Bucks Advertiser and Aylesbury News*, April 6, 1850, 4.

28. See HOTC, First Report, q. 3873 (Charles Freeth).

29. 11 & 12 Vict., c. 63, Interpretation of Terms; 11 & 12 Vict., c. 112, s. 147.

30. The HOTC Second Report indiscriminately referred to surface, main, branch and minor drains, with "minor" drains apparently signifying the household connection; PP 1845 (602), 3–33.

31. The 1846 Health of Towns' Bill and the 1847 Towns Improvement Clauses Act (10 & 11 Vict., c. 34) seemingly assumed that drains were private and sewers public, although neither bill defined the two terms. Neither the 1847 Westminster Commission of Sewers Act (10 & 11 Vict., c. lxx) nor the 1847 Surrey and Kent Commission of Sewers Act (10 & 11 Vict., c. ccxvii) included these definitions.

32. Reports of Surveyors of Metropolitan Commissioners of Sewers . . . as to the Difficulties Experienced by the Surveyors in Executing Improved Works of House Drainage, PP 1854–55 (282), 11.

33. The HOTC explored the high cost of private improvements, yielding one of the few rating recommendations in the report; HOTC, Second Report, PP 1845 (602), 27–28. See D. Fraser, *Urban Politics*, 156–57; Hamlin, *Public Health and Social Justice*, 255. Lawes claimed that the drainage of property and the provision of a sufficient privy was largely the owner's expense; Lawes, *Act for Promoting the Public Health*, 82, note *f*, 88, note *m*. In an effort to ease the financial strain, Parliament allowed individuals to amortize the costs of private improvements over thirty years via a private improvement rate (PIR) (11 & 12 Vict., c. 63, s. 90), but for various reasons this remedy was less than ideal. Loans for private improvement rates had to be raised on the security of something, and because the rate for poor households unable to pay for the connection in one installment was the only security, local boards of health found it difficult to raise money for the PIR. This issue gave local boards of health considerable trouble during the 1850s; see the correspondence between Bangor and the GBH from May 1855 to February 1856 for an example. In London, the cost of private house drainage could be spread over thirty years as well, but here too that did not answer the purpose. For the 1848 MCS Act, see 11 & 12 Vict., c. 112, s. 82. The 1855 MMA gave twenty years: 18 & 19 Vict., c. 112, s. 216. See also Wilson, "Finance of Municipal Capital," 35.

34. 11 & 12 Vict., c. 63, s. 51.

35. Johnson, *Acts for Promoting*, 89, note *t*.

36. The PHA (11 & 12 Vict., c. 63, s. 86) permitted local boards of health to credit premises adequately drained before the board constructed a sewer. According to Edward Lawes (who drafted the PHA), this provision was taken from the 1847 Towns Improvement Clauses Act; Lawes, *Act for Promoting the Public Health*, 135, note *b*. The provision in the TICA (10 & 11 Vict., c. 34, s. 28) was somewhat more elaborate.

37. 11 & 12 Vict., c. 63, s. 120. This appeal covered summary expenses and private improvement rates levied by the local board of health, such as the cost of making a drain into the sewers or the maintenance of privy accommodation: Lawes, *Act for Promoting the Public Health*, 169, note *t*, lists the eligible expenses. The 1855 MMA gave the right of appeal to the MBW: s 211.

38. The files at HLG/19/1, NA contain some orders made by the GBH under appeals levied against the private improvement rate (PIR) (11 & 12 Vict., c. 63, s. 120). One order for the Nantwich Local Board of Health concerns an order to construct a proper drainage ditch (drafted on March 29, 1852); another for the Kendal Local Board of Health details the sums to be collected from multiple owners for the combined drainage of particular properties (July 19, 1852). These protections were, of course, in addition to the right of all individuals to seek an injunction in Chancery restraining local authority action if they believed the injury to their property was serious enough—an option several individuals successfully pursued, as we shall see below.

39. The examples chosen in this section were collected at different times in the course of different research objectives and projects and are intended to be illustrative only. For more on Eton, Hertford, Ware, and Windsor, see Hanley, "All Actions."

40. On qualifications of rights of property, see Hoppit, "Compulsion, Compensation and Property Rights."

41. E. Eton to GBH, June 27, 1855, MH/13/71/2667/55, NA; September 4, 1855, MH/13/71/3438/55, NA.

42. E. Eton to GBH, June 27, 1855, MH/13/71/2667/55, NA.

43. C. S. Voules, Clerk to Eton LBH, to GBH, September 5, 1855, MH/13/71/3450/55, NA; A. Dickens to GBH, September 10, 1855, MH/13/71/3559/55, NA.

44. GBH to Dr. Eton, draft, September 15, 1855, MH/13/71/3559/55, NA.

45. E. Eton to GBH, September 4, 1855, MH/13/71/3438/55, NA. In a compulsory drainage case in London, the courts allowed the local authority discretion in judgments about the ways and means of drainage: "Austin *v.* the Vestry of the Parish of St. Mary, Lambeth," *Justice of the Peace*, February 20, 1858, p. 111; *Law Journal* 27 (1858): 388–92.

46. It seems extraordinary to contemplate that the drainage of one resident's property was a matter fit for ministerial review. Yet when we recall the degree to which the Home Secretary intervened in the production of local bylaws during the 1830s, we have less cause for surprise.

47. E. Eton to GBH, minute, June 27, 1855, MH/13/71/2667/55, NA; A. Dickens to GBH, minute, September 10, 1855, MH/13/71/3559/55, NA.

48. Johnson, *Acts for Promoting*, 133, note *i*. Section 86 of the PHA is not annotated in Lawes's 1849 book, but it was written before local boards of health had much experience (or any) with the statute. Johnson, in contrast, was the chair of an active LBH.

49. "Bucks Police," *Windsor and Eton Express*, October 19, 1850, 4.

50. The rationale for this restriction was that any building on top of the sewer would inhibit access to it in the event of an emergency. The LBH, furthermore, had twenty-four-hour access to the property in order to examine or repair the structure.

51. "Berlin v. Local Board of Health," *Windsor and Eton Express*, December 1, 1860, 4.

52. When we consider the inconvenience to which local board of health actions put other residents, the magistrates' reactions to Berlin's claim makes more sense. The Windsor Local Board of Health served notice on several occupiers of houses that it would be entering their premises in order to flush the sewers. For all that an Englishman's home was his castle was a rhetorical byword, it was nonetheless true for a small sector of the population. The board's action was a complete violation of it: "Windsor Local Board of Health," *Windsor and Eton Express*, June 28, 1862, 4.

53. 11 & 12 Vict. c. 63, s. 53 governed new houses. The board had to ensure that the level of the cellar was consistent with the district's drainage and that the house had appropriate sanitary accommodation. This power was also granted in the TICA (10 & 11 Vict., c. 34, s. 40).

54. "The Health of Towns' Bill," *Hertford Mercury and Reformer*, January 27, 1849, 2. Sworder was of course aware that dilapidated houses could be torn down; this section of the law concerned brand-new houses.

55. Ware LBH Minute Book, May 25, 1850, June 1, 1850, June 8, 1850, LBH/5/1/1, Hertfordshire Archives and Local Studies (HALS).

56. W. Hitch, Surveyor to Ware LBH, to LBH, June 1, 1850, LBH/5/3/16/36, HALS. Reason later complied (LBH/5/3/16/39) on June 22, 1850.

57. John Francis to LBH, June 21, 1850, LBH/5/3/142/64, HALS. T. Webb to GBH, June 15, 1850, MH/13/195/1884/50, NA, and draft reply, June 20, 1850.

58. "Ware. Prosecution under the Health of Towns Act," *Hertford Mercury and Reformer*, June 29, 1850, 3.

59. Builder ambivalence toward the Ware Local Board of Health is also clearly reflected in the letters the builders wrote to the board seeking permission for their projects. George Hitch, who had obviously had a run-in with the board's surveyor, wrote to the board, "I am not digging the foundations of my house yet. I am merely taking out some land for mortar and to fill in the ground again with gravel." Though Hitch accepted the board's control over his actions—he wrote to the board to justify them—he obviously resented it and was determined to resist it as far as possible. Yet in the very next sentence, Hitch wrote, "I shall lay proper plans before the board on Saturday." G. Hitch to LBH, November 1850, LBH/5/3/136/95, HALS. For further instances see W. Hitch to LBH, items 63 and 86, LBH 5/3/16, HALS; Ware LBH Minute Book, April 29, 1851, September 21, 1852, July 26, 1853, LBH/5/1/1, HALS. For instances of the Windsor Local Board of Health's enforcement of the builder provisions, see accounts in the *Windsor and Eton Express*, June 28, 1862, 4; July 5, 1862, 4; August 16, 1862, 4; January 30, 1864, 4; February 27, 1864, 4.

60. Ware LBH Minute Book, September 5, 1854, LBH/5/1/1, HALS.

61. 18 & 19 Vict., c. 120 s. 76 was the main clause. The vestries and district boards of works were authorized to control building for a variety of purposes, including obstructions, but my interest lies with the sections related to drainage and health.

62. The facts may be found in *The Board of Works for the Poplar District, Appellants, and Nicholas Knight and Henry Weitzell, Respondents*, 120 English Reports 561–70.

63. "The Poplar District Board of Works v. Knight and Weitzell," *East London Observer*, September 26, 1857, 3; "Poplar Board of Works and the Demolition of Property," *East London Observer*, October 31, 1857, 3. The paper opened its pages to the aggrieved builders: "Correspondence: The Poplar Board of Wrong," *East London Observer*, July 3, 1858, 3.

64. "Clarke *v.* The Vestry of Paddington," *Justice of the Peace*, January 29, 1859, pp. 69–70.

65. *Cooper v. The Board of Works for the Wandsworth District*, 143 English Reports 417, 420.

66. *Cooper v. The Board of Works for the Wandsworth District*, 143 English Reports 417–21. This case is discussed in Benidickson, *Culture of Flushing*, 85–89. Burn claimed that the holding was weakened in early twentieth-century cases: Burn, *Age of Equipoise*, 145–47. On *ultra vires*, see De Smith and Brazier, *Constitutional and Administrative Law*, 518–25.

67. *Cooper v. The Board of Works for the Wandsworth District*, 143 English Reports 420. It seems odd, however, that Parliament, so jealous of the power of local governments, would neglect a safeguard that was as obvious as the bench implied. The section (76) passed in 1855, and the apparent defect was not remedied in the amending acts that passed in 1856, 1858, or 1862, the last of which was a substantial revision. The 1862 amending act provided only for the application of a penalty for any house built without a permit (s. 88); section 76 of the 1855 act was not repealed until 26 Geo. 5 and 1 Edw. 8, c. 50.

68. Litigants such as Cooper or Tinkler, who were willing to go to the superior courts, could accomplish much. One of the most striking late-century decisions in favor of the rights of property is explored in Taggart, *Private Property*; see also Simpson, *Leading Cases*.

69. Other kinds of local board activity, such as nuisance prosecutions, probably yielded different outcomes. In any area of the law the outcomes may have varied by place even over time. For discussion of magisterial recalcitrance over nuisances in one location, see Kearns, "Cholera, Nuisances, and Environmental Management." For later in the century, see Crook, "Sanitary Inspection"; Hamlin, "Sanitary Policing."

70. Reports of Surveyors, PP 1854–55 (282). This problem was very common in the provinces as well. See, for example, the draft letter to the Bangor LBH (February 22, 1856, MH/13/13/560/56, NA) or the minute on Swansea's letter to the LGAO (March 17, 1859, MH/13/178/531/59, NA). Robert Rawlinson strongly supported empowering local boards of health to execute works of combined drainage: Royal Sanitary Commission [hereafter RSC], First report, 1868–69 (4218), q. 571.

71. Sanitary accommodation was often provided at the back of the house. Therefore, individual drainage required that the house drain come from the back and pass under the entire house. Back drainage meant that a common drain to which all houses would connect (and which itself then connected to a sewer) ran along the back of the property, significantly reducing the labor associated with draining the property. The PHA did not, however, permit local boards to run what was essentially a private drain for one property through the property of another. The back drain into which all properties fed thus had to be declared a sewer (rather than a drain) under the act in order for the local board to be allowed to build it, and that meant it had to be financed differently. This issue was inevitably entangled with the controversial issue of combined surface water–household waste drainage. For an analysis of this last issue, see Hamlin, "Edwin Chadwick and the Engineers." However, back drainage posed a distinct set of legal, in addition to engineering, difficulties.

72. In the 1848 Metropolis Sewers Act, the procedures for making a sewer were different from those for making a drain, hence the difficulty in executing combined drainage: Reports of Surveyors, PP 1854–55 (282), 3.

73. The 1855 Sewers (House Drainage) Act allowed the Metropolitan Commission of Sewers to order various private drainage works in an expedited fashion, bypassing some of the normal safeguards built into the process: 18 Vict., c. 30, s. 2. This was especially intended for low-value property: "Metropolitan Commission of Sewers," *Morning Chronicle*, October 18, 1855, 7. This power was continued in the 1855 MMA: 18 & 19 Vict., c. 120, s. 74. Section 215 of this statute also gave the vestries and district boards of works and the Metropolitan Board of Works the power to apportion as they saw fit.

74. Papers Relating to Metropolitan Drainage, PP 1854 (180), 177–83. On pipe versus brick sewers, see Hamlin, *Public Health and Social Justice*, 320–32. Notwithstanding the surveyors' reports, the MCS showed little interest in changing the system. In early 1852, the commissioners ordered that "as a general rule," separate drains were required for separate houses but permitted an unstated modification where advisable. Later that year, the General Committee reiterated this instruction, stressing that combined drainage be permitted only "exceptionally and for special reasons" and requiring the sanction of the court or MCS committee. See Copy of Orders of Courts and Committees as to House Drainage and Sewers, April 3, 1852, August 10, 1852, SC/PPS/031/192, LMA. Neither the MCS nor property owners were unanimously in favor of combined back drainage even once it was explicitly

legal: see "Metropolitan Sewers Commission," *Morning Chronicle,* November 8, 1855, 2; "Metropolitan Commission of Sewers," *Morning Chronicle,* November 22, 1855, 3.

75. The GBH dealt with this issue very early on. The Kendal LBH lost an appeal from a resident contesting his portion of the charge for a back drain into which his house drained: GBH Minutes, July 6, 1852, MH/5/6, NA. The GBH report on the matter can be found at Draft Orders, Kendal, July 19, 1852, HLG/19/1, NA. The St. Thomas LBH was likewise urged to understand properly the distinction between a drain and a sewer: GBH Minutes, September 20, 1852, MH/5/6, NA.

76. Despite the GBH caution, local boards were not entirely forthcoming to residents. The Croydon LBH ordered mass conversion in early 1852; in response to a complaint from a local property owner, the GBH was silent on the limited powers the LBH possessed: J. Davoson to GBH, March 1, 1852, and draft reply, MH/13/662/52, NA.

77. 11 & 12 Vict., c. 63, s. 51. Johnson, *Acts for Promoting,* 88–91, note *t,* cites this opinion. Lawes did not annotate this section, which suggests that the matter had not yet come up when he prepared his edition.

78. The GBH certainly danced around the issue and quoted Johnson's edition of the Public Health Act when confronted by local boards of health. The Bangor Local Board of Health solicited the opinion of the GBH on the compulsory substitution of water closets for privies in 1853 and again in 1854: Bangor LBH to GBH, December 16, 1853, MH/13/13/5706/53, NA; LBH to GBH, October 23, 1854; draft GBH to LBH, October 24, 1854, MH/13/13/5378/54, NA. The draft reply is a monument to bureaucratic equivocation. The GBH noted that the relevant section (s. 51) of the PHA was "in some degree" uncertain and for that reason suggested that the Bangor Local Board might "allay the exercise of their power." That phrase was, however, immediately crossed out. The GBH suggested instead that it might be well for the Bangor Local Board "not to insist on the powers they may have." This, too, was crossed out, and the GBH ended by suggesting that the Bangor Local Board "refrain from the exercise of the powers that they appear to possess" until the act was considered in Parliament.

79. Wohl, *Endangered Lives,* 107, describes this difficulty in the case of one small town during the 1880s.

80. GBH to Bangor LBH, October 24, 1854, draft, plus "Private" letter," MH/13/13/5378/54, NA. The hoped-for reconsideration of the Public Health Act did not happen in 1854; the 1855 amending bill did not even contain any provision radically different from the PHA: The Public Health Bill, 1855 (17 July 1855), PP 1854–55 (253), ss. 83, 93. This was still an issue in 1869: RSC, First Report, PP 1868–69 (4218), q. 5843. See Benidickson, *Culture of Flushing,* 90–91 for later in the century.

81. *Tinkler v. The Board of Works for the Wandsworth District,* 65 English Reports 979–82. The case is discussed in Benidickson, *Culture of Flushing,* 85–87.

82. *Tinkler v. The Board of Works for the Wandsworth District,* 44 English Reports 989–94.

83. *Tinkler v. The Board of Works for the Wandsworth District,* 65 English Reports 981–82.

84. *Tinkler v. The Board of Works for the Wandsworth District,* 44 English Reports 992–93.

85. The *Justice of the Peace* wrote a leading article about the case: "Metropolis Local Management Act and Nuisances Removal Act," *Justice of the Peace*, April 3, 1858, p. 205. It is important to recognize that the courts did not deny that local authorities had the power to order conversions. In 1860, the Vestry of St. Luke's ordered two privies converted into water closets in one court, and the owner (Lewis) of the houses neglected to do the work. The Vestry did it and sued to recover the charge (a not insubstantial 12/10). At a hearing, the magistrate declined to enforce payment. On appeal, the three QB judges all agreed that the magistrate got it wrong, notwithstanding the magistrate's and the respondent's reliance on Tinkler; in this case, the vestry had carefully stayed within the bounds of the statute. That is, it had not made a policy but had only investigated particular situations. See *The Vestry of St. Luke's, Middlesex, Appellants, against Lewis, Respondent*, 121 English Reports 934–39.

86. After an extraordinary number of minutes and counterminutes, Henry Austin provided a list of twenty-two towns that had done the work: Swansea LBH to LGAO, minute, December 16, 1858, MH13/178/2280/58, NA. See also RSC, First Report, PP 1868–69 (4218), q. 3131. For Swansea's later correspondence, see LB to LGAO, November 7, 1864, MH/13/178/3247/64, NA; LB to LGAO, December 12, 1864, MH/13/178/4092/64, NA; LB to LGAO, December 13, 1865, MH/13/178/4752/65, NA.

87. RSC, First Report, PP 1868–69 (4218), qq. 2909–14. Croydon reported that only one party had to be compelled to carry out private improvement: Croydon LBH to GBH, April 23, 1853, MH/13/56/1263/53, NA.

88. RSC, First Report, PP 1868–69 (4218), qq. 7394, 7405. But see G. Roberts, *Municipal Development*, 49. Richards presumably referred to sewered and watered districts.

89. RSC, First Report, PP 1868–69 (4218), qq. 2909–14. For a description of the Croydon board's somewhat casual attitude to its statutory limitations, see Johnson, *Acts for Promoting*, 89, note *t*.

90. Liverpool's medical officer of health was scathing about Manchester's situation, noting that water closets were found in Manchester's high-value housing but not in the homes of the poor: RSC, First Report, PP 1868–69 (4218), qq. 7725, 7804, 7828. Daunton, *House and Home*, 255 quotes the Manchester Corporation's efforts to "discountenance to the utmost extent possible the introduction of water closets in small tenements."

91. RSC, First Report, PP 1868–69 (4218), q. 2229. James Newlands, the borough engineer, was also firmly in favor of water closets: Hamlin, "James Newlands," 133.

92. "Town Council," *Liverpool Mercury*, January 7, 1864, 5; "The Health Committee and the Government," *Liverpool Mercury*, December 7, 1866, 8. The 1863 conversions coincided with a public campaign, led by Hugh Shimmin, about the state of the town's courts and alleys: D. Fraser, *Power and Authority*, 41–43; Wohl, *Endangered Lives*, 102. Trench also wrote a report on the issue: Scott, "Dr. William Stewart Trench."

93. See the description of the committee's practice in "Health Committee," *Liverpool Mercury*, January 4, 1867, 6.

94. I base this claim on the Health Committee's statement that if the case of Rook *v.* Higgins went against it, a new strategy would be necessary to order conversions: "The Health Committee and the Water Closet Question," *Liverpool Mercury*, February 20, 1868, 8); its subsequent claim of victory ("The Town Council and the

Water-Closet Question," *Liverpool Mercury*, June 18, 1868, 8); and the clerk's 1869 testimony before the RSC that Rook *v.* Higgins authorized the conversion. The Health Committee evidently won the case: RSC, First Report, PP 1868–69 (4218), q. 2227. The clerk noted to the RSC that a metropolitan case had concluded in the same manner. He was likely referring to *The Vestry of St. Luke's, Middlesex, Appellants, against Lewis, Respondent,* 121 English Reports 934–39.

95. RSC, First Report, PP 1868–69 (4218), q. 2227. This was a concern of some Health Committee members and the *Liverpool Mercury*: "Health Committee," *Liverpool Mercury*, January 4, 1867, 6; "The Water Closet Question," *Liverpool Mercury*, June 17, 1868, 6. These musings may well have triggered the Rook *v.* Higgins case, which was decided in 1868. Newcastle claimed to be able to convert under the 1866 Sanitary Act: RSC, First Report, PP, 1868–69, qq. 2824–26.

96. *Third Annual Report of the Local Board of Health, Sandgate* (Hythe: T. Shrewsbury, 1853), 3, MH/13/161/3404/53, NA.

97. J. R. Lonsdale to GBH, November 25, 1854, MH/5971/54, NA. The GBH obtained the opinion of the Law Officers of the Crown in early 1855.

98. Compare A Bill to Empower the Commissioners of Sewers to expend on house drainage a certain sum . . . , PP 1854–55 (111) and the same section as amended in committee, PP 1854–55 (119). Before the bill passed, this clause was again changed, requiring the MCS to recover the full cost: An Act to empower the Commissioners of Sewers to expend on House Drainage a certain sum . . . , 18 Vict., c. 30, s. 2. This minor episode recalls Parliament's determination to make house drainage a private expense in the 1847 Westminster Commission of Sewers Act.

99. The Sewers (House Drainage) Act flew through Parliament, having first reading on May 7 and receiving royal assent on June 15. *Hansard* records very little debate on this measure: *Hansard Parliamentary Debate*, 3rd ser., vol. 138 (May 7, 1855), cols. 227–29. It was effectively temporary and imposed a ceiling on expenditure; thus, members may have thought there was no point in engaging in lengthy debates over this measure. An online search of the British Newspaper Archive found little more in newspapers of the time (britishnewspaperarchive.co.uk, July 5, 2012).

100. *Hansard Parliamentary Debate*, 3rd ser., vol. 138 (May 7, 1855), cols. 227–29. Of course not all owners of low-value housing were poorer; plenty of such houses were owned by wealthy individuals and corporate bodies.

101. It may well be the case that Sir John Shelley's objection in Parliament that the money for this work was to come from loans that the MCS had specifically raised for other purposes was a decisive objection to repurposing it. But creative accounting was stock-in-trade for activist local boards of health.

102. On paying for private improvements, see Lyon Playfair, Report on the Sanatory Condition of the Large Towns in Lancashire, in HOTC, Second Report, Appendix, part II, PP 1845 (610), 3–4. The Liverpool Town Council was authorized to raise a sanitary rate, but it believed that under the local acts it was not authorized to raise a private improvement rate and amortize the cost over thirty years. In 1868, the Liverpool Health Committee received legal opinion that it could spread the private expenses over thirty years: "The Town Council and the Water-Closet Question," *Liverpool Mercury*, June 18, 1868, 8. Liverpool's MOH, Dr. Trench, professed frustration at laying the expense of the conversion at the feet of the poor. In addition to all the other objections that were raised to water-closet conversion in Liverpool, Dr.

Trench believed that cost was paramount: RSC, First Report, PP 1868–69 (4218), q. 7804.

103. "National Association for the Promotion of Social Science," *Liverpool Mercury*, October 15, 1863, 5; "Town Council," *Liverpool Mercury*, February 4, 1864, 5.

104. See the discussion in "Town Council," *Liverpool Mercury*, February 4, 1864, 5; "Town Council," *Liverpool Mercury*, July 7, 1864, 5; "Health Committee," *Liverpool Mercury*, January 4, 1867, 6; "The Health Committee and the Water-Closet Question," *Liverpool Mercury*, January 21, 1867, 3.

105. For the house owners' frustration, see "The Sanitary Bill and the Houseowners," *Liverpool Mercury*, March 17, 1864, 5; "The Water Closet Question," *Liverpool Mercury*, January 14, 1867, 7; D. Fraser, *Power and Authority*, 45. See also "Health Committee," *Liverpool Mercury*, December 7, 1866, 6.

106. "Health Committee," *Liverpool Mercury*, January 4, 1867, 6.

107. "The Water Closet Question," *Liverpool Mercury*, January 14, 1867, 7; "The Health Committee and the Water-Closet Question," *Liverpool Mercury*, January 21, 1867, 3.

108. "Health Committee," *Liverpool Mercury*, January 4, 1867, 6; "The Health Committee and the Water-Closet Question," *Liverpool Mercury*, January 21, 1867, 3.

109. "Health Committee," *Liverpool Mercury*, December 7, 1866, 6; "The Water Closet Question," *Liverpool Mercury*, January 14, 1867, 7.

110. Health Committee," *Liverpool Mercury*, January 4, 1867, 6. The council also subsidized the installation of water closets and baths by removing extra water charges for them: Sheard, "Water and Health," 155.

111. "Health Committee," *Liverpool Mercury*, December 7, 1866, 6. Opponents of public money for water-closet conversions, most of whom supported public payment for the drains, had no real answer to this. They had endorsed public support for the drains, though they were worried that when members of the public heard about it they would be unhappy. See the description of the committee's practice in "Health Committee," *Liverpool Mercury*, January 4, 1867, 6.

112. The water-closet question in Liverpool got mixed up with the town's scavenging system, nuisance prosecutions for town night-soil dumps, the pollution of the Mersey, and the water supply: see, for example, "The Health Committee and the Government," *Liverpool Mercury*, December 7, 1866, 7; "The Government and the Health Committee," *Liverpool Mercury*, January 25, 1867, 6. On the difficulties of Liverpool's water supply, see D. Fraser, *Urban Politics*, 160–69; Sheard, "Water and Health."

113. D. Fraser, *Power and Authority*, 41; D. Fraser, *Urban Politics*, 133–42.

114. The RSC asked Trench how far would he go with public funding, and he replied that it would only be for privies and water closets. The questioner seemed worried about possible corruption, because the electors were the owners of this kind of property. RSC, First Report, PP 1868–69 [4218], qq. 7824–26.

115. There is no doubt that Liverpool's ability to finance these works was a function of the surplus funds the council had at its disposal. But nobody forced the council to use the funds for these purposes. On Liverpool's wealth at this time, see Beckert, *Empire of Cotton*, especially 199–224.

116. "The Health Committee and the Government," *Liverpool Mercury*, December 7, 1866, 7.

117. RSC, First Report, PP 1868–69 (4218), q. 7712; Daunton, *House and Home,* 255.

118. In the case of public sewers, the money came from the sewers rate, levied initially under an 1830 statute on all property in the district: An Act for the better Paving and Sewerage of the Town of Liverpool (11 Geo. 4, c. xv, s. 62). In the case of household drainage and water-closet conversions, the money came from the sanitary rate and from the surplus funds of the borough. Only in the case of public sewers was the money specifically authorized for the purpose. On sewerage work in Liverpool at this time, see Muir, *History of Municipal Government in Liverpool,* 145–50; White, *History of the Liverpool Corporation,* 14, 34, 49. The commissioners established under this act had built fifty-three miles of sewers before 1846.

119. Playfair, Report on the Sanatory Condition, PP 1845 (610), paragraphs 8–10, 16–19.

120. Notwithstanding Trench's efforts, which the Town Council did not necessarily support, the RSC did not recommend that local authorities be allowed to use public funds for private drainage.

121. From a question asked of Trench at the RSC, it appears that another unnamed place believed or had done the same: RSC, First Report, PP 1868–69 (4218), q. 7824. According to Liverpool's clerk in 1868, no other town assisted with conversions: "The Health Committee and the Water Closet Question," *Liverpool Mercury,* February 20, 1868, 8. Daunton notes that Manchester and Leicester underwrote conversions around the turn of the twentieth century: Daunton, *House and Home,* 254. So did Sheffield: Taylor and Trentmann, "Liquid Politics," 233. For similar payments in cases of nuisances, see Hamlin, "Nuisances and Community," 375.

122. Liverpool's example is particularly instructive. The Health Committee endorsed a plan to convert water closets as a policy, but that report was never accepted by the full Town Council. Instead, the council acted on the recommendation of its MOH under the 1855 Nuisances Removal Act. The council was careful to do it piecemeal, one group of insanitary privies at a time. In light of the Tinkler ruling, this looks very astute. See "Town Council," *Liverpool Mercury,* February 4, 1864, 5; "Health Committee," *Liverpool Mercury,* March 11, 1864, 6.

123. Wohl, *Eternal Slum,* 74–75. Amanda Vickery discusses various kinds of lodging in the eighteenth century, particularly for bachelors, in *Behind Closed Doors,* 49–82. See also Hitchcock, *Down and Out,* 23–48.

124. Children could lodge on their own. For a description of young Charles Dickens's lodgings while the family was in the Marshalsea, see Richardson, *Dickens and the Workhouse,* 152–54. For Darwin, see Bowler, *Charles Darwin,* 68.

125. For the nineteenth century, see Burnet, *Social History of Housing,* 74; Gauldie, *Cruel Habitations,* 239, 244–46; Samuel, "Comers and Goers," 223–24; Wohl, *Eternal Slum,* 74–75.

126. Parliament first granted statutory control over lodging houses in the permissive 1847 Towns Improvement Clauses Act (10 & 11 Vict., c. 34, ss. 116–18). Further permissive control of common lodging houses came in the 1848 Public Health Act (11 & 12 Vict., c. 63, s. 66). In 1851, the discretion implied in the 1847 and 1848 acts was abandoned. The Common Lodging House Act (14 & 15 Vict., c. 28) required local authorities to undertake some oversight. This law was amended in 1853 (16 & 17 Vict., c. 41) and became the foundation of common lodging-house regulation

until 1875. Common lodging houses were also controlled in some local laws before 1847.

127. Crook, "Accommodating the Outcast."

128. The 1824 Vagrancy Act (5 Geo. 4, c. 83, s. 13) allowed police to obtain warrants to search houses "kept for the reception, lodging, or entertainment of travellers." M. J. D. Roberts has written persuasively about the vagrancy acts and the boundaries between public and private space: "Public and Private." For an early bylaw dealing with vagrancy and common lodging houses, see the St. Albans bylaws (enacted November 9, 1836): bye law no. 9, HO/70/5, NA. The 1839 Royal Commission on Constabulary, of which Edwin Chadwick was a member, also noted the importance of bylaws from a police perspective. Chadwick claimed that local authorities wanted to control these establishments, but the absence of any provision concerning lodging houses in bylaws submitted by town councils up to this time is striking. Some councils tried to control houses of ill fame or other public establishments, but I have not seen regulations about lodging houses per se. For an example of brothel control, see Shrewsbury's 1842 extensive bylaw code: *Bye Laws for the Good Rule and Government of the Borough of Shrewsbury* (Shrewsbury: R. Davies, [1842]), 20–21, HO/45/os 4416, NA. This lack of attention stands in marked contrast to that given other matters, in which town councils were pioneers (the health hazard, for example) and suggests that Chadwick may have oversold the extent of local concern. An online search of "lodging houses" turns up only nine references in *Hansard* from 1840 to 1846. On haunts, see Crook, "Accommodating the Outcast."

129. On cholera in 1831–32 and vagrants, see Brown, *Performing Medicine*, 151; Hart, *History of Cheltenham*, 283–84; Lees, *Solidarities of Strangers*, 127–28. This link did not go away; in 1855, there was a report on cholera and common lodging houses; see Report on the Common and Model Lodging Houses of the Metropolis, PP 1854–55 (1892).

130. Chadwick, *Report on the Sanitary Condition*, 419–21. For the Act, see 3 Vict., c. xxviii, ss. 20–22. Liverpool controlled lodging houses in its 1846 local act, taking a section from Glasgow's local act: Laxton, "Fighting for Public Health," 79.

131. Wohl claimed that the low standard of accommodation meant that few of the regularly employed would have used them: *Eternal Slum*, 74–75. That they had a cost at all, even if minimal, meant that the clients differed from those found in the casual wards of workhouses or night refuges. No doubt there was slippage between casual wards and what contemporaries called "low" lodging houses, with individuals moving back and forth as circumstances dictated. As Mayhew noted, the low lodging houses were not monolithic, and even within them some gradations existed: Mayhew, *London Labour and the London Poor*, 251–52. The first report of Captain William Hay ("one of the commissioners of the Metropolitan Police") on lodging-house control in the metropolis noted that some lodgers were "industrious . . . labourers, with their wives and children." They fell under the new rules: PP 1852–53 (237), 1.

132. Chadwick, *Report on the Sanitary Condition*, 419.

133. Second Report of the HOTC, PP 1845 (602), 66–67.

134. A Bill for the Improvement of the Sewerage and Drainage of Towns and Populous Districts, PP 1845 (574), s. 179. The bill did not pass, and it is impossible to know how the description would have been interpreted. These houses all had annual values under £15.

135. See 10 & 11 Vict., c. 34, s. 116 for the definition of a "public lodging-house."

136. Some local authorities, at least initially, used this definition: Crook, "Accommodating the Outcast," 430.

137. With one (largely irrelevant) exception, no future legislative or official definition made any explicit reference to vagrants or tramps. The 1853 Common Lodging House Bill briefly defined lodging houses in terms of "Wayfarers, Vagrants, or Mendicants": PP 1852–53 (573), s. 20. In this case, these terms were introduced for a very different purpose; see discussion below. The 1853 act included a separate section dealing with any common lodging house "in which beggars or vagrants are received," suggesting that they were a subset of the category of common lodging houses: 16 & 17 Vict. c., 41, s. 8. All other future bills and official opinions (see table 5.1) referred only to "persons" or "persons of the lowest classes." See Hundred House Division magistrates to HO, November 28, 1851, minute, HO/45/os4427/138, NA; Udsey Petty Sessional Division to HO, January 21, 1852, minute, HO/45/os4427/103, NA.

138. 10 & 11 Vict., c. 34, s. 117; 11 & 12 Vict. c. 63, s. 66.

139. To be sure, Lord Lincoln's 1845 bill had emphasized the public health significance of lodging houses: A Bill for the Improvement of the Sewerage and Drainage of Towns and Populous Districts, PP 1845 (574), s. 179. Lodging houses were certainly an object of local complaint, and in 1850 the General Board of Health received multiple letters from Whitechapel. See May 31, 1850, MH/13/268/1684/50, NA; August 4, 1850, MH/13/268/2664/50, NA; August 9, 1850, MH/13/268/2767/50, NA.

140. Even some matters thought to be related to health got no attention. The regulations ignored space as a metric for overcrowding and insalubrity. This was an issue at the time: Second Report of the HOTC, PP 1845 (602), 66–67. Some local authorities certainly asked about space requirements (Peterborough Improvement Commission to HO, October 28, 1851, HO/45/os4427/111, NA), and some included it in their draft regulations and bylaws (Hastings Local Board of Health Bye Laws and Regulations, made November 10, 1851, no. 22, HO/45/os4427/65, NA).

141. See Poovey, "Domesticity and Class Formation," 122–23.

142. Mort was not particularly interested in lodging houses and saw the Contagious Diseases Acts as the genesis of sanitary prescriptions around sex: Mort, *Dangerous Sexualities*, 73. On moral reform, see A. Hunt, *Governing Morals*, 57–76.

143. 14 & 15 Vict., c. 28, s. 9. The first version of the bill prohibited opposite sexes from sleeping in the same room, except for married couples and children under eight years of age: A Bill . . . Common Lodging Houses, PP 1851 (272) s. 27.

144. This omission is surprising. Certainly the 1845 Health of Towns Committee alluded to the inability to preserve decency in overcrowded common lodging houses, as did many of Chadwick's informants in the *Report on the Sanitary Condition*. Chadwick, it is worth noting, did not explicitly call for the separation of sexes in the *Report*. According to Mayhew, low lodging houses typically included rooms for children (under twenty years old in some cases). Others had separate male and female rooms, but there is no way to generalize: Mayhew, *London Labour and the London Poor*, 1: 257. Workhouses, as is well known, segregated husbands and wives as part of a larger system of classification: see Higginbotham, *Workhouse Encyclopedia*, s.v. "Classification."

145. See regulations for London [Report of Captain Hay on the operation of the Common Lodging House Act; PP 1852–53 (237), pp. 16–17] and the provinces; see, for example, the draft code sent by the Devizes Town Council, June 7, 1852, HO/45/os4416, NA. The Home Office reported to the GBH that it did not intend to disseminate the regulations beyond sending them to those authorities in need of them, and they do not seem to have been published: GBH Minutes, October 27, 1851, MH/13/5/5, NA.

146. Samuel, "Comers and Goers."

147. "Lodging Houses," *Quarterly Review* 82 (1847): 142–53; *Hansard Parliamentary Debate*, 3rd ser., vol. 99 (June 6, 1848), cols. 429–55, esp. 432–37. On the character of Ashley's philanthropy, see Koven, *Slumming*, 42; F. D. Roberts, *Social Conscience*, 210–11, 251–57. Robert Slaney and Blandford cosponsored the 1851 bill.

148. GBH to HO, October 10, 1850, regulation no. 14, HO/45/3406, NA. This regulation anticipated the provision found in the first printed version of the 1851 Lodging House Bill but struck out in the act. A Bill . . . Common Lodging Houses, PP 1851 (272) s. 27.

149. As late as 1890, the courts were still struggling with the lack of a definition: *Booth v. Ferrett*, 59 LJR (MC) 136–37.

150. The process can be followed in successive printed versions of the Public Health Bill. See PP 1847–48, (83), s. 49; (325), s. 57; (354), s. 57.

151. Lawes, *Act for Promoting the Public Health*, 104–5, note *d*. Lawes claimed that the definition—"any public lodging-house, not being a licensed victualling house, in which persons are harboured or lodged for hire for a single night, or less than a week at one time, or in which any room is let for hire, to be occupied by more than one family at one time"—in the Public Health Bill was derived from that in the Towns Improvement Clauses Act. The difference between these two definitions, however, was not trivial. The Lords added the stipulation about rooms let to more than one family, the first time this formulation appeared in a general bill. As Lawes also noted, the definition that the Commons rejected for the Public Health Bill was incorporated into the City Sewers Act, debated shortly after the Public Health Act passed.

152. Compare the interpretation clauses in PP 1851 (272) and PP 1851 (359). In the act, a common lodging house includes any house of which only a part is used as a common lodging house.

153. In the opinion of the central government, magistrates did not always use their discretion wisely. Permanent Under-Secretary Horatio Waddington called one magisterial decision a piece of "sad nonsense": Hastings Town Clerk to HO, November 30, 1852, minute, HO/45/os4427/65, NA.

154. The 1853 Act (16 & 17 Vict., c. 41) permitted local authorities to require a certificate of character (s. 4) for keepers and permitted the authorities to prohibit triple violators of the act from operating a common lodging house (s. 12).

155. Shaftesbury may have been inspired by Glasgow's 1840 local act, which permitted the removal of the infectious sick not only from lodging houses but from a much wider range of working-class housing: 3 Vict., c. xxviii, s. 22. When Liverpool's nuisance inspector commented on the GBH's lodging-house regulations, he noted that Liverpool was trying to promote a bill to allow the local board of health to inspect houses let as lodgings in addition to common lodging houses.

Chadwick minuted that the passage should be copied to Ashley, who would shortly bring in the first Common Lodging House Bill: J. Fresh to GBH, February 4, 1851, MH/13/268/466/51, NA. The bill was brought in on May 7, 1851: PP 1851 (272).

156. *Hansard Parliamentary Debate*, 3rd ser., vol. 127 (May 13, 1853), cols. 294–99, (May 26, 1853), cols. 553–56. Lord Redesdale (col. 297) drew attention to the fact that any house let in single rooms to persons on weekly wages would be open to inspection, and the Marquess of Clanricarde (col. 297) objected that the bill would seriously injure occupiers of small houses in Ireland.

157. PP 1852–53 (573), s. 20. *Hansard Parliamentary Debate*, 3rd ser., vol. 127 (May 13, 1853), cols. 294–99, (May 26, 1853), cols. 553–56. Beaumont's comment is at col. 555.

158. 16 & 17 Vict. c. 41. The clause in the bill that had exercised some Lords (PP 1852–53 [573], s. 4) allowed any constable or officer of a local authority to report any (presumably previously unregistered) house for common lodging-house inspection.

159. The 1855 Nuisance Act (18 & 19 Vict., c. 121, s. 29) allowed overcrowding of any house to be controlled if two medical practitioners certified it to be "dangerous or prejudicial to the health of the inhabitants." On the control of overcrowding, see Wohl, *Endangered Lives*, 310–13; Wohl, "Housing of the Working Classes," 13–54; Wohl, "Unfit for Human Habitation," 603–24. This section was difficult to enforce. The parliamentary draughtsman Henry Thring thought that most if not all poor people's houses in London were in some sense prejudicial to health: RSC, First Report, PP 1868–69 (4218), qq. 483–87.

160. PP 1857 Sess. 2 (160), s. 3; (187), s. 2.

161. Gauldie, *Cruel Habitations*, 254–56; Wohl, *Eternal Slum*, 75. The liberty of the subject was a standard objection if, in the words of one member, a hackneyed one. See the comments of Mr. [Arthur] Kinnaird, *Hansard Parliamentary Debate*, 3rd ser., vol. 146 (August 17, 1857), col. 1768. Other members objected because of the power the bill granted the police to inspect homes, which would make the situation worse for some people and would attack the symptom rather than the cause of the disease. See the comments, respectively, of Mr. [Joseph] Henley (col. 1768), Sir John Trelawny (col. 1772), and Mr John Locke (col. 1769). This last objection, articulated by the metropolitan MP John Locke, was the most radical, asserting that people could not afford accommodation in large part because houses had been destroyed in the name of improvement with nothing provided in their stead. On Locke, see Hamilton, "Locke, John (1805–1880)."

162. Although Shaftesbury got support from a local Devonshire paper, leader writers were more or less unsympathetic: *Morning Chronicle*, August 20, 1857, 4; *Manchester Courier*, August 22, 1857, 6; "A Villainous Act of Parliament," *Reynold's Newspaper*, August 23, 1857, 1; *North Devon Journal*, August 27, 1857, 4. A more sympathetic piece was "Overcrowded Dwellings," *Tait's Edinburgh Magazine* 24 (September 1857): 559–63, which rejected the "Englishman's castle mania" and thought the bill did not go nearly far enough in prohibiting the construction of inferior dwellings.

163. *Hansard Parliamentary Debate*, 3rd ser., vol. 146 (August 18, 1857), cols. 1856–63.

164. The 1866 Sanitary Act (s. 35) provided some control of houses with lodgers, but it was widely seen as ineffective, and in any event it preserved the (undefined) family exemption. Hardy, *Epidemic Streets*, 243–45 describes the post-1855 and

post-1866 situations in London. The houses in question were, under this section, explicitly not common lodging houses.

165. For an incisive analysis of the way in which legal and disciplinary mechanisms worked together even though seemingly opposed, see Ogborn, "Law and Discipline."

166. The Home Office's regulations were prepared without any input from the General Board of Health, to which the Home Office refused even to send a copy: GBH Minutes, October 22, 1851, October 27, 1851, MH/5/5, NA.

167. Quoted in Husband, *Sanitary Law*, 53.

168. See Hundred House Division magistrates to HO, November 28, 1851, minute, HO/45/os4427/138, NA. On beer shops and pubs, see Udsey Petty Sessional Division to HO, January 21, 1852, minute, HO/45/os4427/103, NA; Romsey Pavement Commissioners to HO, November 17, 1851, minute, HO/45/os4427/120, NA; Stroud IC to HO, December 30, 1852, minute, HO/45/os4427/140, NA. This formulation carefully avoided the wider implication of the Lords' 1848 definition.

169. Quoted in Husband, *Sanitary Law*, 54.

170. London's working class had a large proportion of weekly wage earners: Hardy, *Epidemic Streets*, 198–99.

171. See Hundred House Division magistrates to HO, November 28, 1851, minute, HO/45/os4427/138, NA. But these transitory workers were clearly not the "vagrants, trampers and other such wayfarers" whom the HOTC wanted to control.

172. Leicestershire districts to HO, April 15, 1852, minute, HO/45/os 4427/80, NA.

173. Leek IC to HO, March 2, 1852, no. 9, HO/45/os4427/128, NA.

174. Salisbury Clerk to HO, August 17, 1852, minute, HO/45/os4427128, NA.

175. Devizes Corporation to HO, June 7, 1852, June 14, 1852, minute, HO/45/os4427/42, NA.

176. Second Report . . . on the Operation of the Common Lodging Houses Act, PP 1854 (1780), 9.

177. Mayhew, *London Labour and London Poor*, 1: 253.

178. These were the same sorts of regulations that applied to indoor paupers. The common lodging-house regulations were not so elaborate as workhouse regulations, or so harsh. On workhouse classifications, see Higginbotham, *Workhouse Encyclopedia*, s.v. "Classification"; Lees, *Solidarities of Strangers*, 134–45.

179. Lees, *Solidarities of Strangers*, 150.

180. Poovey, "Domesticity and Class Formation."

181. Himmelfarb, *Idea of Poverty*, 312–400; Lees, *Solidarities of Strangers*; Luckin, "Revisiting the Idea."

182. Mayhew is of particular significance here, because his *Morning Chronicle* letters highlighted the lodging-house system and its supposed nefarious effects. In his letters, Mayhew also proposed a rudimentary taxonomy of the poor, classifying them along moral (honest versus dishonest; will work, can't work, won't work) or functional axes (artisans, labourers, petty traders), which each type subdivided further: Himmelfarb, *Idea of Poverty*, 316.

183. The GBH preempted independent local board of health control of lodging houses very early on. In the Ware Local Board of Health's December 1849 bylaws, the common lodging house provision was completely crossed out: LBH5/3/154/1, HALS.

184. The Northampton County Quarter Sessions apparently went its own way and did not use the official form. The HO records do not include the originals, but the letter transmitting them noted that "many of these regulations cannot be approved of. Suggest the official form": November 2, 1852, HO/45/os/4427/101, NA. Ramsgate's improvement commissioners experienced the same situation: December 3, 1851, HO/45/os/4427/115, NA. See also Rotherham and Kimberworth Local Board of Health to HO, October 5, 1852, HO/45/os4427/122, NA. The Metropolitan Police, charged with enforcing the Common Lodging Houses Act in the metropolis, prepared the regulations for London.

185. I base this claim on an analysis of lodging house regulations and bylaws contained in HO/45/os/4427, NA. This box contains several different folders. I randomly chose and reviewed files 41–80 and 101–40 from 1851–52. I also reviewed applications in HO/45/os/5152, NA from 1853, including regulations promoted before and after the 1853 Amending Act received royal assent (August 4, 1853).

186. First Annual Report of the Local Government Act Office, appendix C, pp. 30–55, PP 1859 Sess 2 (2585).

187. Royston Lambert noted that the Local Government Act Office examined over fifteen hundred bylaw codes during its existence. Its "'suggestions' became standards": Lambert, "Central and Local Relations," 130. To some extent, the Home Office was the predecessor of the LGAO.

Conclusion

1. The best evaluation of metropolitan health authorities is Anne Hardy's study of London's experience of disease during the second half of the nineteenth century. She has demonstrated that sanitary interventions interrupted the chain of contagion for several infectious diseases: Hardy, *Epidemic Streets*. For a recent review of the mortality debate, see Szreter, "Rethinking McKeown"; Szreter and Hardy, "Urban Fertility," 631–49. The most important determinant not fully under local control for the duration of this study was housing.

2. Daunton, *Trusting Leviathan*, 246–85; Luckin, "Pollution in the City"; Szreter, "Economic Growth."

3. Thompson, "Peculiarities of the English," 358–59.

4. Of course, poor ratepayers in rich parishes would have to contribute to this redistribution, but equalization would not have been fought so vehemently if it did not cause a redistribution of wealth toward poverty.

5. Public health was hardly the only service associated with this kind of reimagining. It had a parallel in changing conceptions of poor relief: Lees, *Solidarities of Strangers*. Ideas of community were of course not monolithic; any given notion simultaneously included and excluded individuals from full membership.

6. Redlich and Hirst, *History of Local Government*, 160–66.

7. This support included half payment of medical officer of health and sanitary officer salaries and, even more important, loan guarantees at below-market rates: Daunton, *Trusting Leviathan*, 277–78; J. F. Wilson, "Finance of Municipal Capital." The Treasury changed the interest rate from 3.5 percent to 5 percent in 1875.

8. Daunton, *Trusting Leviathan*; Matthew, "Disraeli." The cost of improvement during the second half of the century was not only controversial in sum but also controversial in incidence. Whether the occupier or the owner bore the cost and received the benefits of urban improvement was highly contested. Even if the occupier paid the rates, contemporaries were deeply divided over the "ultimate" incidence, and the debate was constitutive of party positions on local affairs. See Offer, *Property and Politics*. I am less concerned with this issue than with the redistribution of rates among areas, irrespective of whether owners or occupiers paid those rates.

Bibliography

Ackerknecht, Erwin. "Anticontagionism between 1821 and 1867." *Bulletin of the History of Medicine* 22 (1948): 562–93.

Adams, Annmarie. *Architecture in the Family Way: Doctors, Houses, and Women, 1870–1900.* Montreal: McGill–Queen's University Press, 1996.

Allen-Emerson, Michelle, ed. *Sanitary Engineering.* Part I, vol. 3 of *Sanitary Reform in Victorian Britain.* Brookfield, VT: Pickering & Chatto, 2012.

Arnot, Margaret L. "Infant Death, Child Care and the State: The Baby-Farming Scandal and the First Infant Life Protection Legislation of 1872." *Continuity and Change* 9, no. 2 (1994): 271–311.

Ashbridge, Pauline. "Paying for the Poor: A Middle-Class Metropolitan Movement for Rate Equalization 1857–67." *London Journal* 22, no. 2 (December 1997): 107–22.

Atkins, Peter. *Liquid Materialities: A History of Milk, Science and the Law.* Burlington, VT: Ashgate, 2010. Kindle edition.

Atkinson, Logan. "The Impact of Cholera on the Design and Implementation of Toronto's First Municipal By-Laws, 1834." *Urban History Review* 30 (2002): 3–15.

Austin, Henry. *Report on the Proceedings of the Local Board of Health of Taunton.* London: W. Clowes, 1850.

Ayers, Gwendoline M. *England's First State Hospitals and the Metropolitan Asylums Board, 1867–1930.* London: Wellcome, 1971.

Baker, J. *An Introduction to English Legal History.* 4th ed. London: Butterworths, 2002.

Baker, J. H., and S. F. C. Milsom, eds. *Sources of English Legal History: Private Law to 1750.* London: Butterworths, 1986.

Baldwin, Peter. *Contagion and the State in Europe, 1830–1930.* Cambridge: Cambridge University Press, 1999.

Barnet, Margaret C. "The 1832 Cholera Epidemic in York." *Medical History* 16, no. 1 (January 1972): 27–39.

Bartrip, P. W. J. *The Home Office and the Dangerous Trades: Regulating Occupational Disease in Victorian and Edwardian Britain.* Amsterdam: Clio Medica/Rodopi, 2002.

Bashford, Alison. *Imperial Hygiene: A Critical History of Colonialism, Nationalism and Public Health.* New York: Palgrave Macmillan, 2004.

Beales, Derek. "The Electorate Before and After 1832: The Right to Vote, and the Opportunity." *Parliamentary History* 11, no. 1 (February 1992): 139–50.

Beaven, Brad, and John Griffiths. "Creating the Exemplary Citizen: The Changing Notion of Citizenship in Britain 1870–1939." *Contemporary British History* 22, no. 2 (June 2008): 203–25. doi:10.1080/13619460701189559.

———. "Urban Elites, Socialists and Notions of Citizenship in an Industrial Boomtown: Coventry, c. 1870–1914." *Labour History Review* 69, no. 1 (April 2004): 3–18.

Beckert, Sven. *Empire of Cotton: A Global History.* New York: Knopf, 2014.

Beckett, J. V. *Local Taxation: National Legislation and the Problems of Enforcement.* London: Bedford Square Press, 1980.

Bell, Frances, and Robert Millward. "Public Health Expenditures and Mortality in England and Wales, 1870–1914." *Continuity and Change* 13, no. 2 (1998): 221–49.

Bellamy, Christine. *Administering Central-Local Relations, 1871–1919: The Local Government Board in Its Fiscal and Cultural Context.* Manchester: Manchester University Press, 1988.

Benidickson, Jamie. *The Culture of Flushing: A Social and Legal History of Sewage.* Vancouver: University of British Columbia Press, 2007.

Bernhardt, Christoph. "At the Limits of the European Sanitary City: Water-related Environmental Inequalities in Berlin-Brandenburg, c. 1900–39." In *Environmental and Social Justice in the City: Historical Perspectives,* edited by Geneviève Massard-Guilbaud and Richard Rodger, 155–70. Cambridge: White Horse Press, 2011.

Blackstone, William. *Commentaries on the Laws of England.* 4 vols. Chicago: University of Chicago Press, 1979.

Blake, Steven. *Pittville, 1824–1860: A Scene of Gorgeous Magnificence.* Cheltenham: Cheltenham Art Gallery and Museums, 1988.

Borough of Great Yarmouth, *Bye-Laws made and passed by the Town Council on the ninth day of November, 1837, the Fourteenth day of May, 1840, and the Twenty-Sixth day of November, 1850.* Yarmouth: Charles Barber, n.d.

Borough of Kingston-upon-Hull. *Bye-Laws ordained by the Town Council, 22nd day of June, 1848.* Hull, 1848.

Bowler, Peter J. *Charles Darwin: The Man and His Influence.* Cambridge, MA: Blackwell, 1990.

Brand, Jeanne L. *Doctors and the State: The British Medical Profession and Government Action in Public Health, 1870–1912.* Baltimore: Johns Hopkins University Press, 1965.

Brenner, Joel F. "Nuisance Law and the Industrial Revolution." *Journal of Legal Studies* 3 (1974): 403–33.

Briggs, Asa. *Victorian Cities.* New York: Harper & Row, 1965.

Brock, M. G. *The Great Reform Act.* London: Hutchinson, 1973.

Brockington, C. Fraser. *Public Health in the Nineteenth Century.* London: E. & S. Livingstone, 1965.

Brown, Michael. "From Foetid Air to Filth: The Cultural Transformation of British Epidemiological Thought, ca. 1780–1848." *Bulletin of the History of Medicine* 82, no. 3 (Fall 2008): 515–44.

———. *Performing Medicine: Medical Culture and Identity in Provincial England, c. 1760–1850.* Manchester: Manchester University Press, 2011.

Brundage, Anthony. *England's "Prussian Minister": Edwin Chadwick and the Politics of Government Growth, 1832–1854.* University Park, PA: Pennsylvania State University Press, 1988.

———. *The English Poor Laws, 1700–1930.* Basingstoke, UK: Palgrave Macmillan, 2001.

———. *The Making of the New Poor Law: The Politics of Inquiry, Enactment, and Implementation, 1832–1839.* New Brunswick, NJ: Rutgers University Press, 1978.

Brunton, Deborah. "Policy, Powers and Practice: The Public Response to Public Health in the Scottish City." In *Medicine, Health and the Public Sphere in Britain, 1600–2000*, edited by Steve Sturdy, 171–88. New York: Routledge, 2002.

———. *The Politics of Vaccination: Practice and Policy in England, Wales, Ireland, and Scotland, 1800–1874*. Rochester, NY: University of Rochester Press, 2008.

Burn, William Laurence. *The Age of Equipoise: A Study of the Mid-Victorian Generation*. New York: W. W. Norton, 1965.

Burnett, John. *A Social History of Housing, 1815–1970*. London: Methuen, 1978.

Burney, Ian A. "A Poisoning of No Substance: The Trials of Medico-Legal Proof in Mid-Victorian England." *Journal of British Studies* 38, no. 1 (January 1999): 59–92.

———. *Bodies of Evidence: Medicine and the Politics of the English Inquest, 1830–1926*. Baltimore: Johns Hopkins University Press, 2000.

———. "Medicine in the Age of Reform." In *Rethinking the Age of Reform: Britain, 1780–1850*, edited by Arthur Burns and Joanna Innes, 163–81. New York: Cambridge University Press, 2003.

Burrell, S., and G. Gill, "The Liverpool Cholera Epidemic of 1832 and Anatomical Dissection—Medical Mistrust and Civil Unrest." *Journal of the History of Medicine and Allied Sciences* 60, no. 4 (October 2005): 478–98.

Bynum, W. F. *Science and the Practice of Medicine in the Nineteenth Century*. New York: Cambridge University Press, 1994.

Cannon, John Ashton. *Parliamentary Reform 1640–1832*. Cambridge: Cambridge University Press, 1973.

Caplan, Maurice. "The New Poor Law and the Struggle for Union Chargeability." *International Review of Social History* 23, no. 2 (August 1978): 267–300.

Carroll, P. "Medical Police and the History of Public Health." *Medical History* 46, no. 4 (2002): 461–94.

Chadwick, Edwin. *Report on the Sanitary Condition of the Labouring Population of Great Britain*. Edited with an introduction by M. W. Flinn. Edinburgh: Edinburgh University Press, 1965.

Chambers, George F. *A Digest of the Law Relating to Public Health and Local Government, with the Statutes in Full, Various Precedents, Various Official Documents, Brief Notes of 1260 Leading Cases, a Table of Offences and Punishments, and Ample Indexes: The Whole Forming an Exhaustive Index to the "Public Health Act, 1875."* 8th ed. London: Stevens and Sons, 1881.

Chapman, H. *The Act for the Regulation of Municipal Corporations in England and Wales*. London: Charles Ely, 1835.

Chapman, Stanley D., ed. *The History of Working-Class Housing: A Symposium*. Newton Abbot, UK: David & Charles, 1971.

Charlesworth, Lorie. *Welfare's Forgotten Past: A Socio-Legal History of the Poor Law*. London: Routledge-Cavendish, 2011.

Chase, Malcolm. *Chartism: A New History*. New York: Manchester University Press, 2007.

Cherry, Steven. "Before the National Health Service: Financing the Voluntary Hospitals, 1900–1939." *Economic History Review* 50, no. 2 (May 1997): 305–26.

City & Borough of Worcester. *Bye Laws made by the Council of the City and Borough of Worcester*. Worcester: T. Hayes, 1837.

Clark, George Thomas. *Report to the General Board of Health on a Further Inquiry held in the Borough of Swansea.* London: W. Clowes, 1850.

———. *Report to the General Board of Health on a Preliminary Inquiry into the Sewerage, Drainage, and Supply of Water, and the Sanitary Condition of the Inhabitants of the Borough of Bangor.* London: W. Clowes, 1849.

———. *Report to the General Board of Health on a Preliminary Inquiry into the Sewerage, Drainage, and Supply of Water, and the Sanitary Condition of the Inhabitants of the Borough of Taunton.* London: W. Clowes, 1849.

———. *Report to the General Board of Health on a Preliminary Inquiry into the Sewerage, Drainage, and Supply of Water, and the Sanitary Condition of the Inhabitants of the Town and Borough of Swansea.* London: W. Clowes, 1849.

Clark, Michael, and Catherine Crawford, eds. *Legal Medicine in History.* Cambridge: Cambridge University Press, 1994.

Claus, Peter. "Languages of Citizenship in the City of London 1848–1867." *London Journal* 24, no. 1 (June 1999): 23–37.

Clifford, Frederick. *A History of Private Bill Legislation.* 2 vols. 1885. Reprint, New York: Augustus M. Kelley, 1968.

Clifton, Gloria C. *Professionalism, Patronage and Public Service in Victorian London.* Atlantic Highlands, NJ: Athlone Press, 2002.

Clinton, A., and P. Murray. "Reassessing the Vestries: London Local Government, 1855–1900." In *Government and Institutions in the Post-1832 United Kingdom,* edited by Alan O'Day, 51–84. Lewiston, NY: Edwin Mellen Press, 1995.

Cocks, Raymond. "Statutes, Social Reform, and Control." In *The Oxford History of the Laws of England,* edited by William Cornish et al., 13: 465–619. Oxford: Oxford University Press, 2010.

Coleman, William. *Death Is a Social Disease: Public Health and Political Economy in Early Industrial France.* Madison: University of Wisconsin Press, 1982.

Comyns, Sir John. *A Digest of the Laws of England.* 4th ed. 6 vols. Dublin: Luke White, 1793.

Cook, Chris. *The Routledge Companion to Britain in the Nineteenth Century, 1815–1914.* New York: Routledge, 2005.

Cooter, Roger. "Anticontagionism and History's Medical Record." In *The Problem of Medical Knowledge: Examining the Social Construction of Medicine,* edited by Peter Wright and Andrew Treacher, 87–108. Edinburgh: Edinburgh University Press, 1982.

Cottrell, P. L. "Resolving the Sewage Question: Metropolis Sewage & Essex Reclamation Company, 1865–81." In *Cities of Ideas: Civil Society and Urban Governance in Britain 1800–2000,* edited by Robert Colls and Richard Rodger, 67–95. Burlington, VT: Ashgate, 2004.

Cox, Pamela. "Compulsion, Voluntarism, and Venereal Disease: Governing Sexual Health in England after the Contagious Diseases Acts." *Journal of British Studies* 46, no. 1 (January 2007): 91–115.

Crawford, Catherine. "Patients' Rights and the Law of Contract in Eighteenth-Century England." *Social History of Medicine* 13, no. 3 (December 1, 2000): 381–410.

Cresy, Edward. *Report to the General Board of Health on a Preliminary Inquiry into the Sewerage, Drainage, and Supply of Water, and the Sanitary Condition of the Inhabitants of the Town of Cheltenham.* London: W. Clowes, 1849.

———. *Report to the General Board of Health on a Preliminary Inquiry into the Sewerage, Drainage, and Supply of Water, and the Sanitary Condition of the Inhabitants of the Town of Eton.* London: W. Clowes, 1849.

———. *Report to the General Board of Health on a Second Inquiry to Extend the Boundaries of the District of the Town of Eton.* London: W. Clowes, 1851.

Croll, Andy. "Street Disorder, Surveillance and Shame: Regulating Behavior in the Public Spaces of the Late Victorian British Town." *Social History* 24 (1999): 250–68.

Cromwell, Valerie. "Interpretations of Nineteenth-Century Administration: An Analysis." *Victorian Studies* 9, no. 3 (Winter 1966): 245–55.

Crook, Tom. "Accommodating the Outcast: Common Lodging Houses and the Limits of Urban Governance in Victorian and Edwardian London." *Urban History* 35, no. 3 (December 2008): 414–36. doi:10.1017/S0963926808005713.

———. "Putting Matter in Its Right Place: Dirt, Time and Regeneration in Mid-Victorian Britain." *Journal of Victorian Culture* 13, no. 2 (September 2008): 200–222. doi:10.3366/E1355550208000313.

———. "Sanitary Inspection and the Public Sphere in Late Victorian and Edwardian Britain: A Case Study in Liberal Governance." *Social History* 32, no. 4 (November 2007): 369–93. doi:10.1080/03071020701616654.

Crowther, M. A., and Brenda M. White. "Medicine, Property and the Law in Britain, 1800–1914." *Historical Journal* 31, no. 4 (December 1988): 853–70.

———. *On Soul and Conscience: The Medical Expert and Crime: 150 Years of Forensic Medicine in Glasgow.* Aberdeen: Aberdeen University Press, 1988.

Cunningham, Hugh. "The Metropolitan Fairs: A Case Study in the Social Control of Leisure." In *Social Control in Nineteenth Century Britain*, edited by A. P. Donajgrodzki, 163–84. Totowa, NJ: Rowman and Littlefield, 1977.

Daunton, Martin. *House and Home in the Victorian City: Working Class Housing, 1850–1914.* Baltimore, MD: Edward Arnold, 1983.

———. Introduction to *The Cambridge Urban History of Britain*, vol. 3, *1840–1950*, 1–56. New York: Cambridge University Press, 2000.

———. "The Material Politics of Natural Monopoly: Gas in Victorian Britain." In *State and Market in Victorian Britain: War, Welfare and Capitalism*, 111–27. Rochester, NY: Boydell and Brewer, 2008.

———. "Payment and Participation: Welfare and State Formation in Britain, 1900–1951." In *State and Market in Victorian Britain: War, Welfare and Capitalism*, 254–89. Rochester, NY: Boydell and Brewer, 2008.

———. "Taxation and Representation in the Victorian City." In *State and Market in Victorian Britain: War, Welfare and Capitalism*, 89–110. Rochester, NY: Boydell and Brewer, 2008.

———. "Trusting Leviathan: The Politics of Taxation, 1815–1914." In *State and Market in Victorian Britain: War, Welfare and Capitalism*, 61–88. Rochester, NY: Boydell and Brewer, 2008.

———. *Trusting Leviathan: The Politics of Taxation in Britain, 1799–1914.* New York: Cambridge University Press, 2001.

Davies, Celia. "The Health Visitor as Mother's Friend: A Woman's Place in Public Health, 1900–14." *Social History of Medicine* 1, no. 1 (April 1, 1988): 39–59.

Davies, Megan J. "Night Soil, Cesspools, and Smelly Hogs on the Streets: Sanitation, Race, and Governance in Early British Columbia." *Histoire Sociale: Social History* 38, no. 75 (May 2005): 1–35.

Davis, Jennifer. "Jennings' Buildings and the Royal Borough: The Construction of the Underclass in Mid-Victorian England." In *Metropolis London: Histories and Representations*, edited by David Feldman and Gareth Stedman Jones, 11–39. New York: Routledge, 1989.

Davis, John. "Central Government and the Towns." In *The Cambridge Urban History of Britain*, ed. Martin Daunton, vol. 3, *1840–1950*, 261–86. New York: Cambridge University Press, 2000.

———. *Reforming London: The London Government Problem, 1855–1900*. Oxford: Oxford University Press, 1988.

Dennis, Richard. "Modern London." In *The Cambridge Urban History of Britain*, ed. Martin Daunton, vol. 3, *1840–1950*, 95–131. New York: Cambridge University Press, 2000.

De Smith, S. A., and Rodney Brazier. *Constitutional and Administrative Law*. 8th ed. London: Penguin Books, 1998.

Devine, Rosemary. *Index to the Local and Personal Acts, 1797–1849*. London: Stationery Office Books, 1999.

Dicey, Albert Venn. *Lectures on the Relation between Law & Public Opinion in England during the Nineteenth Century*. 2nd ed. 1914. Reprinted with preface by E. C. S. Wade. London: Macmillan, 1962.

Digby, Ann. *Pauper Palaces*. Studies in Economic History. London: Routledge & Kegan Paul, 1978.

Dingle, A. E. "'The Monster Nuisance of All': Landowners, Alkali Manufacturers, and Air Pollution, 1828–64." *Economic History Review* 35, no. 4 (1982): 529–48.

Dobraszczyk, Paul. *Into the Belly of the Beast: Exploring London's Victorian Sewers*. Reading, UK: Spire Books, 2009.

Drescher, Seymour. *Abolition: A History of Slavery and Antislavery*. New York: Cambridge University Press, 2009.

Dunsford, Deborah. "Principle versus Expediency: A Rejoinder to F. B. Smith." *Social History of Medicine* 5, no. 3 (December 1992): 505–13.

Durbach, Nadja. *Bodily Matters: The Anti-Vaccination Movement in England, 1853–1907*. Durham: Duke University Press, 2005.

Durey, Michael. *The Return of the Plague: British Society and the Cholera, 1831–2*. Dublin: Gill and Macmillan, 1979.

Dyos, H. J. *Victorian Suburb: A Study of the Growth of Camberwell*. Leicester: Leicester University Press, 1966.

Dyos, H. J., and D. A. Reeder. "Slums and Suburbs." In *The Victorian City: Images and Realities*, edited by H. J. Dyos and Michael Wolff, 1: 359–86. London: Routledge & Kegan Paul, 1973.

Dyos, H. J., and Michael Wolff, eds. *The Victorian City: Images and Realities*. Vol. 1. London: Routledge & Kegan Paul, 1973.

Eastwood, David. *Government and Community in the English Provinces, 1700–1870*. New York: St. Martin's Press, 1997.

———. "Men, Morals and the Machinery of Social Legislation, 1790–1840." *Parliamentary History* 13, no. 2 (June 1994): 190–205.

Emsley, Clive, Tim Hitchcock, and Robert B. Shoemaker. "London History—A Population History of London." Old Bailey Proceedings Online (version 7.0, 05 October 2015). http://www.oldbaileyonline.org/static/Population-history-of-london.jsp. Accessed November 13, 2015.

Evans, Richard J. "Epidemics and Revolutions: Cholera in Nineteenth-Century Europe." *Past & Present*, no. 120 (August 1988): 123–46.

Everest-Phillips, Max. "William Everest of Epsom." *Surrey History* 6 (2003): 258–73.

Eyler, John M. *Victorian Social Medicine: The Ideas and Methods of William Farr.* Baltimore: Johns Hopkins University Press, 1979.

Farrant, John H. "Cooper, William Durrant (1812–1875), antiquary." In *Oxford Dictionary of National Biography*. Oxford: Oxford University Press, 2004. Online ed., Jan 2008. http://www.oxforddnb.com/index/6/101006236. Accessed November 13, 2015.

Fee, Elizabeth, and Roy M. Acheson, eds. *A History of Education in Public Health: Health That Mocks the Doctors' Rules.* Oxford: Oxford University Press, 1991.

Fee, Elizabeth, and Dorothy Porter. "Public Health, Preventive Medicine and Professionalization: England and America in the Nineteenth Century." In *Medicine in Society: Historical Essays*, edited by Andrew Wear, 249–75. Cambridge: Cambridge University Press, 1992.

Finer, Samuel. *The Life and Times of Sir Edwin Chadwick.* London: Methuen, 1952.

Fissell, Mary Elizabeth. *Patients, Power, and the Poor in Eighteenth-Century Bristol.* New York: Cambridge University Press, 2002.

Flinn, Michael. "Medical Service under the New Poor Law." In *The New Poor Law in the Nineteenth Century*, edited by Derek Fraser, 45–66. London: Macmillan, 1976.

Forbes, Thomas. *Surgeons at the Old Bailey: English Forensic Medicine to 1878.* New Haven: Yale University Press, 1985.

Foulkes, David. *Introduction to Administrative Law.* London: Butterworths, 1964.

Fraser, Antonia. *Perilous Question: Reform or Revolution? Britain on the Brink, 1832.* New York: Public Affairs, 2014.

Fraser, Derek. "Areas of Urban Politics: Leeds, 1830–80." In *The Victorian City*, edited by Harold James Dyos and Michael Wolff, 763–88. London: Routledge & Kegan Paul, 1973.

———. *The Evolution of the British Welfare State: A History of Social Policy since the Industrial Revolution.* 2nd ed. Basingstoke, UK: Palgrave, 1984.

———. *Power and Authority in the Victorian City.* Oxford: Blackwell, 1979.

———. *Urban Politics in Victorian England: The Structure of Politics in Victorian Cities.* Leicester, UK: Leicester University Press, 1976.

Fraser, Hamish. "Municipal Socialism and Social Policy." In *The Victorian City: A Reader in British Urban History*, edited by R. J. Morris and Richard Rodger, 258–80. New York: Longman, 1993.

Fraser, W. Hamish, and Irene Maver. *Glasgow*, vol. 2, *1830–1912*. Manchester: Manchester University Press, 1996.

Frazer, W. M. *A History of English Public Health, 1834–1939.* London: Baillière, Tindall and Cox, 1950.

———. *Duncan of Liverpool: An Account of the Work of Dr. W. M. Duncan, Medical Officer of Health of Liverpool, 1847–1863.* Preston, UK: Carnegie, 1997.

Freeman, Thomas Walter. *Geography and Regional Administration, England and Wales, 1830–1968.* London: Hutchinson, 1968.

Fullmer, June Z. "Technology, Chemistry and the Law in Early Nineteenth-Century England." *Technology and Culture* 21 (1980): 1–28.

Garrard, John. *Democratisation in Britain: Elites, Civil Society, and Reform since 1800.* Basingstoke, UK: Palgrave, 2002.

———. *Leadership and Power in Victorian Industrial Towns, 1830–80.* Manchester: Manchester University Press, 1983.

Gash, Norman. *Politics in the Age of Peel: A Study in the Technique of Parliamentary Representation, 1830–1850.* Toronto: Longmans, Green, 1953.

Gaskell, S. Martin. *Building Control: National Legislation and the Introduction of Local Byelaws in Victorian England.* Somersal Herbert, UK: British Association for Local History, 1983.

Gatrell, V. A. C. "Crime, Authority and the Policeman-state." In *The Cambridge Social History of Britain, 1750–1950,* ed. F. M. L. Thompson, vol. 3, *Social Agencies and Institutions,* 245–310. New York: Cambridge University Press), 1990.

Gauldie, Enid. *Cruel Habitations: A History of Working-Class Housing 1780–1918.* London: Allen & Unwin, 1974.

Getzler, Joshua. *A History of Water Rights at Common Law.* Oxford: Oxford University Press, 2004.

Gilbert, David. "Community and Municipalism: Collective Identity in Late-Victorian and Edwardian Mining Towns." *Journal of Historical Geography* 17, no. 3 (July 1991): 257–70.

Gilbert, Pamela K. *Cholera and Nation: Doctoring the Social Body in Victorian England.* Albany: State University of New York Press, 2008.

———. *The Citizen's Body: Desire, Health, and the Social in Victorian England.* Columbus: Ohio State University Press, 2007.

———. "Producing the Public: Public Medicine in Private Spaces." In *Medicine, Health and the Public Sphere in Britain, 1600–2000,* edited by Steve Sturdy, 43–59. New York: Routledge, 2002.

Golan, Tal. "The History of Scientific Expert Testimony in the English Courtroom." *Science in Context* 12 (1999): 7–32.

Goold, Imogen, and Catherine Kelly, eds. *Lawyers' Medicine: The Legislature, the Courts, and Medical Practice, 1760–2000.* Oxford: Hart Publishing, 2009.

Gray, Robert. "Medical Men, Industrial Labour and the State in Britain, 1830–50." *Social History* 16, no. 1 (1991): 19–43.

Green, David R. *Pauper Capital: London and the Poor Law, 1790–1870.* Burlington, VT: Ashgate, 2010.

Guldi, Jo. *Roads to Power: Britain Invents the Infrastructure State.* Cambridge, MA: Harvard University Press, 2012.

Gunn, Simon. "From Hegemony to Governmentality: Changing Conceptions of Power in Social History." *Journal of Social History* 39, no. 3 (Spring 2006): 705–20.

Hall, Catherine, Keith McClelland, and Jane Rendall. *Defining the Victorian Nation: Class, Race, Gender and the British Reform Act of 1867.* Cambridge: Cambridge University Press, 2000.

Halliday, Stephen. *The Great Stink of London: Sir Joseph Bazalgette and the Cleansing of the Victorian Metropolis.* Stroud, UK: History Press, 2001.

Hamilton, John Andrew, and Colin Matthew. "Locke, John (1805–1880), legal writer and politician." In *Oxford Dictionary of National Biography*, Oxford: Oxford University Press, 2004. Online ed., May 2005. http://oxfordindex.oup.com/view/10.1093/ref:odnb/16886?rskey=emQzuM&result=1. Accessed November 13, 2015.

Hamlin, Christopher. *Cholera: The Biography*. New York: Oxford University Press, 2009.

———. "Edwin Chadwick and the Engineers, 1842–1854: Systems and Antisystems in the Pipe-and-Brick Sewers War." *Technology & Culture* 33, no. 4 (October 1992): 680–709.

———. "Edwin Chadwick, 'Mutton Medicine,' and the Fever Question." *Bulletin of the History of Medicine* 70 (1996): 233–65.

———. "Environmental Sensibility in Edinburgh, 1839–1840." *Journal of Urban History* 20, no. 3 (May 1994): 311.

———. "James Newlands and the Boundaries of Public Health." *Transactions of the Historic Society of Lancashire and Cheshire* 143 (1994): 117–39.

———. *More than Hot: A Short History of Fever*. Baltimore: Johns Hopkins University Press, 2000. Kindle edition.

———. "Muddling in Bumbledom: On the Enormity of Large Sanitary Improvements in Four British Towns, 1855–1885." *Victorian Studies* 32, no. 1 (1988): 55–83.

———. "Nuisances and Community in Mid-Victorian England: The Attractions of Inspection." *Social History* 38, no. 3 (August 2013): 346–79. doi:10.1080/03071022.2013.817061.

———. "Predisposing Causes and Public Health in Early Nineteenth-Century Medical Thought." *Social History of Medicine* 5, no. 1 (April 1992): 43–70.

———. *Public Health and Social Justice in the Age of Chadwick: Britain, 1800–1854*. New York: Cambridge University Press, 1998.

———. "Public Sphere to Public Health: The Transformation of Nuisance." In *Medicine, Health and the Public Sphere in Britain, 1600–2000*, edited by Steve Sturdy, 189–204. London: Routledge, 2002.

———. "Sanitary Policing and the Local State, 1873–1874: A Statistical Study of English and Welsh Towns." *Social History of Medicine* 18, no. 1 (April 2005): 39–61.

———. *A Science of Impurity: Water Analysis in Nineteenth Century Britain*. Berkeley: University of California Press, 1990.

———. "Scientific Method and Expert Witnessing: Victorian Perspectives on a Modern Problem." *Social Studies of Science* 16, no. 3 (1986): 485–513.

———. "State Medicine in Great Britain." In *The History of Public Health and the Modern State*, edited by Dorothy Porter, 132–64. Amsterdam: Clio Medica/Rodopi, 1994.

———. "William Pulteney Alison, the Scottish Philosophy, and the Making of a Political Medicine." *Journal of the History of Medicine & Allied Sciences* 61, no. 2 (April 2006): 144–86. doi:10.1093/jhmas/jrj036.

Hamlin, Christopher, ed. *Sanitary Reform in the Provinces*. Part I, vol. 2 of *Sanitary Reform in Victorian Britain*. Brookfield, VT: Pickering & Chatto, 2012.

Hammond, John Lawrence, and Barbara Bradby Hammond. *The Bleak Age*. West Drayton, UK: Penguin Books, 1947.

Hanley, James G. "All Actions Great and Small: English Sanitary Reform, 1840–1865." PhD diss., Yale University, 1998.

———. "Bye Laws, the Environment, and Health before Chadwick, 1835–1840." In *Lawyers' Medicine: The Legislature, The Courts and Medical Practice, 1760–2000*, edited by Imogen Goold and Catherine Kelly, 39–59. Portland, OR: Hart Publishing, 2009.

———. "The Metropolitan Commissioners of Sewers and the Law, 1812–1847." *Urban History* 33, no. 3 (December 2006): 350–68. doi:10.1017/S0963926806004020.

———. "Parliament, Physicians, and Nuisances: The Demedicalization of Nuisance Law, 1831–1855." *Bulletin of the History of Medicine* 80, no. 4 (Winter 2006): 702–32.

———. "Public Health, London's Levels and the Politics of Taxation, 1840–1860." *Social History of Medicine* 20, no. 1 (April 2007): 21–38. doi:10.1093/shm/hkl084.

Hardy, Anne. "Cholera, Quarantine and the English Preventive System, 1850–1895." *Medical History* 37, no. 3 (July 1993): 250–69.

———. *The Epidemic Streets: Infectious Disease and the Rise of Preventive Medicine, 1856–1900*. Oxford: Clarendon, 1993.

———. "The Medical Response to Epidemic Disease during the Long Eighteenth Century." In *Epidemic Disease in London*, edited by J. A. I. Champion, 65–70. London: Centre for Metropolitan History, 1993.

———. "Public Health and the Expert: The London Medical Officers of Health, 1856–1900." In *Government and Expertise: Specialists, Administrators and Professionals, 1860–1919*, edited by Roy MacLeod, 128–42. Cambridge: Cambridge University Press, 2003.

———. *Salmonella Infections, Networks of Knowledge, and Public Health in Britain, 1880–1975*. Oxford: Oxford University Press, 2015.

———. "Urban Famine or Urban Crisis? Typhus in the Victorian City." *Medical History* 32, no. 4 (October 1988): 401–25.

Harling, Philip. "The Centrality of Locality: The Local State, Local Democracy, and Local Consciousness in Late-Victorian and Edwardian Britain." *Journal of Victorian Culture* 9, no. 2 (2004): 216–34.

———. "The Powers of the Victorian State." In *Liberty and Authority in Victorian Britain*, edited by Peter Mandler, 25–50. Oxford: Oxford University Press, 2006.

Harling, Philip, and Peter Mandler. "From 'Fiscal-Military' State to Laissez-Faire State, 1760–1850." *Journal of British Studies* 32, no. 1 (January 1993): 44–70.

Harper, Roger H. *Victorian Building Regulations: Summary Tables of the Principal English Building Acts and Model By-laws*. London: Mansell, 1985.

Harris, Jose. "Introduction: Civil Society in British History: Paradigm or Peculiarity?" In *Civil Society in British History: Ideas, Identities, Institutions*, edited by Jose Harris, 1–12. Toronto: Oxford University Press, 2005.

Harrison, J. F. C. *Early Victorian Britain, 1832–51*. London: Fontana, 1988.

Harrison, Mark. *Disease and the Modern World: 1500 to the Present Day*. Cambridge: Polity, 2004.

Hart, Gwen. *A History of Cheltenham*. Leicester, UK: Leicester University Press, 1965.

Hassan, J. A. "The Growth and Impact of the British Water Industry in the Nineteenth Century." *Economic History Review* 38, no. 4 (November 1985): 531–47.

Hennock, E. P. "Finance and Politics in Urban Local Government in England, 1835–1900." *Historical Journal* 6, no. 2 (1963): 212–25.

———. *Fit and Proper Persons: Ideal and Reality in Nineteenth-Century Urban Government.* Montreal: McGill–Queen's University Press, 1973.

———. "Urban Sanitary Reform a Generation before Chadwick?" *Economic History Review* 10, no. 1 (1957): 113. doi:10.2307/2600066.

Higginbotham, Peter. *The Workhouse Encyclopedia.* Stroud, UK: History Press, 2012.

Hilton, Boyd. "Whiggery, Religion and Social Reform: The Case of Lord Morpeth." *Historical Journal* 37, no. 4 (December 1994): 829.

Himmelfarb, Gertrude. *The Idea of Poverty: England in the Early Industrial Age.* New York: Knopf, 1984.

Hitchcock, Tim. *Down and Out in Eighteenth-Century London.* London: Hambledon Continuum, 2007.

Hobsbawm, E. J. *Industry and Empire: An Economic History of Britain since 1750.* London: Penguin Books, 1990.

Hobsbawm, Eric, and George Rude. *Captain Swing.* 1969. Reprint, New York: Verso, 2014.

Hodgkinson, Ruth G. *The Origins of the National Health Service: The Medical Services of the New Poor Law, 1834–1871.* London: Wellcome, 1967.

Hoppit, Julian. "Compulsion, Compensation and Property Rights in Britain, 1688–1833." *Past & Present* 210, no. 1 (February 2011): 93–128.

———. "Patterns of Parliamentary Legislation, 1660–1800." *Historical Journal* 39, no. 1 (March 1996): 109–31.

Howell, Philip. "A Private Contagious Diseases Act: Prostitution and Public Space in Victorian Cambridge." *Journal of Historical Geography* 26, no. 3 (July 2000): 376–402.

Humphries, Jane. *Childhood and Child Labour in the British Industrial Revolution.* 2010. Reprint, Cambridge: Cambridge University Press, 2011.

Hunt, Alan. *Governing Morals: A Social History of Moral Regulation.* Cambridge: Cambridge University Press, 1999.

Hunt, Tristram. *Building Jerusalem: The Rise and Fall of the Victorian City.* London: Phoenix, 2005.

Husband, Henry Aubrey. *Sanitary Law: A Digest of the Sanitary Acts of England and Scotland.* Edinburgh: Livingstone, 1883. E-book.

Innes, Joanna. *Inferior Politics: Social Problems and Social Policies in Eighteenth-Century Britain.* Oxford ; New York: Oxford University Press, 2009.

———. "The Local Acts of a National Parliament: Parliament's Role in Sanctioning Local Action in Eighteenth-Century Britain." *Parliamentary History* 17, no. 1 (1998): 23–47.

Innes, Joanna, and Nicholas Rogers. "Politics and Government, 1700–1840." In *The Cambridge Urban History of Britain,* ed. Peter Clark, vol. 2, *1540–1840,* 529–74. New York: Cambridge University Press, 2000.

Jenkins, Terry. "Freshfield, James William (1775–1864), of The Manor House, Stoke Newington and 9 Upper Wimpole Street, Mdx." The History of Parliament Online, http://www.historyofparliamentonline.org/volume/1820-1832/member/freshfield-james-1775-1864. Accessed November 12, 2015.

Jenner, Mark S. R. "Monopoly, Markets and Public Health: Pollution and Commerce in the History of London Water 1780–1830." In *Medicine and the Market in England and Its Colonies, c. 1450–c. 1850*, edited by Mark S. R. Jenner and Patrick Wallis, 216–37. Basingstoke, UK: Palgrave, 2007.

Jenson, Jane. "Getting to Sewers and Sanitation: Doing Public Health within Nineteenth-Century Britain's Citizenship Regimes." *Politics & Society* 36, no. 4 (December 2008): 532–56.

Johnson, Cuthbert William. *The Acts for Promoting the Public Health, 1848 to 1851.* London: Charles Knight, 1852. E-book.

Jones, Carol. *Expert Witnesses: Science, Medicine, and the Practice of Law.* Oxford: Clarendon Press, 1994.

Jones, Eric L., and Malcolm E. Falkus. "Urban Improvement and the English Economy in the Seventeenth and Eighteenth Centuries." In *The Eighteenth-Century Town: A Reader in English Urban History, 1688–1820*, edited by Peter Borsay, 116–58. London: Longman, 1990.

Jones, Gareth H., and Vivienne Jones. "Campbell, John, first Baron Campbell of St Andrews (1779–1861)." In *Oxford Dictionary of National Biography.* Oxford: Oxford University Press, 2004. Online ed., Jan 2008. http://www.oxforddnb.com/view/article/4521. Accessed November 13, 2015.

Jones, Greta, and Elizabeth Malcolm. *Medicine, Disease and the State in Ireland 1650–1940.* Portland, OR: Cork University Press, 1998.

Jones, Ieuan Gwynedd. "The People's Health in Mid-Victorian Wales." *Transactions of the Honourable Society of Cymmrodorion*, 1984, 115.

Joyce, Patrick. *The Rule of Freedom: Liberalism and the Modern City.* London: Verso, 2003.

Jupp, Peter. *The Governing of Britain, 1688–1848: Parliament and the People.* New York: Routledge, 2006.

Kay, James Phillips. *The Moral and Physical Condition of the Working Classes Employed in the Cotton Manufacture in Manchester.* 2nd ed. 1832. Reprint, Manchester: E. P. Morten, 1969.

Kearns, Gerry. "Cholera, Nuisances and Environmental Management in Islington, 1830–55." *Medical History* Supplement no. 11 (1991): 94–125.

———. "Private Property and Public Health Reform in England 1830–70." *Social Sciences and Medicine* 26 (1988): 187–99.

———. "Town Hall and Whitehall: Sanitary Intelligence in Liverpool, 1840–63." In *Body and City: Histories of Urban Public Health*, edited by Sally Sheard and Helen Power, 89–108. Burlington, VT: Ashgate, 2000.

Keith-Lucas, Bryan. "Some Influences Affecting the Development of Sanitary Legislation in England." *Economic History Review* 6, no. 3 (1954): 290–96.

———. *The Unreformed Local Government System.* London: Croom Helm, 1980.

Keith-Lucas, Bryan, and Peter G. Richards. *A History of Local Government in the Twentieth Century.* London: G. Allen & Unwin, 1978.

Kellett, J. R. "Municipal Socialism, Enterprise and Trading in the Victorian City." *Urban History Yearbook* (1978): 36–45.

Kelly, Catherine. "'Not from the College, but Through the Public and the Legislature': Charles Maclean and the Relocation of Medical Debate in the Early Nineteenth Century." *Bulletin of the History of Medicine* 82, no. 3 (Fall 2008): 545–69.

Kessel, Anthony. *Air, the Environment and Public Health.* New York: Cambridge University Press, 2006.

Kidd, Alan, and Terry Wyke. "The Cholera Epidemic in Manchester 1831–32." *Bulletin of the John Rylands University Library of Manchester* 87, no. 1 (April 2005): 43–56.

King, Peter. *Crime and Law in England, 1750–1840: Remaking Justice from the Margins.* Cambridge: Cambridge University Press, 2006.

King, Walter. "How High Is Too High: Disposing of Dung in Seventeenth-Century Prescot." *Sixteenth Century Journal* 23, no. 3 (Fall 1992): 443–57.

Kirby, Peter. *Child Workers and Industrial Health in Britain, 1780–1850.* Rochester, NY: Boydell and Brewer, 2013.

Koven, Seth. *Slumming: Sexual and Social Politics in Victorian London.* Princeton, NJ: Princeton University Press, 2004.

La Berge, Ann Elizabeth Fowler. *Mission and Method: The Early Nineteenth-Century French Public Health Movement.* New York: Cambridge University Press, 1992.

Lambert, Royston. "Central and Local Relations in Mid-Victorian England: The Local Government Act Office, 1858–71." *Victorian Studies* 6 (1962): 121–50.

———. *Sir John Simon, 1816–1904, and English Social Administration.* London: MacGibbon & Kee, 1963.

Lancaster, Brian. "Thwaites, Sir John (1815–1870)." In *Oxford Dictionary of National Biography,* Oxford: Oxford University Press, 2004. Online ed., May 2008. http://www.oxforddnb.com/index/52/101052332. Accessed November 13, 2015.

Large, David. "Proceedings of the Bristol Local Board of Health." In *A Bristol Miscellany,* edited by Patrick McGrath. Bristol: Bristol Record Society, 1985.

Large, David, and Patrick McGrath, eds. "Records of the Bristol Local Board of Health 1851–1872." In *A Bristol Miscellany.* Bristol: Bristol Record Society, 1985.

Latimer, John. *Annals of Bristol: The Nineteenth Century.* 3 vols. 1887. Reprint, Bath: Kingsmead Reprints, 1970.

Lawes, Edward. *The Act for Promoting the Public Health: With Notes, an Analytical Index, and (by Way of Appendix) The Nuisances Removal and Diseases Prevention Act, 1848, Some Additional Forms, and a Table of Rates Leviable under the Public Health Act.* London: Shaw and Sons, 1849. E-book.

Lawrence, Christopher. *Medicine in the Making of Modern Britain, 1700–1920.* London: Routledge, 1994.

———. "Sanitary Reformers and the Medical Profession in Victorian England." In *Public Health: Proceedings of the 5th International Symposium on the Comparative History of Medicine, East and West: October 26th–November 1st, 1980, Susono-Shi, Shizuoka, Japan,* 145–68. Tokyo: Saikon, 1981.

Laxton, Paul. "Fighting for Public Health: Dr. Duncan and His Adversaries, 1847–1863." In *Body and City: Histories of Urban Public Health,* edited by Sally Sheard and Helen Power, 59–88. Burlington, VT: Ashgate, 2000.

Laxton, Paul, and Richard Rodger. *Insanitary City: Henry Littlejohn and the Condition of Edinburgh.* Lancaster, UK: Carnegie, 2014.

Lee, William. *Report to the General Board of Health on a Preliminary Inquiry into the Sewerage, Drainage, and Supply of Water, and the Sanitary Condition of the Inhabitants of the Parish of Epsom.* London: W. Clowes, 1849.

Lees, Lynn Hollen. *The Solidarities of Strangers: The English Poor Laws and the People, 1700–1948.* Cambridge: Cambridge University Press, 1998.

Lewes, Fred. "The GRO and the Provinces in the Nineteenth Century." *Social History of Medicine* 4, no. 3 (December 1991): 479–96.

Lewis, Richard A. *Edwin Chadwick and the Public Health Movement, 1832–1854.* London: Longmans, Green, 1952.

Lilienfeld, David E. "'The Greening of Epidemiology': Sanitary Physicians and the London Epidemiological Society (1830–1870)." *Bulletin of the History of Medicine* 52, no. 4 (Winter 1978): 503–28.

Lipman, V. D. *Local Government Areas, 1834–1945.* Westport, CT: Greenwood, 1976.

Lobban, Michael. "Phillipps, Samuel March (1780–1862)." In *Oxford Dictionary of National Biography,* Oxford: Oxford University Press, 2004. Online ed., Jan 2008. http://www.oxforddnb.com/index/22/101022142/. Accessed November 13, 2015.

Longmate, Norman. *King Cholera: The Biography of a Disease.* London: Hamish Hamilton, 1966.

LoPatin-Lummis, Nancy. "The 1832 Reform Act Debate: Should the Suffrage Be Based on Property or Taxpaying?" *Journal of British Studies* 46, no. 2 (April 2007): 320–45.

Lubenow, William C. *The Politics of Government Growth: Early Victorian Attitudes toward State Intervention, 1833–1848.* Library of Politics and Society. Devon, UK: David & Charles, 1971.

Luckin, Bill. "The Metropolitan and the Municipal: The Politics of Health and the Environment in London, 1860–1920." In *Cities of Ideas: Civil Society and Urban Governance in Britain, 1800–2000,* edited by Robert Colls and Richard Rodger, 46–66. Burlington, VT: Ashgate, 2004.

———. "Pollution in the City." In *The Cambridge Urban History of Britain,* ed. Martin Daunton, vol. 3, *1840–1950,* 207–28. Cambridge: Cambridge University Press, 2000.

———. "Revisiting the Idea of Degeneration in Urban Britain, 1830–1900." *Urban History* 33, no. 2 (August 2006): 234–52.

———. "The Shaping of a Public Environmental Sphere in Late Nineteenth-Century London." In *Medicine, Health and the Public Sphere in Britain, 1600–2000,* edited by Steve Sturdy, 24–40. New York: Routledge, 2002.

Lumley, W. G. *The Act for the More Speedy Removal of Nuisances and the Prevention of Contagious Diseases, 9 & 10 Vic. c. 96.* London: Charles Knight, 1846.

Macdonagh, Oliver. *O'Connell: The Life of Daniel O'Connell, 1775–1847.* London: Weidenfeld and Nicolson, 1991.

MacLeod, Roy M. "The Anatomy of State Medicine: Concept and Application." In *Medicine and Science in the 1860s,* edited by F. N. L. Poynter, 199–227. London: Wellcome, 1968.

MacLeod, Roy M., ed. *Government and Expertise: Specialists, Administrators and Professionals, 1860–1919.* Cambridge: Cambridge University Press, 2003.

MacRaild, Donald M. *The Irish Diaspora in Britain, 1750–1939.* 2nd ed. Basingstoke, UK: Palgrave Macmillan, 2010.

Malcolm, Rosalind, and John Pointing. *Statutory Nuisance: Law and Practice.* New York: Oxford University Press, 2002.

Malone, Carolyn. "The Gendering of Dangerous Trades: Government Regulation of Women's Work in the White Lead Trade in England, 1892–1898." *Journal of Women's History* 8, no. 1 (1996): 15–35.

Mandler, Peter. "After the Welfare State." *Journal of British Studies* 39, no. 3 (July 2000): 382–88.

———. *Aristocratic Government in the Age of Reform: Whigs and Liberals, 1830–1852.* Oxford: Clarendon, 1990.

———. "Cain and Abel: Two Aristocrats and the Early Victorian Factory Acts." *Historical Journal* 27, no. 1 (March 1984): 83–109.

———. "Introduction: State and Society in Victorian Britain." In *Liberty and Authority in Victorian Britain,* edited by Peter Mandler, 1–24. Oxford: Oxford University Press, 2006.

Manitoba Hydro, Find Ways to Save Energy. http://www.hydro.mb.ca/your_home/power_smart/index.shtml (accessed November 2, 2015).

Marks, Lara. *Model Mothers: Jewish Mothers and Maternity Provision in East London, 1870–1939.* Oxford Historical Monographs. Oxford: Clarendon Press, 1994.

Marland, Hilary. *Medicine and Society in Wakefield and Huddersfield, 1780–1870.* Cambridge: Cambridge University Press, 1987.

Massard-Guilbaud, Geneviève, and Richard Rodger, eds. *Environmental and Social Justice in the City: Historical Perspectives.* Cambridge: White Horse Press, 2011.

Matthew, H. C. G. "Disraeli, Gladstone, and the Politics of Mid-Victorian Budgets." *Historical Journal* 22, no. 3 (September 1979): 615–44.

Mayhew, Henry. *London Labour and the London Poor: A Cyclopaedia of the Condition and Earnings of Those That Will Work, Those That Cannot Work, and Those That Will Not Work.* Enlarged ed. 4 vols. 1861–62. Reprint, London: Frank Cass, 1967.

McLaren, John P. S. "Nuisance Law and the Industrial Revolution: Some Lessons from Social History." *Oxford Journal of Legal Studies* 3, no. 2 (1983): 155–221.

Meller, Helen. "Urban Renewal and Citizenship: The Quality of Life in British Cities, 1890–1990." *Urban History* 22, no. 1 (May 1995): 63–84.

Melosi, Martin V. *The Sanitary City: Urban Infrastructure in America from Colonial Times to the Present.* Creating the North American Landscape. Baltimore: Johns Hopkins University Press, 2000.

Merewether, H. A., and A. J. Stephens. *The History of the Boroughs and Municipal Corporations of the United Kingdom.* 3 vols. Brighton: Harvester Press, 1972.

Mill, John Stuart. *Considerations on Representative Government.* In *Collected Works of John Stuart Mill,* edited by J. M. Robson, 19: 371–577. Toronto: University of Toronto Press, 1977.

Millward, Robert. "The Political Economy of Urban Utilities." In *The Cambridge Urban History of Britain,* ed. Martin Daunton, vol. 3, *1840–1950,* 315–49. New York: Cambridge University Press, 2000.

Millward, Robert, and Sally Sheard. "The Urban Fiscal Problem, 1870–1914: Government Expenditure and Finance in England and Wales." *The Economic History Review* 48, no. 3 (1995): 501–35.

Millward, Robert, and Robert Ward. "From Private to Public Ownership of Gas Undertakings in England and Wales, 1851–1947: Chronology, Incidence and Causes." *Business History* 35, no. 3 (July 1993): 1–21.

Miskell, Louise. *Intelligent Town: An Urban History of Swansea, 1780–1855.* Studies in Welsh History 24. Cardiff: University of Wales Press, 2006.

———. "Urban Power, Industrialisation and Political Reform: Swansea Elites in the Town and Region, 1780–1850." In *Who Ran the Cities? City Elites and Urban Power Structures in Britain and North America, 1750–1940,* edited by Ralf Roth and Robert Beachy, 21–36. Burlington, VT: Ashgate, 2007.

Moir, Esther. *The Justice of the Peace.* British Institutions. London: Penguin, 1969.

Molina, Natalia. *Fit to Be Citizens? Public Health and Race in Los Angeles, 1879–1939.* Berkeley: University of California Press, 2006.

Mooney, Graham. *Intrusive Interventions: Public Health, Domestic Space, and Infectious Disease Surveillance in England, 1840–1914.* Rochester, NY: University of Rochester Press, 2015.

———. "Public Health versus Private Practice: The Contested Development of Compulsory Infectious Disease Notification in Late Nineteenth-Century Britain." *Bulletin of the History of Medicine* 73, no. 2 (Summer 1999): 238–67.

Moore, James, and Richard Rodger. "Who Really Ran the Cities? Municipal Knowledge and Policy Networks in British Local Government, 1832–1914." In *Who Ran the Cities? City Elites and Urban Power Structures in Britain and North America, 1750–1940,* edited by Ralf Roth and Robert Beachy, 37–68. Historical Urban Studies. Burlington, VT: Ashgate, 2007.

Morris, R. J. *Cholera, 1832: The Social Response to an Epidemic.* New York: Holmes and Meier, 1976.

———. "Externalities, the Market, Power Structure and the Urban Agenda." *Urban History Yearbook* 17 (1990): 99–109.

Morris, R. J, and Richard H. Trainor, eds. *Urban Governance: Britain and Beyond since 1750.* Historical Urban Studies. Aldershot, UK: Ashgate, 2000.

Mort, Frank. *Dangerous Sexualities: Medico-Moral Politics in England since 1830.* London: Routledge & Kegan Paul, 1987.

Mosley, Stephen. *The Chimney of the World: A History of Smoke Pollution in Victorian and Edwardian Manchester.* Cambridge: White Horse Press, 2001.

Muir, Ramsay. *A History of Municipal Government in Liverpool from the Earliest Times to the Municipal Reform Act of 1835.* 2 parts. London: Williams and Norgate, for the University Press of Liverpool, 1906.

Mumford, Lewis. *The City in History: Its Origins, Its Transformations, and Its Prospects.* New York: Harcourt, Brace & World, 1961.

Nicholls, George. *A History of the Irish Poor Law, in Connexion with the Condition of the People.* London: J. Murray, 1856.

Norton, C. E., and F. C. Allworth. *Borough Boundaries.* London: Butterworth, 1926.

Novak, Steven J. "Professionalism and Bureaucracy: English Doctors and the Victorian Public Health Administration." *Journal of Social History* 6, no. 4 (1973): 440–62.

Offer, Avner. *Property and Politics, 1870–1914: Landownership, Law, Ideology, and Urban Development in England.* Cambridge: Cambridge University Press, 1981.

Ogborn, Miles. "Law and Discipline in Nineteenth Century English State Formation: The Contagious Diseases Acts of 1864, 1866 and 1869." *Journal of Historical Sociology* 6, no. 1 (March 1993): 28–55.

———. "Ordering the City: Surveillance, Public Space and the Reform of Urban Policing in England 1835–56." *Political Geography* 12, no. 6 (November 1993): 505–22.

———. *Spaces of Modernity: London's Geographies 1680–1780*. New York: Guilford Press, 1998.

O'Gorman, Frank. "Reply: The Electorate Before and After 1832." *Parliamentary History* 12, no. 2 (June 1993): 171–83.

Olien, Diana Davids. *Morpeth: A Victorian Public Career*. Washington, DC: University Press of America, 1983.

O'Reilly, Carole. "From 'the People' to 'the Citizen': The Emergence of the Edwardian Municipal Park in Manchester, 1902–1912." *Urban History* 40, no. 1 (February 2013): 136–55.

Osborne, Thomas. "Security and Vitality: Drains, Liberalism and Power in the Nineteenth Century." In *Foucault and Political Reason: Liberalism, Neo-Liberalism and Rationalities of Government*, edited by Andrew Barry, Thomas Osborne, and Nikolas Rose, 99–121. Chicago: University of Chicago Press, 1996.

Otter, Christopher. "Cleansing and Clarifying: Technology and Perception in Nineteenth-Century London." *Journal of British Studies* 43, no. 1 (January 2004): 40–64.

———. "Making Liberalism Durable: Vision and Civility in the Late Victorian City." *Social History* 27, no. 1 (2002): 1–15.

Owen, David. *The Government of Victorian London, 1855–1889: The Metropolitan Board of Works, the Vestries, and the City Corporation*, edited by Roy MacLeod. Cambridge, MA: Harvard University Press, 1982.

Paris, John A., and John S. M. Fonblanque. *Medical Jurisprudence*. 3 vols. London: W. Phillips, 1823.

Pellew, Jill. *Home Office, 1848–1914: From Clerks to Bureaucrats*. East Brunswick, NJ: Associated University Presses, 1982.

Pelling, Margaret. *Cholera, Fever and English Medicine, 1825–1865*. Oxford: Oxford University Press, 1978.

Perren, Richard. "The Meat and Livestock Trade in Britain, 1850–70." *Economic History Review* 28, no. 3 (1975): 385–400.

———. *The Meat Trade in Britain, 1840–1914*. London: Routledge and Kegan Paul, 1978.

Petrow, Stefan. *Policing Morals: The Metropolitan Police and the Home Office, 1870–1914*. Oxford: Clarendon, 1994.

Pickstone, John V. "Dearth, Dirt and Fever Epidemics: Rewriting the History of British 'Public Health,' 1750–1850." In *Epidemics and Ideas: Essays on the Historical Perception of Pestilence*, edited by Terence Ranger and Paul Slack, 124–48. New York: Cambridge University Press, 1992.

———. "Ferrier's Fever to Kay's Cholera: Disease and Social Structure in Cottonopolis." *History of Science* 22, no. 4 (June 1984): 410–19.

Piketty, Thomas. *Capital in the Twenty-First Century*. Translated by Arthur Goldhammer. Cambridge, MA: Belknap Press, 2014. Kindle edition.

Platt, Harold L. *Shock Cities: The Environmental Transformation and Reform of Manchester and Chicago*. Chicago: University of Chicago Press, 2005.

Polanyi, Karl. *The Great Transformation: The Political and Economic Origins of Our Time*. 2nd ed. Boston: Beacon Press, 2001.

Pooley, Colin G. "Patterns on the Ground: Urban Form, Residential Structure and the Social Construction of Space." In *The Cambridge Urban History of Britain*, vol. 2, *1830–1912*, edited by Martin Daunton, 429–65. New York: Cambridge University Press, 2000.

Poovey, Mary. "Curing the Social Body in 1832: James Phillips Kay and the Irish in Manchester." In *Making a Social Body: British Cultural Formation, 1830–1864*, 55–72. Chicago: University of Chicago Press, 1995.

———. "Domesticity and Class Formation: Chadwick's 1842 Sanitary Report." In *Making a Social Body: British Cultural Formation, 1830–1864*, 115–31. Chicago: University of Chicago Press, 1995.

Porter, Dale H. *The Thames Embankment: Environment, Technology, and Society in Victorian London.* Technology and the Environment. Akron, OH: University of Akron Press, 1998.

Porter, Dorothy. *Health, Civilization and the State: A History of Public Health from Ancient to Modern Times.* New York: Routledge, 1999.

———. Introduction. In *The History of Public Health and the Modern State*, 1–44. Amsterdam: Clio Medica/Rodopi, 1994.

———. "Public Health." In *Companion Encyclopedia of the History of Medicine*, edited by W. F. Bynum and Roy Porter, 1231–61. New York: Routledge, 1993.

Porter, Dorothy, ed. *The History of Public Health and the Modern State.* Amsterdam: Clio Medica/Rodopi, 1994.

Porter, Dorothy, and Roy Porter, eds. Introduction to *Doctors, Politics, and Society: Historical Essays*, 1–29. Amsterdam: Clio Medica/Rodopi, 1993.

Porter, R. "Cleaning up the Great Wen: Public Health in Eighteenth-Century London." *Medical History.* Supplement no. 11 (1991): 61–75.

Porter, Roy. "The Gift Relation: Philanthropy and Provincial Hospitals in Eighteenth-Century England." In *The Hospital in History*, edited by Lindsay Granshaw and Roy Porter, 149–78. New York: Routledge, 1989.

———. *London: A Social History.* Toronto: Penguin, 2000.

Poynter, J. R. *Society and Pauperism: English Ideas on Poor Relief, 1795–1834.* London: Routledge & Kegan Paul, 1969.

Prest, John. *Liberty and Locality: Parliament, Permissive Legislation and Ratepayers' Democracies in the Nineteenth Century.* New York: Oxford University Press, 1990.

Rammell, T. W. *Report to the General Board of Health on a Further Inquiry as to the Boundaries which may be most Advantageously Adopted for the Purposes of the PHA, 1848, in the Borough of Bangor.* London: Eyre and Spottiswoode, 1852.

Rares, Steven. "Blind Justice: The Pitfalls for Administrative Decision-making." http://www.austlii.edu.au/au/journals/FedJSchol/2006/13.html. Accessed November 2, 2015.

Redlich, Josef, and Francis Wrigley Hirst. *The History of Local Government in England: Being a Reissue of Book 1 of Local Government in England.* Edited by Bryan Keith-Lucas. 2nd ed. London: Macmillan, 1970.

Rees, John, and Lindsey German. *A People's History of London.* London: Verso Books, 2012.

Rees, Ronald. "The South Wales Copper-Smoke Dispute, 1833–95." *Welsh History Review* 10 (1980–81): 480–96.

Reid, D. "Praying and Playing." In *The Cambridge Urban History of Britain*, ed. Martin Daunton, vol. 3, *1840–1950*, 758–67. New York: Cambridge University Press, 2000.

Reinarz, Jonathan, and Leonard Schwarz, eds. *Medicine and the Workhouse*. Rochester, NY: University of Rochester Press, 2013.

Richardson, Ruth. *Death, Dissection, and the Destitute*. London: Routledge & Kegan Paul, 1987.

———. *Dickens and the Workhouse: Oliver Twist and the London Poor*. Toronto: Oxford University Press, 2012.

Richardson, Ruth, and Brian Hurwitz. "Joseph Rogers and the Reform of Workhouse Medicine." *History Workshop Journal*, no. 43 (April 1997): 218–25.

Ringen, Knut. "Edwin Chadwick, the Market Ideology, and Sanitary Reform: On the Nature of the 19th-Century Public Health Movement." *International Journal of Health Services* 9, no. 1 (1979): 107–20.

Risse, Guenter B. "'Typhus' Fever in Eighteenth-Century Hospitals: New Approaches to Medical Treatment." *Bulletin of the History of Medicine* 59, no. 2 (Summer 1985): 176–95.

Roberts, F. David. *The Social Conscience of the Early Victorians*. Stanford: Stanford University Press, 2002.

Roberts, Glyn. *The Municipal Development of the Borough of Swansea to 1900*. Swansea: University of Wales Press Board, 1940.

Roberts, Matthew. *Political Movements in Urban England, 1832–1914*. Basingstoke, UK: Palgrave Macmillan, 2009.

Roberts, M. J. D. *Making Victorian Morals: Voluntary Associations and Moral Reform in England, 1787–1886*. New York: Cambridge University Press, 2004.

———. "Public and Private in Early Nineteenth-Century London: The Vagrant Act of 1822 and Its Enforcement." *Social History* 13, no. 3 (October 1988): 273–94.

Rodger, Richard. "The 'Common Good' and Civic Promotion: Edinburgh 1860–1914." In *Cities of Ideas: Civil Society and Urban Governance*, edited by Robert Colls and Richard Rodger, 144–77. Burlington, VT: Ashgate, 2004.

———. "Political Economy, Ideology and the Persistence of Working-Class Housing Problems in Britain, 1850–1914." *International Review of Social History* 32, no. 2 (August 1987): 109–43.

———. "Slums and Suburbs: The Persistence of Residential Apartheid." In *The English Urban Landscape*, edited by Philip Waller, 233–68. New York: Oxford University Press, 2000.

———. "Taking Stock: Perspectives on British Urban History." *Urban History Review / Revue d'Histoire Urbaine* 32, no. 1 (Fall 2003): 54–63.

Rodger, Richard, and Robert Colls. "Civil Society and British Cities." In *City of Ideas: Civil Society and Urban Governance in Britain, 1800–2000*, edited by Robert Colls and Richard Rodger, 1–20. Burlington, VT: Ashgate, 2004.

Roe, John. *To the Provost and Fellows of the College of the Blessed Mary of Eton*. London: J. Rider [1845].

Rose, Michael E. "The Doctor in the Industrial Revolution." *British Journal of Industrial Medicine* 28 (January 1971): 22–26.

Rosen, George. *A History of Public Health*. New York: MD Publications, 1958.

Salmon, Philip. *Electoral Reform at Work: Local Politics and National Parties, 1832–1841*. Woodbridge, UK: Royal Historical Society Press, 2002.

Samuel, Ralph. "Comers and Goers." In *The Victorian City: Images and Realities*, edited by H. J. Dyos and Michael Wolff, 1: 123–60. Boston: Routledge & Kegan Paul, 1973.

Savage, James. *The History of Taunton . . . originally written by the Late Joshua Toulmin.* New ed., enlgd. Taunton: John Poole and James Savage, 1822.

Schwarz, L. D. *London in the Age of Industrialisation: Entrepreneurs, Labour Force, and Living Conditions, 1700–1850.* Cambridge: Cambridge University Press, 1992.

Scott, Rita. "Dr William Stewart Trench, Medical Officer of Health for Liverpool, 1863–1876: From Middens to WCs." *Bulletin of the Liverpool Medical History Society* 13 (2002–3): 12–21. http://www.lmi.org.uk/LiverpoolMedicalHistorySociety/Medical-Historian-No-13-2002-2003-Session.aspx. Accessed November 13, 2015.

Shah, Nayan. *Contagious Divides: Epidemics and Race in San Francisco's Chinatown.* Berkeley: University of California Press, 2001.

Shapter, Thomas. *The History of the Cholera in Exeter in 1832.* 1849. Reprint, Wakefield: S. R. Publishers, 1971.

Sheard, Sally. "Water and Health: The Formation and Exploitation of the Relationship in Liverpool, 1847–1900." *Transactions of the Historic Society of Lancashire and Cheshire* 143 (1993): 141–64.

Sheard, Sally, and Helen J. Power, eds. *Body and City: Histories of Urban Public Health.* Aldershot, UK: Ashgate, 2000.

Sheppard, F. H. W. *London, 1808–1870: The Infernal Wen.* London: Secker and Warburg, 1971.

Sheppard, Francis. "The Crisis of London's Government." In David Owen, *The Government of Victorian London, 1855–1889: The Metropolitan Board of Works, the Vestries, and the City Corporation*, edited by Roy MacLeod, 23–30. Cambridge, MA: Harvard University Press, 1982.

———. "St. Leonard, Shoreditch." In David Owen, *The Government of Victorian London, 1855–1889: The Metropolitan Board of Works, the Vestries, and the City Corporation*, edited by Roy MacLeod, 324–45. Cambridge, MA: Harvard University Press, 1982.

Siena, Kevin. "Hospitals for the Excluded or Convalescent Homes? Workhouses, Medicalization and the Poor Law in Long Eighteenth-Century London and Pre-Confederation Toronto." *Canadian Bulletin of Medical History* 27, no. 1 (June 2010): 5–25.

Sigsworth, Michael. "Cholera in the Large Towns of the West and East Ridings, 1848–1893." PhD diss., Sheffield City Polytechnic, 1991.

Simpson, A. W. Brian. *Leading Cases in the Common Law.* New York: Oxford University Press, 1995.

Smellie, K. B. *A History of Local Government.* London: George Allen and Unwin, 1946.

Smith, F. B. "The Contagious Diseases Acts Reconsidered." *Social History of Medicine* 3, no. 2 (August 1990): 197–215.

Smith, H. J. Introduction. In *Urban and Rural Social Conditions: The Local Reports to the General Board of Health, 1848–1857*, 3–14. Hassocks, UK: Harvester Press, 1978.

Smith, John. "Urban Elites c. 1830–1930 and Urban History." *Urban History* 27, no. 2 (August 2000): 255–75.

Smith, Joshua Toulmin. *The Laws of England Relating to Public Health, Including an Epitome of the Law of Nuisances.* London: S. Sweet, 1848.

Smith, Peter Jefferson. "Before Bazalgette: The Surrey and Kent Commissioners of Sewers, 1800–1847." *Transactions of the Newcomen Society* 74 (2004): 131–46.

Smith, Stanley. "Page, Thomas (1803–1877), civil engineer." In *Oxford Dictionary of National Biography*, Oxford: Oxford University Press, 2004. Online ed., Jan. 2008. http://www.oxforddnb.com/index/21/101021096/. Accessed November 13, 2015.

Spencer, Frederick. *Municipal Origins: An Account of English Private Bill Legislation Relating to Local Government, 1740–1835*. London: Constable, 1911.

Spongberg, Mary. *Feminizing Venereal Disease: The Body of the Prostitute in Nineteenth-Century Medical Discourse*. London: Macmillan, 1997.

Stedman Jones, Gareth. *Outcast London: A Study in the Relationship between Classes in Victorian Society*. Oxford: Clarendon Press, 1971.

———. "Rethinking Chartism." In *Languages of Class: Studies in English Working Class History, 1832–1982*, 90–178. New York: Cambridge University Press, 1983.

Stebbings, Chantal. *The Victorian Taxpayer and the Law: A Study in Constitutional Conflict*. New York: Cambridge University Press, 2009.

Stippak, Marcus. "German Cities and Their Sewage Systems: Darmstadt and Dessau in the Nineteenth and Twentieth Centuries." In *Environmental and Social Justice in the City: Historical Perspectives*, edited by Geneviève Massard-Guilbaud and Richard Rodger, 155–70. Cambridge: White Horse Press, 2011.

Storch, Robert. "The Policeman as Domestic Missionary: Urban Discipline and Popular Culture in Northern England, 1850–80." *Journal of Social History* 9 (1976): 481–509.

Sunderland, David. "'A Monument to Defective Administration'? The London Commissions of Sewers in the Early Nineteenth Century." *Urban History* 26, no. 3 (December 1999): 349–72.

Supplementary Bye Laws, Passed by the Council of the Borough of Devonport on Friday, the 5th of April, 1839. Devonport: W. Picken and Son, n.d.

Sutcliffe, Anthony. "The Growth of Public Intervention in the British Urban Environment During the Nineteenth Century: A Structural Approach." In *The Structure of Nineteenth Century Cities*, edited by James Johnson and Colin Poovey, 107–24. London: Croom Helm, 1982.

Szreter, Simon. "Economic Growth, Disruption, Deprivation, Disease, and Death: On the Importance of the Politics of Public Health for Development." *Population & Development Review* 23, no. 4 (December 1997): 693–728.

———. "The GRO and the Public Health Movement in Britain, 1837–1914." *Social History of Medicine* 4, no. 3 (December 1, 1991): 435–63. doi:10.1093/shm/4.3.435.

———. "The Importance of Social Intervention in Mortality Decline c. 1850–1914: A Re-Interpretation of the Role of Public Health." *Social History of Medicine* 1, no. 1 (1988): 1–38.

———. "Rethinking McKeown: The Relationship Between Public Health and Social Change." *American Journal of Public Health* 92, no. 5 (2002): 722–29.

Szreter, Simon, and Anne Hardy. "Urban Fertility and Mortality Patterns." In *The Cambridge Urban History of Britain*, ed. Martin Daunton, vol. 3, *1840–1950*, 629–72. New York: Cambridge University Press, 2000.

Taggart, Michael. *Private Property and Abuse of Rights in Victorian England: The Story of Edward Pickles and the Bradford Water Supply*. Oxford: Oxford University Press, 2002.

Taylor, David. "Crime and Policing in Early Victorian Middlesbrough, 1835–55." *Journal of Local and Regional Studies* 11 (1991): 48–67.

———. "Melbourne, Middlesbrough and Morality: Policing Victorian 'New Towns' in the Old World and the New." *Social History* 31, no. 1 (February 2006): 15–38. doi:10.1080/03071020500424409.

Taylor, Vanessa, and Frank Trentmann. "Liquid Politics: Water and the Politics of Everyday Life in the Modern City." *Past & Present* 211, no. 1 (May 2011): 199–241.

Thane, Pat. "Government and Society in England and Wales, 1750–1914." In *The Cambridge Social History of Britain, 1750–1950*, ed. F. M. L. Thompson, vol. 3, *Social Agencies and Institutions*, 1–61. New York: Cambridge University Press, 1990.

Thompson, Dorothy. *The Chartists*. Aldershot, UK: Wildwood, 1986.

Thompson, E. P. *The Making of the English Working Class*. 1963. Reprinted with a new preface, Harmondsworth, UK: Pelican Books, Penguin, 1980.

———. "The Peculiarities of the English." *Socialist Register* 2, no. 2 (March 19, 1965). http://socialistregister.com/index.hp/srv/article/view/5963. Accessed November 13, 2015.

Thompson, F. M. L. "The Rise of Suburbia." In *The Victorian City: A Reader in British Urban History, 1820–1914*, edited by R. J. Morris and Richard Rodger, 149–80. New York: Longman, 1993.

Vickery, Amanda. *Behind Closed Doors: At Home in Georgian England*. New Haven, CT: Yale University Press, 2010.

Waddington, Keir. "Paying for the Sick Poor: Financing Medicine under the Victorian Poor Law – the Case of the Whitechapel Union, 1850–1900." In *Financing Medicine: The British Experience since 1750*, edited by M. Gorsky and S. Sheard, 95–111. New York: Routledge, 2006.

Walkowitz, Judith R. *Prostitution and Victorian Society: Women, Class, and the State*. Cambridge: Cambridge University Press, 1980.

Waller, P. J. *Town, City, and Nation: England in 1850–1914*. New York: Clarendon, 1984.

Ward, David. "Environs and Neighbours in the 'Two Nations': Residential Differentiation in Mid-Nineteenth-Century Leeds." *Journal of Historical Geography* 6, no. 2 (April 1980): 133–62.

Ward, Tony. "Law, Common Sense and the Authority of Science: Expert Witnesses and Criminal Insanity in England, ca. 1840–1940." *Social & Legal Studies* 6, no. 3 (September 1997): 343–62.

Webb, R. K., "Southwood Smith: The Intellectual Sources of Public Service." In *Doctors, Politics, and Society: Historical Essays*, edited by Dorothy Porter and Roy Porter, 46–80. Amsterdam: Clio Medica/Rodopi, 1993.

Webb, Sidney, and Beatrice Potter Webb. *The Manor and the Borough*. 11 vols. *English Local Government*. Hamden, CT: Archon Books, 1963.

Webb, Sidney, and Beatrice Webb. *Statutory Authorities for Special Purposes*. London: Longmans, Green & Co., 1922.

———. *The Story of the King's Highway*. London: Longmans, Green & Co., 1913.

Weinstein, Ben. "'Local Self-Government Is True Socialism': Joshua Toulmin Smith, the State and Character Formation." *English Historical Review* 123, no. 504 (October 2008): 1193–1228.

White, Brenda M. "Medical Police. Politics and Police: The Fate of John Roberton." *Medical History* 27, no. 4 (October 1983): 407–22.

White, Brian D. *A History of the Liverpool Corporation, 1835–1914.* Liverpool: University of Liverpool Press, 1951.

Whyte, Rebecca. "Changing Approaches to Disinfection in England, 1848–1914." PhD diss., Cambridge University, 2012.

Wiener, Martin J. "The Unloved State: Twentieth-Century Politics in the Writing of Nineteenth-Century History." *Journal of British Studies* 33, no. 3 (July 1, 1994): 283–308. doi:10.2307/176074.

Williams, A. W., trans. and ed. *Public Health in Mid-Victorian Wales*, 3. Cardiff: University of Wales, Board of Celtic Studies, 1983.

Williams, Michael. *The Draining of the Somerset Levels.* Cambridge: Cambridge University Press, 1970.

Wilson, John F. "The Finance of Municipal Capital Expenditure in England and Wales, 1870–1914." *Financial History Review* 4 (1997): 31–50.

Wilson, Leonard G. "Fevers and Science in Early Nineteenth Century Medicine." *Journal of the History of Medicine & Allied Sciences* 33, no. 3 (July 1978): 386–407.

Winnipeg. Water Conservation. http://www.winnipeg.ca/waterandwaste/water/conservation/toiletreplacement/. Accessed November 2, 2015.

Wohl, Anthony. *Endangered Lives: Public Health in Victorian Britain.* London: J. M. Dent, 1983.

———. *The Eternal Slum: Housing and Social Policy in Victorian London.* London: Edward Arnold, 1977.

———. "The Housing of the Working Classes in London, 1815–1914." In *The History of Working-Class Housing: A Symposium*, edited by Stanley D. Chapman, 13–54. Newton Abbot, UK: David & Charles, 1971.

———. "Unfit for Human Habitation." In *The Victorian City: Images and Realities*, edited by H. J. Dyos and Michael Wolff, 2: 603–24. London: Routledge & Kegan Paul, 1973.

Wolfenstein, Gabriel K. "Recounting the Nation: The General Register Office and Victorian Bureaucracies." *Centaurus* 49, no. 4 (2007): 261–88.

Wood, Peter. "Finance and the Urban Poor Law: Sunderland Union, 1836–1914." In *The Poor and the City: The English Poor Law in Its Urban Context, 1834–1914*, edited by M. Rose. Leicester: Leicester University Press, 1985.

Worboys, Michael. *Spreading Germs: Disease Theories and Medical Practice in Britain, 1865–1900.* New York: Cambridge University Press, 2006.

Wrigley, E. A. "Coping with Rapid Population Growth: How England Fared in the Century Preceding the Great Exhibition of 1851." In *Structures and Transformations in Modern British History*, edited by David Feldman and Jon Lawrence. New York: Cambridge University Press, 2011. Kindle edition.

Young, Kenneth George, and Patricia L. Garside. *Metropolitan London: Politics and Urban Change, 1837–1981.* London: Edward Arnold, 1982.

Index

Aldgate. *See* St. Botolph without Aldgate
anticentralization, 90
Ashley, Lord. *See* Shaftesbury, Earl of
   (Anthony Ashley-Cooper)

Bazalgette, Sir Joseph, 100–101
Beche, Sir Henry Thomas de la, 56–57
benefit, 11, 13, 40, 44, 46, 54, 56–57,
   63, 68, 70, 72, 75–76, 80–87, 89,
   93–95, 97–101, 108–9, 142n89,
   167n103, 186n113, 202n96; health,
   11, 63, 110; indirect, 9, 11, 41, 63, 67,
   78–82, 84–88, 93, 107, 133, 176n198,
   186n122, 207n146; redefinition, 47,
   53, 67, 78–79, 80–81, 88
Benidickson, Jamie, 4
bills, private, 6
Birmingham, 3, 7, 16, 39
boundaries, 55–62, 65–67, 142n86;
   financial, 67, 75; of health, 70, 72–82,
   143n96; LBH, 178n18; municipal,
   66–67, 71, 177n10; parliamentary,
   65–66; physical, 67–72; poor law, 65,
   177n6. *See also* drainage: areas
Bristol, 76, 110
bylaws, 147n30; common lodging house,
   129–31, 221n128; nuisance, 6–8, 12,
   14, 18–19, 26–37. *See also* Liverpool;
   nuisances; health hazard; Pwllhelli;
   Shrewsbury; Worcester

Camberwell (St. Giles), 108–9
Campbell, John, first Baron Campbell of
   St. Andrews, 51, 74–75, 93–94
central-local relations, 7–8, 14, 19, 135,
   140n59, 140n60

Chadwick, Edwin, 1, 3, 15, 17, 33–34,
   68, 77, 124–25, 127, 131, 134–35,
   171n141, 186n123
Chancery, 118, 120
Chelmsford, 73, 75
Cheltenham, 13, 23–25, 85–86, 88:
   Improvement Commission, 44; local
   act, 190n156; Sewer Company, 23–24,
   44–45
cholera, 6, 9, 11–12, 15, 17, 19, 28–29,
   36–37, 43, 90, 119, 124; bylaws and,
   23–25; influence, 23–25, 41, 50–54,
   90
Clark, George Thomas, 71–72, 83
Coleridge, Sir John Taylor, 80–81, 86,
   93
common lodgers, 11, 112, 124–27,
   130–31
common lodging houses, 14; bylaws,
   129–31, 221n128 ; control, 112–13,
   124; definition, 111, 124–28,
   223n151; regulation, 129–31
Common Lodging Houses Act (1851),
   8, 127–29; amendment, 128
Common Lodging Houses Act (1853),
   128
communities, 66–67, 99; of health, 11,
   65, 68, 87–88, 99
conversions, 115, 120–23, 216n78,
   217n85
Cresy, Edward, 69–70, 85, 115
Crompton, Sir Charles John, 75, 93,
   107–8
Crook, Tom, 124, 130
Crowded Dwellings Bill, 128
Croydon, 120–21, 124

Daunton, Martin, 10–11, 91, 180n43, 208n165

Davis, John, 91, 110, 193n22, 209n167

democracy, 15, 19, 25, 30, 71; fear of, 27, 70, 179n35

Dicey, Albert Venn, 5, 81

disease, 9–10, 15, 41; prevention of, 47, 52

districts boards of works, 90–92, 103, 109

dock companies, 93–94, 102, 104–5

domesticity, 13, 111, 127–30

Dorling, 79–87, 93, 207n146

Dorling, Henry, 79–80

drainage: areas, 39–40, 55, 59–64; combined, 119, 215n71, 215n74; compulsory, 113–14, 120–23; houses, 13, 46, 111, 119. *See also* boundaries

drains: branch, 85–86; definition, 114–15

Duncan, Dr. William, 8

Durrant Cooper, William, 104, 198n66

Dyos, Henry J, 62–63

effluvia, 24, 28–29, 152n92, 171n141

Epsom, 6, 13, 68, 72, 74–75, 77–88, 133, 135

Epsom case, 72. See also *Dorling*

equalization, 13, 71, 75–76, 88, 91–92, 98–99, 101–7, 110, 206n139

Erle, Sir William, 93, 95

Eton, 67–72, 116–17

Eton, Dr. Edward, 116–17

Eton College, 68–71

Farr, Dr. William, 8

franchise, local, 26–27; plural, 26–27, 70

General Board of Health (GBH), 7–8, 15, 67, 69–70, 75–78, 82–83, 85–86, 90, 115–16, 120, 129, 131

General Register Office, 8

Gilbert, Pamela, 9

Glasgow, 124, 157n2, 221n130, 223n155

goods: private, 12, 40, 42–43, 46, 209n5, 210n7; public, 11, 39–40, 42, 44, 78

Green, David, 91

Hall, Benjamin, Baron Llanover, 79–80, 90, 97

Hardy, Anne, 8, 199n77, 208n160, 224n164, 226n1

Hamlin, Christopher, 3, 10, 21, 59, 156n126

health: 25, 41, 51–54, 58, 61, 63; benefits of, 11, 63, 110; communities of, 11, 65, 87–88, 99; liability for, 91, 93, 99, 101, 143n91; nuisances to, 23–24; right to, 11, 81, 88, 99

health hazard, 6, 8, 10, 12, 15, 18–19. *See also* bylaws; nuisances

Health of Towns Bill (1845), 55–57, 90, 125

Health of Towns Commission (HOTC), *See* Royal Commission on the State of Large Towns and Populous Districts

Hennock, Peter, 3

Hertford, 114, 117

Hertslet, Lewis, 56–57

Home Office, 7–8, 19, 29, 34–37, 129–30

Home Secretary, 34, 154n104

house drainage, 13, 46–47, 111, 119; cost, 115, 119–23; Sewers (House Drainage) Bill, 121–22

houses, demolition of, 117–19

Huddersfield, 60–62

improvement commissions, 7, 15, 20–21

improvement, private, 114–15

Innes, Joanna, 20, 140n60, 156n124, 159n19

inquiries: further, 72; preliminary, 56–62, 68, 70–71

inspection inquest, 29–30, 32, 35–36, 153n95

Johnson, Cuthbert William, 76, 183n73, 213n48

Joyce, Patrick, 3–4

Kearns, Gerry, 10, 142n81, 153n93, 157n4

Kelly, Sir Fitzroy Edward, 91, 94, 101, 105–7

Lambert, Royston, 2
law, judge-made, 5–6, 74–75, 81–82, 106–9, 118–20
law officers, 51, 79, 81, 129
Leeds, 59, 62
legal history, 4–7, 82–83
liability: dock companies, 93–94, 102, 104–5; politics of, 96; railways, 72, 74, 94
Lighting and Watching Act, 77–78
Lincoln, Lord. *See* Newcastle, Duke of (Henry Pelham-Clinton)
Liverpool, 121–24; bylaws, 30–35; health committee, 121–23; local act, 24–25, 30, 32; lodging houses, 223n155
local acts, 6, 18, 20–21, 85, 147n25, 159n19; drainage, 42, 44–45, 57–64; nuisances, 19–23
local boards of health, 10, 13, 15
Local Government Act (1858), 86, 131
Local Government Act Office, 87, 131
Local Government Board Act (1871), 15
local initiative, 7–8, 63, 74, 77, 82, 112–13
lodgers, 11, 112, 124–26, 130–31
London, 2, 12–14; drainage, 12–13, 90; government, 89–91, 109–10; main drainage of, 90, 98–99
Long Acre, 50–52, 54

Masters v. Scroggs, 48, 50, 165n90
Mayhew, Henry, 130–31
medical participation: at trials, 49, 165n87; in nuisance proceedings, 36, 146n12, 151n82; in preliminary inquiries, 58–59, 61; in select committees, 80, 186n117, 202n94
medics, 8–9
Metropolis Local Management Act (1855), 5–7, 90, 107; amending bill (1860), 99–101, 104; amendments, 6, 13, 92, 96–97, 99, 199n81, 200n82, 201n86; section 159, 93–94, 101–7, 110, 194n32; section 170, 92, 97–101
Metropolis Local Management Act (1858), 97–100, 113, 115, 118–19, 120, 123

Metropolis Local Management Amendment Act (1862), 202n96
Metropolis Sewers Act, 113, 115
Metropolitan Board of Works (MBW), 8, 13, 90–101, 104–6, 108–10, 119
Metropolitan Board of Works v. the Vauxhall Bridge Company. See *Vauxhall Bridge*
Metropolitan Commission of Sewers, 90–92, 94–96, 98–99, 109–10, 115, 119, 121, 193n12
miasmatism, 4, 9–10, 25, 38, 49, 53, 63–64, 85, 134–35, 164n83, 202n94
model clauses acts. *See* Towns Improvement Clauses Act (1847)
Mooney, Graham, 138n22, 143n97, 145n116, 209n3
municipal corporations, 20–21, 26–27. *See also* Liverpool; Pwllhelli; Shrewsbury; Worcester
Municipal Reform Act (1835), 6–8, 12, 19, 26–28, 31, 34
municipalization, 12, 39–40, 54, 56–58
municipal socialism, 63

Newcastle, Duke of (Henry Pelham-Clinton), 55
nuisances: common law, 18, 22–23, 146n11; common, 22, 31; to health, 12, 23–24; local acts, 19–23; medical certification, 23–25, 36; "particular," 21–22, 28; private, 22; public, 22, 31; sanitary, 6, 17, 21; sewer, 48. *See also* bylaws; health hazard
Nuisances Removal Act (1846), 14, 17, 35–37

Overseers of the Poor of the Parish of St. Botolph Without Aldgate v. Whitechapel District Board of Works. See St. Botolph without Aldgate

Paddington, 47, 94, 104, 118
Pew v. MBW, 108–9
Poovey, Mary 127, 210n8
poor law, 11, 15, 88, 92, 101–6
Poplar, 118
Porter, Dorothy, 9, 140n59, 143n91

Preliminary Inquiries Act (1846), 56–57; surveying officers, 56, 58–62
private land, 14, 22–23, 28, 30–31
Privy Council, 19, 24, 34–35
property: liability of, 10–11, 40–47, 49–51, 53, 55, 60–65, 67, 73, 75, 78, 93–94, 107–8, 207n151; protection of, 10, 19, 28, 30–34, 63; rights of 111, 114, 116–19, 124; taxation of, 10–13, 180n43. *See also* liability; rates; rating
public health, historiography, 1–4, 7–12, 14, 40, 82–83, 109–12, 123–24
Public Health Act (1848), 1, 5, 8, 12, 91, 113–15, 117, 120, 123, 125, 128
Public Health Act (1872), 16
Public Health Act (1875), 2
Pwllheli, 28, 30, 33–34

Queen's Bench, 68, 74, 76, 79–81, 92, 94–95, 103, 107, 119
Quarter Sessions, 74, 78–79, 81, 86
Queen v. Head, 107–8

railways, 72, 74, 94
Rammell, Thomas W, 72
ratepayers, 10–11, 44; as consumers, 77, 158n10
rates: general district, 73–74; highway, 69–70, 77, 82; main drainage, 98–99, 110; metropolitan, 91–92, 98–100; poor, 92, 101–7; private improvement, 55, 212n33; special district, 76, 78–79, 85, 189n138
rating: exemptions, 55, 198n60, 201n87; frontage, 44, 53, 123; rateable value, 4, 95–96, 123, 197n54, 197n55; reductions, 55–57, 59, 60–62, 175n183, 187n125
redistribution, 11–13, 41, 47, 49, 52–54, 68, 73, 75–77, 81–82, 85–86, 88, 91, 96, 99, 109, 206n137
Reeder, David, 62–63
reform, political, 15, 26–27
R v. Head, 107–8
Report on the Sanitary Condition of the Labouring Population of Great Britain, 1, 17, 37, 54, 68, 124–25

rights: to health, 11, 81, 88, 99, 143n93; to privacy, 13–14, 125, 130; of property, 111, 114, 116–19, 124
Royal Commission on the State of Large Towns and Populous Districts, 37, 54–55, 113, 123–25, 128
Royal Commission on the Health of the Metropolis (1847), 90
Royal Sanitary Commission, 15, 87

Sanitary Report. See *Report on the Sanitary Condition*
Select Committees, 6, 8–9; Cheltenham Improvement Bill, 85–86; Contagious Fever in London (1818), 49; Metropolis Sewers (1834), 166n100, 175n184, 176n198; Metropolis Local Management Amendment Bill (1860), 100–101, 104–5; Metropolitan Commissioners of Sewers (1823), 50; Public Health Bill (1854), 79–80
sewer law, Tudor (23 Hen. 8, c. 5), 39–41, 46, 53, 58, 93, 95
sewers, building, 47, 50–52, 165n94; definition, 114–15; metropolitan commissions of, 15, 70, 84, 109, 113; private, 39–40, 42, 44–46, 57, 157n5; tax, 40–41. *See also* property; liability
Shaftesbury, Earl of (Anthony Ashley-Cooper), 127–28
Shrewsbury, 32–33
Simon, Sir John, 2, 8, 15
Smith, Joshua Toulmin, 37, 41, 147n28
Smith, Dr. Thomas Southwood, 8
St. Botolph without Aldgate, 102–4, 106–7
St. Giles (Camberwell), 108–9
St. Katharine Dock Precinct, 102, 104
St. Marylebone, 95–96
St. Pancras, 104
Stafford v. Hamston, 48–50
Stuart, Sir John, 118, 120
Sturges-Bourne, William, 26
subdivision, 55–57, 59–61, 75–76, 78, 86–87, 100, 103, 110, 201n89

suburbs, 12–13, 15, 40, 42, 55, 62–63, 70, 72, 78, 176n190

superintending inspectors, 67, 69, 76

Surrey and Kent Commission of Sewers, 60–64, 108–9

Swansea, 13, 71–72, 74–75, 83–85, 88, 120–21, 124

Szreter, Simon, 7, 176n190, 191n168

Taunton, 22, 40, 174n178; drainage, 42–46, 58–62; Market Trustees, 42–46

taxation, 10–11, 135; indirect, 43–44

Thwaites, Sir John, 98–99, 110

Tinkler v. Wandsworth, 120, 210n10, 217n85

Towns Improvement Clauses Act (1847), 57–60, 212n36, 213n53

Trench, Dr. William, 121, 123

typhus, 9, 12, 15, 41, 48–49, 134, 164n77, 164n80

vagrants, 124–25, 128, 222n137

Vauxhall Bridge, 92–95, 107–9

vestries, 90–92, 109

Wandsworth, 94, 120, 210n10, 217n85

Ware, 117–18

Westminster Commissioners of Sewers, 9, 12, 41, 46–54, 63–64, 99

Whitechapel, 92, 102–7

Windsor, 117

Woolrych, Edmund Humphrey, 96

Woolwich, 86

Worcester, 28–30, 32–35

Printed in the United States
By Bookmasters